I'm Mad as Hell, and I'm Not Going to Eat It Anymore!

I'm Mad as Hell, and I'm Not Going to Eat It Anymore!

TAKING CONTROL OF YOUR HEALTH AND YOUR LIFE— ONE VEGAN RECIPE AT A TIME

Christina Pirello

A PERIGEE BOOK

A PERIGEE BOOK
Published by the Penguin Group
Penguin Group (USA) Inc.
375 Hudson Street, New York, New York 10014, USA
Penguin Group (Canada), 90 Eglinton Avenue East, Suite 700, Toronto, Ontario M4P 2Y3, Canada
(a division of Pearson Penguin Canada Inc.)
Penguin Books Ltd., 80 Strand, London WC2R 0RL, England
Penguin Group Ireland, 25 St. Stephen's Green, Dublin 2, Ireland (a division of Penguin Books Ltd.)
Penguin Group (Australia), 250 Camberwell Road, Camberwell, Victoria 3124, Australia
(a division of Pearson Australia Group Pty. Ltd.)
Penguin Books India Pvt. Ltd., 11 Community Centre, Panchsheel Park, New Delhi—110 017, India
Penguin Group (NZ), 67 Apollo Drive, Rosedale, Auckland 0632, New Zealand
(a division of Pearson New Zealand Ltd.)
Penguin Books (South Africa) (Pty.) Ltd., 24 Sturdee Avenue, Rosebank, Johannesburg 2196,
South Africa

Penguin Books Ltd., Registered Offices: 80 Strand, London WC2R 0RL, England

While the author has made every effort to provide accurate telephone numbers and Internet addresses at the time of publication, neither the publisher nor the author assumes any responsibility for errors or for changes that occur after publication. Further, the publisher does not have any control over and does not assume any responsibility for author or third-party websites or their content.

First edition: January 2012

Library of Congress Cataloging-in-Publication Data

Pirello, Christina.
    I'm mad as hell, and I'm not going to eat it anymore! : taking control of your health and your life—one vegan recipe at a time / Christina Pirello.
        p.   cm. — (A Perigee book)
    Includes bibliographical references and index.
    ISBN 978-0-399-53724-0 (pbk.)
    1. Vegan cooking.   2. Health.   3. Diet—Health aspects—United States.   4. Cookbooks.   I. Title.
    TX837.P558   2012
    641.5'636—dc23   2011035180

PRINTED IN THE UNITED STATES OF AMERICA

10   9   8   7   6   5   4   3   2   1

PUBLISHER'S NOTE: The recipes contained in this book are to be followed exactly as written. The publisher is not responsible for your specific health or allergy needs that may require medical supervision. The publisher is not responsible for any adverse reactions to the recipes contained in this book.

Most Perigee books are available at special quantity discounts for bulk purchases for sales promotions, premiums, fund-raising, or educational use. Special books, or book excerpts, can also be created to fit specific needs. For details, write: Special Markets, Penguin Group (USA) Inc., 375 Hudson Street, New York, New York 10014.

"Christina Pirello tells the truth about what is in our food that creates health and gives some simple recipes to set people on their paths. She is a sincere advocate for health—for all of us."

—T. Colin Campbell, Jacob Gould Schurman Professor Emeritus of Nutritional Biochemistry at Cornell University and author of *The China Study*

To Dennis Tice

For twenty-five years, your friendship has inspired,
supported, comforted, and confounded me. You're family, and
we both know what that means. I love you, your spirit, and
all that you have brought to my life.

CONTENTS

FOREWORD

No choice I've made in my life has had the effects that were as immediate and as dramatic as going veggie. It was like my whole body suddenly screamed, "Thank you, Alicia!" Because my original motivation for changing my diet was out of compassion for animals, I wasn't fully prepared for how much of a difference it would make in the way I felt physically. But going from steak and cheese to vegetables, fruits, whole grains, and beans will do that for you. In no time, my extra weight melted away, my skin cleared up, my energy level soared, and my troublesome digestion smoothed itself out. No more trips to the allergists for shots once a week and no more need for the inhaler for asthma, to name just two of the noticeable differences. It was only then that I realized that the choice I'd made for the lives of other creatures wound up changing my own life as much.

If you're looking for these kinds of changes, the information, advice, and recipes that Christina shares in this book will have an impact on your life and well-being in dramatic ways. It's already happening to countless others. People are waking up to this kind of diet and lifestyle—and overcoming many forms of cancer, diabetes, and obesity, and a range of other diseases that plague our society.

Since launching my website, *The Kind Life* (www.thekindlife.com), I've had the remarkable privilege of reading the emails from readers about the amazing changes they are experiencing, from conquering migraines and PMS to improvements in their lupus and thyroid conditions. These people are happy and energized by the changes in their lives as a result of adopting a vegan diet. It has freed them from the constant battle of yo-yo dieting, counting calories, and the bathroom scale seesaw. Eating a plant-based diet, like the one you will find in these pages, will give you health, wellness, and vitality, along with the peace of mind to turn your attention back to the things that are really important to you.

I've called on Christina's expertise, both as an advisor and as a regular guest blogger at *The Kind Life*. But she's become more like a big sister mentor to me personally. Feisty, smart, and incredibly knowledgeable, Christina is often the person I call when I get stumped on a health question or when the nutritional science babble goes over my head. She also is the creator of some of my favorite recipes, a few of which I used in my own book, *The Kind Diet*.

Together, Christina and I share a mission to influence people all over the world to make it a happier, healthier place. Much of this book is about encouraging us to leave behind our old ways of doing things, which are based on beliefs and information that is obsolete, outmoded, discredited, and false. It's a sad truth that we're told a lot of lies every day by those whose self-interests come before our health. Christina stands apart from those voices, but she doesn't reject conventional thinking for its own sake. She's neither anti-medicine nor anti-Western. In fact, in some cases, her views are very much in line with mainstream thinking and conventional wisdom. For her, it's less about who's saying it and more about getting to the heart of the facts about what is truly healthful and even lifesaving—for us and for the planet.

So, yes, some of this book is passionate in its condemnation of the companies and agencies that compromise our health for profit. What else would you expect from a fiery redhead? You can read this book knowing that the woman who is guiding you is fair-minded, incredibly well informed, and extraordinarily committed to making the world a better place. The information that she gives in these pages should become a tool that you can use to shape your own journey on a path that—I promise you—will change your life.

—Alicia Silverstone,
actress and author of *The Kind Diet*

INTRODUCTION

As my mother used to say, I'm so mad I could spit. The collapsing dollar, recession, lost jobs, multiple wars and political unrest, global natural disasters, and, as Peter Finch's character declared in the 1976 film *Network*, "air you can't breathe, water you can't drink, and food you can't eat."

I can't tell you what to do about the economy, terrorism, or global warming (although I have a few opinions about that), but I surely can tell you what we can do about the food we eat.

When it comes to our health and well-being, I'm mad as hell and I'm not going to take it anymore. And neither should you.

I grew up surrounded by strong, self-reliant, resourceful people who worked hard and lived vital lives. I don't see many of those kinds of people anymore. What happened to us? When did we give away our power—and our health? When did we allow others to dictate what we'll buy, wear, read—and eat?

We live in a country founded on revolution; on taking personal responsibility; on throwing out what doesn't work and replacing it with what does. Americans have always seen themselves as the masters of their destiny.

This country is in a health crisis, and nothing short of a revolution will change the course we find ourselves on. It's time to get off the sofa and fight for our lives.

Eating healthfully has become complicated in our modern life. "Experts" advise us on our food choices. From television chefs to nutrition scientists to news anchors to government advisory committees—there is no shortage of opinions on what we should be eating. They have filled our heads with facts, figures, and statistics. Many of these are as familiar as our own names. Concepts like antioxidants, polyphenols, saturated fats, omega-3, and, of course, calories are common currency in our daily discussions. But in this barrage of information, we lost our way to real food and our inherent wisdom about what eating healthfully means.

It's as though we don't even see food as food anymore, just the sum of its nutritional parts. We have lost touch with our intuition and fallen victim to the science of nutrition—and marketing. We have become victims of the biggest con in human history. Marketers, lobbyists, and their well-paid experts, through the smoke and mirrors of dazzling packaging, checkmarks, seals of approval, and dubious health claims, have slowly and consistently robbed us of our well-being. And it seems to me, made us stupid in the process. It's as though we don't think for ourselves anymore—about anything.

We have lost sight of the simplest of truths: whole, unprocessed plant foods give us all the nutrition we require.

Food is simple. Nature is simple. But misleading marketing has caused us to lose sight of some basic truths about human nutrition.

First, populations that consume the typical modern Western diet, i.e., large volumes of refined foods, added sugar, fat, salt, and very few veggies, fruits, and whole grains, invariably suffer from what we now call "lifestyle" diseases such as obesity, type II diabetes, stroke, heart disease, and cancer. We all know this. But nutrition science isn't making this connection, or at least they are not talking about it. Instead, they spend millions of dollars on studies to find the one key, the one nutrient that is the culprit; the one thing that is making us fat and unhealthy and killing us in record numbers.

There is no one singular nutrient—or lack of it—that is responsible for our declining health.

Second, populations that eat the traditional diets of their respective cultures—whatever they might be—don't seem to suffer from these same lifestyle illnesses. And those diets are widely varied: from the high-fat diets of the Eskimos, whose consumption of whale fat sustained them for thousands of years before "civilization" caught up with them, to the high-carb diets of Central Americans, comprised largely of corn and beans, to the high-protein diets of African tribes that included everything from cattle blood to milk, to the now widely acclaimed Mediterranean diet of olive oil, nuts, seeds, lean protein like fish, and lots of vegetables and fruit. Based on the seasonal traditional cooking patterns of the poor regions of the Mediterranean, this diet has shown itself to promote health and wellness by emphasizing healthy fats and other ingredients we now know to be healthy and nutrient dense. This tells us something very important: There is no one diet that serves all of humanity equally well. As humans, we can adapt to a wide variety of foods and eating patterns, except, it seems, to the modern Western diet of processed foods so commonly eaten today. The disastrous results of that diet are all around us.

And here is the real headline grabber and what should get your dander up because there are no headlines about this: When people stop eating a modern Western diet, they experience a dramatic improvement in their health. A departure from this diet shows drastic reductions in the risk of heart disease alone, like 80 percent! The risk of type II diabetes can be reduced by almost 90 percent and the chances of cancer by almost 70 percent. What does that tell you about the impact of the way America eats?

Interestingly, none of these dramatic facts are at the center of the discussion of nutrition research. Why?

Sadly, there's a lot of money to be made by those who support the way we currently eat—and the interests of those commercial organizations come at a great cost to consumers.

Manufacturers love to tweak products in ways that leave our diet largely unchanged but allow for new "hot buttons" to be added to the product packaging to create a "health halo" and seduce us to buy more of whatever junk it may be. Pharmaceutical companies can then develop more and more drugs to cure us of the diseases that our food choices cause. The healthcare industry makes more money treating chronic diseases than it does preventing them. And the circle of business goes round and round, leaving us dizzy with confusion.

Case in point: New research shows that of all the children born in 2010, one in three will develop type II diabetes and over the next forty years, the incidence of type II diabetes will go from one in ten people to one in three to five people. As alarming as these numbers are, pharmaceutical companies are doing the happy dance. That's a lot of blood glucose monitors and other diabetes paraphernalia to market!

In a perfect world, research would be done independently, free of the influence of food manufacturers and pharmaceutical companies. But one only needs read Marion Nestle's *Food Politics* to see that is far from the truth. Funding everything from conventions to professional meetings and training sessions, to studies and research universities themselves, food companies work hard to influence the outcome of any study to be in their favor. According to Nestle, we like to think of universities as ivory towers of knowledge and science, but the reality is that most people have no idea the level at which these universities and their programs are sponsored by companies like PepsiCo and Coca-Cola.

In many cases, according to Nestle, even most of the researchers have no idea how heavily influenced the final outcome of their work will be. So while the "experts" focus on finding the single element in the modern Western diet that is responsible for our ills, they are missing the point. Food manufacturers can recycle the same junk with fresh marketing strategies, and the media has a constant stream of "discoveries" about food and nutrition to write about. Everyone wins.

Except us.

I am not antiscience. In fact, every day I uncover new studies and surveys that show how science actually proves the benefits of eating a whole-foods, plant-based diet But, I am tired of the way commercial interests have twisted science to their favor.

With this book, I would like to take us back to the basics of food; to the fundamental wisdom of eating; and recover the intuitive understanding that food—real food—supports our lives and our health.

I will show how the food industry and its marketing efforts have conspired against people trying their best to be well. In offering their "magic bullets," these for-profit organizations are holding out false hopes instead of supporting the disciplined effort required to make the real and effective changes.

When you get right down to it, we don't need another fad diet, wonder food, or health craze. What we need is a revolution. We must replace the tired, outdated system of lobbyists, special interests, and corporate greed with a "Declaration of Health," a contract that commits us to creating a new and healthy relationship with real food.

That's where I come in.

With information and advice that I am offering in this book—and a willingness to act like grown-ups and let go of the childish behaviors that are destroying our lives—you will be inspired and motivated to make the changes, as difficult as they may seem at first. We can show these pirates that we can accept personal responsibility, get rid of the things that aren't working, and take control of our own destinies—and our own health.

In the end, there is no new advice, really. For us to be a healthy and robust society, with a bright future for generations to come, we must eat real food; food that is truly fit for human consumption.

In my own life, a diet of plant-based foods has been the key to health and wellness. It is the force behind the life I live. It is the source of my strength and stamina. I stepped off the carousel of processed foods years ago and saw the changes that created the health I enjoy today. It took a life-threatening illness to open my eyes, and that led to the mission I have been on for the past two decades: to help people find their way to health, deliciously.

We're mad as hell, and we're not gonna eat it anymore!

PART ONE

Why It's So Hard
Not to Be Fat
and Sick in America

I am perplexed. For the life of me, I cannot figure out how people can go on believing the nonsense being fed to us (pun intended) about food. I cannot figure out why we are not protesting in the streets at the injustices being put on us in the name of profits. It's obvious to me that the bottom line health of food companies has become far more important than the collective health of the people buying food.

People find lots of excuses: Life is difficult. We're entitled to a little pleasure as a reward for surviving our daily challenges—like getting a lollipop for going to the dentist. The science is complicated and we suffer from information overload to the point of paralysis. It takes too much discipline to eat healthfully. Just getting through the day is hard enough. Besides, somebody will invent a pill or treatment, or some diet guru will give us the magical formula that will make us thin, fit, and energetic—someday. In the meantime, what's the point of denying ourselves anything, no matter how bad we know it is for us? Besides, eating fresh, whole foods, fruits, and vegetables is a lot of work and too expensive. We smoke, we drink too much, and we eat stuff that hurts us. We've set a pretty low bar for how we look and feel. There's a disconnect between what we say we want and what we are willing to do to get it. Then we feel guilty and stressed and the cycle just perpetuates itself.

We are in serious trouble. If you think it's too expensive to eat well, just take a good look at the increasing cost of healthcare—much of which could be reduced if we took some pretty simple preventive measures now. Why is no one asking why? Or doing anything about it?

Call me naïve, but I just can't believe that the desire to look and feel our best doesn't give us the motivation to do what we need to do to be strong, vital, and healthy. It's seems to be a no-brainer to me.

What's it going to take for us to change? It's a simple question, but the implications are enormous. How much fatter, sicker, and more exhausted must we become before we have had enough? How much longer will we settle for simply existing and not thriving? How much longer will we let our health be hijacked?

Now before I go off the rails on a rant not unlike so many others I have gone on in my life, I have to ask: How much responsibility for the health crisis is on us and how much is on giant food and pharmaceutical companies? The answer is simple: It's both.

But it appears to me that just a few decades ago, the food industry made a conscious choice to seduce the American public into eating more processed food, which featured fat, sugar, salt, preservatives, and dozens of other unpronounceable ingredients. And we could not have made it easier for them. We've come to love anything fast and convenient. "Heat and eat" or "grab and go" have become the buzzwords of the day. It seems that the less healthy the food, the more we love it. We left the dinner table for dinner in a bucket.

1

Another Nice Mess We've Gotten Ourselves Into

A BRIEF HISTORY OF FOOD

Food is more to us than a means of subsistence. It is deeply steeped in culture, emotion, even religion. It embodies our shared traditions and defines us as societies. In seventeenth- and eighteenth-century Europe, food illustrated class distinctions. How you ate determined your cultural standing. Haute cuisine and elaborate table traditions differentiated the social elite from the masses.

During the nineteenth and twentieth centuries, food became a symbol of national identities; foods were suddenly associated with specific cultures, like Italian pasta or American hamburgers. Food became a symbol of national pride and status within that culture.

During all of this food evolution, the discovery of the New World served as a momentous turning point in the human experience. New ingredients like tomatoes, corn, yams, and beans came on the scene, and the use of pigs, sheep, and cattle for food increased. Sugar, coffee, and cocoa grown in the New World became the first multinational consumer industries. Everything changed.

Prior to the Civil War, the food of America was regionally divided with the austere piety of religion: New Englanders eschewed sensual food, and the Quakers ate plain, boiled foods; Southerners enjoyed the African influence of spices and oil, and westward migration introduced a greater dependence on corn and potatoes. The arrival of the first German immigrants in the nineteenth century brought new influences, with marinated meats, hot dogs, hamburgers, cured meats like wursts, donuts, and barbecue (yup, barbecue). But the biggest change these new immigrants brought to the table, literally, was the idea of food as celebration; that meals were a big part of special occasions. They broke the stranglehold of austerity born of religious zeal that had kept food from being enjoyed in a sensual way.

However, it wasn't until the Industrial Age that we began to see the kinds of changes in food that sparked the trend we still see today. In the late nineteenth century, food began to be mass produced and standardized because now it could be transported long distances as railways expanded into every region of the country. Reliance on the local food of the family farm was diminished.

And, in 1903, trans fats were invented, allowing food to sit on shelves without spoiling for much longer periods of time.

Food became more "exciting" during this period. Processed cereals hit the market, promoted as the first "health food," and fast became the epitome of the American breakfast. The 1920s saw the introduction of techniques for freezing food, as well as the invention of the first preservatives. And everything changed again. Nationally (and internationally) distributed processed and packaged foods began to dominate the way America thought about food—and the way America ate.

While a massive influx of immigrants from all over Europe in the early twentieth century brought new and distinctive foods and traditions to our shores, America really had no food identity of its own. But the American way—now quickly being distinguished by processed, homogenized, and bland foods—was now being urged on these new citizens. To be truly American meant to abandon the traditions of their own food cultures.

At the same time, as the population exploded and food production moved from local farmers to big corporations, questions of food safety, freshness, and purity were being raised by a few crusading journalists and concerned citizens, leading to the first federal laws mandating inspections and banning unsafe additives.

After World War II, the reliance on processed foods saw a dramatic upswing as the result of women leaving the kitchen to work outside the home. At the same time, the war played a major role in creating a more cosmopolitan diet for Americans as servicemen, exposed to a wide variety of cuisines overseas, began returning. On top of that, America was breaking out of its prewar isolationism, and expanded international trade made a wider variety of foods available, including year-round access to exotic fruits and vegetables, creating a more diverse diet for Americans.

In the 1950s, as superhighways were built and cars became more accessible, people shifted from urban living to the suburbs and commuting was born. Television brought daily entertainment into our homes, and as a result, Americans stayed in, and the phenomenon of "snack food"—to be consumed while sitting in front of the boob tube—took hold.

Meanwhile, down on the farm, there was a dramatic increase in the use of pesticides and other chemicals to keep food waste low and the food fresher as it was shipped longer and longer distances. By the 1960s, agricultural subsidies came into play, with the federal government encouraging farmers to grow more specific crops, like corn, to be used as cattle feed and to turn into dextrose, which did nothing short of revolutionizing the fast-food industries.

In the 1970s, dietary pattern shifts accelerated dramatically, creating a new food landscape. Regardless of ancestry, all Americans started to eat bagels, egg rolls, pizza, tacos—and Thanksgiving dinner. With this shift, food again became a class marker, with the more affluent people of America enjoying fine wines and gourmet foods and the middle and underserved classes relying more and more on cheaply produced processed foods.

Urban sprawl and the rise of the use of technology brought the demise of the small family market, which was replaced by gigantic supermarkets with parking lots for your convenience.

By the 1980s, we were driving to malls and loading up our cars with massive amounts of food for a whole week's worth of eating. In supermarkets and big box stores across the country, food—or what passes for it—was being heavily merchandised. Even the well-planned layout of these mammoth stores encouraged consumers to buy canned, bottled, frozen, or dried—every manner of packaged food. And new products continue to hit the shelves with dizzying speed, all cleverly and relentlessly marketed to seduce us away from locally grown, fresh food prepared from scratch.

From Julia Child to the Kitchen Circus

Today's food television–obsessed culture might find food show pioneers like Julia Child to be quaint, almost comical; now it seems we prefer the circus acts of celebrity chefs to the actual art of cooking. Julia gave her viewers much more than a few recipes and an hour of entertainment. Her love of real food and cooking was evident in every show. With her encouraging words and fearlessness, she empowered viewers to venture into the kitchen and cook their hearts out.

But back then, cooking was still considered an important part of life, love, family, and community.

Today, millions are glued to their televisions watching Gordon Ramsay terrify young chefs and *Iron Chef* competitors race around in chaos. We can debate the results of *Top Chef* and discuss what wine Giada paired with the food prepared on her show.

There has been a shift from learning how to prepare and produce food on television to consumption. We have gone from watching Julia and Jacques slice, simmer, and stir their way to a finished meal to a glut of shows about gluttony, watching chef after chef stuff their faces in all sorts of places from diners to cafés to the base of the Eiffel Tower.

It appears that cooking has become a spectator sport. In fact, Americans today spend less than twenty-seven minutes preparing food for their day. That's less than half the time it takes to watch *Top Chef.* In a *New York Times* article ("Out of the Kitchen, Onto the Couch"), Michael Pollan asked, "How is it that we are so eager to watch other people browning beef cubes on screen but so much less eager to brown them ourselves?"

And even as fascination with the stars of these shows rises, the consumption of fast and processed foods has skyrocketed.

This kind of programming only makes it that much harder not to be fat. With cooking transformed to a spectacle that we view from the sidelines, it has become another soporific that keeps us sedentary on the sofa yet leaves us yearning, wanting, craving something, which is exactly what advertisers want.

NO TIME TO COOK

For years, many Americans have devoted more time to their jobs than to their home lives—and that includes cooking. Since 1967, we have added about 167 hours (about a month's worth of work) to our yearly hours of labor. It doesn't sound like much, but Americans now hold the title of working the most hours of any industrialized nation.

"The amount of time spent on food preparation in America," says Michael Pollan, "has fallen at the same precipitous rate among women who don't work outside the home as it has among women who do; in both cases, a decline of about 40 percent since 1965." So we can't just blame the postwar flood of women into the workplace and out of the kitchen.

In *Something from the Oven: Reinventing Dinner in 1950s America*, Laura Shapiro declared that the food industry worked hard to "persuade millions of Americans to develop a lasting taste for meals that were a lot like field rations." Yuck, but accurate. America shifted toward industrialized—everything.

In taking on the herculean job of convincing women to turn to processed and convenience food, marketers have had to overcome generations of women's moral obligation to cook for their families. They have been fabulously successful in seducing consumers to open cans and pop plastic bags of food into boiling pots of water, peel back the foil lids of TV dinners, and, of course, load things into the microwave. Over the years, food companies got better at making processed foods look fresh, real, and beautiful, so we began to think of it as food. This manufactured product has inevitably come to dominate our diets.

In the end, changing lifestyles has led us to a sedentary existence where we are subjected to the relentless marketing of processed and fast foods. No wonder it's so hard not to be fat in America today!

PB&J

The humble peanut butter and jelly sandwich has been hijacked. In its original incarnation, made with natural no-sugar strawberry preserves, peanut butter (the sole ingredient of which is peanuts), and whole-wheat bread, it registers a modest 195 calories. But not content with that, the folks at Smucker's have created "Uncrustables," a frozen dough pocket filled with peanut butter and various flavors of jellies. One 58-gram serving (one 2-ounce pocket) has 210 calories and an ingredient panel that reads like a Russian novel—artificial ingredients that include high-fructose corn syrup (plus two other sugars), hydrogenated oils, and a variety of preservatives. Even the peanut butter contains hydrogenated oils, and the whole-wheat version contains unhealthy, artificial ingredients.

It may not look like you save a lot of calories, but a real sandwich is a lot bigger than two ounces, so chances are you—or your child—will eat only one and avoid consuming loads of chemicals.

Does it take so much time to make a peanut butter and jelly sandwich that we need this product?

HUMANS ARE MEANT TO COOK

If we took cooking seriously, we could change the human condition. French food expert Jean-Anthelme Brillat Savarin held that cooking made us who we were; that the discovery of fire in cooking "had done the most to advance the cause of civilization." In 1964, anthropologist Claude Lévi-Strauss regarded cooking as a way to distinguish humans from other animals. Since then, other anthropology experts, including Richard Wrangham of Harvard University, contend that it was the discovery of cooking with fire, more than anything else, that made us human. Wrangham says that cooking helped create cultures and societies because cooking gave us the meal, the occasion to gather and eat. Sitting around a table (or a campfire), we learned to share food, make eye contact, communicate, show affection. All this served to civilize us.

All that stands to become extinct in the face of the way we eat today. We seem to be regressing, grazing through our days like foragers of the past. We eat at gas stations, fast-food windows, in stadiums, in movie theaters, in our cars, as we walk down the street, sitting on a curb, standing over the sink; skipping meals entirely for daily fare that consists largely of snack food.

Our willingness to outsource our food preparation to food corporations and fast-food joints has taken a huge toll on our health and vitality.

A 2003 study done by Harvard economists revealed that the rise of food preparation outside the home could easily explain the accelerated rise in obesity in this country. And while you think you have heard this before, here's a new twist as to why this is the believed truth. The mass production of food has not only driven down the cost of food, but also the amount of time it takes to get the food. French fries did not become a common food choice in our culture until the JR Simplot Company perfected the process of freezing fried potatoes for the home cook. Before that, we had to buy, wash, peel, boil, pat dry, and then fry the potatoes if we wanted french-fried potatoes. Not anymore.

Similarly, mass-produced cakes, pies, cookies, and other labor-intensive foods have made them so much more accessible in our daily lives. These foods are no longer just for special occasions, but are everyday fare. We can indulge at any moment of any day. How could we do anything but get fat?

It seems that as the time and work factor involved in food preparation falls, obesity rises. If you observe cooking patterns across various cultures, you will see a clear picture emerge. The more time a culture spends on food preparation, the lower their rates of obesity. Turks, for example, spend the most time on cooking each day, about seventy-four minutes (in 2010). Thirteen years ago, these people enjoyed an obesity rate of less than 15 percent. Since 2008, an increased urbanized and hectic society has changed that. People are cooking less and their weight is creeping up—fast—with women gaining thirteen pounds over the last thirteen years and men gaining fifteen pounds during that same period.

Think about it. When you have to prepare all that you eat; when you can't just tear open a package, you think twice before eating.

A 1992 study published in the *Journal of the American Dietetic Association* found that underserved women who cooked meals on a regular basis were far more likely to eat a healthy diet than more affluent women who did not cook. This tells us that the act of cooking matters a great deal to our health and wellness, regardless of our socioeconomic status.

This shouldn't surprise us. When we hand over the task of cooking to food corporations, fast-food companies, and take-out windows, we will be consuming loads of fat, sugar, and salt, the three ingredients that we are hardwired to love, and will keep coming back for more and more processed foods. When special-occasion foods like cake and pies are cheap and available on a daily basis, we'll eat them every day and not only on special occasions.

When cooking takes time and effort, with delayed gratification built right into the process, we can easily keep our appetites under control. Processed foods have removed that control valve, and we have to live with the consequences: obesity, diabetes, heart disease, stroke, and cancer.

But all is not lost. We can reverse this trend and take control of our health and our lives. The question is: Can we re-create a culture of everyday cooking in millions of American households? Can we rebuild a culture in which the art of cooking and life at the dinner table is resurrected?

I believe we can, and we have already seen some evidence of it. While the prime-time hours of the Food Network still look more like ancient Rome's gladiator games and gluttony fests, they have—based on viewer demand—also created a new channel, the Cooking Channel, dedicated to shows that teach us how to cook, taking us step by step through recipes, just like their public television counterparts.

So while America is not actually cooking just yet, there is a spark, a glimmer of hope that we are ready to head back to our kitchens and begin to rebuild a culture of real food and its preparation.

2

How Fast Food Has Changed Our Nation

In order to regain control of our health, we need to let go of our childish attachments to food. I don't mean we are behaving like petulant children who want what they want when they want it. Rather, I mean we have become attached to the food of children.

While hamburgers were introduced to the United States in the early twentieth century, the first fast-food restaurant chain, White Castle, opened its doors in 1921 in Wichita, Kansas, selling burgers for a nickel along with side orders of fries and colas. White Castle thrived, but it wasn't until after World War II that we began the journey to becoming a fast-food nation.

The McDonald brothers designed their fast-food hamburger restaurant in an attempt to streamline the process of making food and to reduce the costs of production. Their octagonal-shaped restaurant, which opened in San Bernardino, California, in 1940, also eliminated the need for waitresses, thus reducing operating costs even further. By 1951, McDonald's grossed $275,000, an unheard of amount of money for any small restaurant at the time.

The decision to franchise their idea along with a distinctive architectural design (the Golden Arches) put McDonald's on the map. By 1960, there were one hundred franchises operating across the country. But it was Ray Kroc, an equipment salesman who serviced McDonald's, who bought the business from the McDonalds and took it to new levels of success.

By 1990, fast-food businesses, including Burger King, Wendy's, and numerous other Johnny-come-latelies, had taken over the American landscape with 11,800 McDonald's, 6,298 Burger Kings, and 3,721 Wendy's.

Today, more than 160,000 fast-food restaurants feed more than fifty million Americans each and every day, generating sales of more than $110 billion annually.

What do all these statistics, facts, and figures mean to us? It is no coincidence that the decline of our health has moved in direct proportion to the rise in the consumption of fast food. Forsaking home-cooked meals for snacks and fast food has more Americans than ever gorging on calorie-rich, nutrient-poor foods, sodas, and sweets. Over the last twenty-five years, we have come to take more of our calories from burgers, fries, pizza, and sweets than we have from home-cooked meals.

U.S. government surveys from 1977–1978, 1989–1991, and 1994–1996 reveal an alarming trend: more and more Americans ate their daily foods in the form of snack food and fast food with each subsequent survey. The surveys also showed that Americans have come to prefer snacks to sit-down meals, and quick, easy, calorically dense treats like pizza, potato chips, and cookies to real food. Among nineteen- to thirty-nine-year-olds, restaurant and fast-food consumption has more than doubled since the 1970s. In one study, Dr. Ashima Kant of City University of New York found that "energy-dense, nutrient-poor foods now account for more than 30 percent of American children's energy (calorie) intake."

On any given day, more than a quarter of all Americans will eat at a fast-food restaurant. This industry has, in a relatively short period of time, transformed not only the way we eat, but also our economic and cultural landscape.

With fast-food restaurants everywhere, from airports to hospital lobbies, Americans are spending more on these foods than they do on higher education, computers, or new cars combined! A generation ago, more than three-quarters of the money spent on food was spent on ingredients to cook at home. Today more than half of money spent on food is spent on food eaten outside the home.

McDonald's opens new restaurants at a rate of two thousand per year and employs more people than any other organization, public or private. It is the largest purchaser of beef, pork, and potatoes and is the largest owner of retail property in the world. Via monster advertising campaigns that leave no demographic untouched, it has become the most famous brand in the world with the Golden Arches more recognized than the Christian cross, according to Eric Schlosser, author of *Fast Food Nation*.

The fast-food industry is the largest employer of minimum-wage workers in the country, with migrant farm workers being the only group of people paid less. With the food prepared in enormous central kitchens and flavors coming from chemical plants along the New Jersey Turnpike, fast-food empires stand on top of huge industrial complexes that have destroyed the family farm, creating in its place industrial farms with absentee corporate owners.

And while this may make you mad as hell in an abstract Peter Finch-ish way, let me bring it home for you.

FAST-FOOD DECEPTION

The current obesity epidemic didn't just happen overnight. According to the National Bureau of Economic Research, the generally persistent upward trend of Americans' weight began just after World War II. In the 1950s less than 10 percent of Americans were overweight or obese. As fast-food restaurants and processed foods took control of our diets, the numbers jumped. By 1975 (about the time McDonald's introduced the drive-through window), the

The Heart Attack Grill (now in Arizona and Texas) is an oasis of gluttony, and claims to be the only restaurant that tells the truth: that restaurant food is bad for your health. But still, the audacity of a restaurant that offers a Quadruple Bypass Burger at 8,000 calories or feeds anyone over 350 pounds for free should give any thinking person pause for thought.

obesity rate in America had climbed to 15 percent. Since then, the over-weight population has ballooned, with obesity rates topping 32 percent.

If the clear evidence of *rising* obesity isn't enough to scare you back to your own kitchen, consider the following statistics related to what have become known as "lifestyle" diseases:

- Diabetes will kill twice as many women as breast cancer each year.

- Heart disease is the leading cause of death in both men and women, and has been for years.

- Cardiovascular disease kills more than one million people each year. That is 42 percent of all deaths.

- Not one state in the United States meets the Healthy People Guidelines of obesity at 15 percent or less.

- In 2010, only one state (Colorado) had an obesity rate of less than 20 percent.

- Nearly 34 percent of adult men and women over the age of twenty are obese.

- Two out of three Americans are overweight (67 percent).

- In less than ten years, a full 75 percent of adult Americans will be overweight.

- Childhood obesity has tripled in the past thirty years, to 25 percent of those under nineteen years of age.

- Americans consume more than five hundred calories more today than we did in the 1960s.

- $150 billion will be spent (and increase) each year on obesity-related illnesses.

- $174 billion (and increasing) will be spent each year on diabetes-related illnesses.

■ In 2009, more than half the cancers diagnosed were cancers of the prostate, female breast, lung, and colon; a direct result of our high-fat diets, according to the National Research Council.

■ According to the National Cancer Institute, 75 percent of cancers are rooted in environmental and lifestyle causes—and can be prevented.

TAKING CONTROL OF OUR FOOD

What the food industry has done to us is criminal. We know that now. The facts speak for themselves. We can choose to ignore it and bury our heads in the sand, but in my view, the price is too high. The time for that kind of thinking is over. I think our very existence is being threatened by junk food's effect on human health.

The "foodlike" substances that Michael Pollan describes so eloquently in his writings have little or nothing to do with food in its natural state and everything to do with why we are so fat and getting fatter. And where are our brains, our ability to think? A study published in *Prevention* magazine (August 2009) tells the sad results of a survey of consumers taken by Duke University. Apparently, just because people see and consider the healthy salad option on a fast-food menu, they feel justified in ordering the unhealthy items, like fries. It's called the "Vicarious Goal Fulfillment Effect." You heard right. Considering the salad leads people to feel better about themselves even when they order the less-than-healthy options on the menu. So, I guess you can plan on seeing gorgeous, seductive photos of salads at each and every fast-food franchise you visit.

The Standard American Diet has to be rethought, and I don't mean going from Kentucky Fried Chicken to Kentucky Grilled Chicken. You won't see the results you need to rescue humanity by reducing your intake of food by a few chips, a soda or two, or paring away the fat on your pork chop. Nothing short of a complete rethinking of how we feed ourselves is going to turn the tide of this epidemic of obesity and disease that threatens the very existence of future generations.

WHO'S CALLING THE SHOTS ON OUR DIETARY GUIDELINES?

One of the problems we face with our modern way of eating is that for many years, no one was telling the whole story. Now we are seeing books by Michael Pollan and Marion Nestle and films like *Food, Inc* and *Forks Over Knives*, but for decades, marketing had free reign over us.

To make matters more complicated, in my view, Americans also have a very naïve view of the world and politics. It's almost sweet. Many of us believe that the men and women in Washington, D.C., who have governance over our food safety are actually working to keep our food safe. Most of us believe that if fast and processed foods were that bad for us, someone would put a stop to it. In reality, our health is for sale to the highest bidder.

I was invited to testify as one of the experts on the benefits of plant-based eating when the U.S. Department of Agriculture (USDA) created new dietary guidelines. My job was to inform the committee of experts who would decide what facts and recommendations would be made public. I did my job, as did my fellow experts who spoke to the positive health impact of plant-based eating. But here is what struck me: We were the only group of experts with no special interest group behind us. There is no lobby with a vested interest in Americans eating broccoli. The rest of the experts were paid to testify, representing businesses and their interests. From the dairy council to the beef, egg, and poultry industries, to the sugar and the grocery lobbies (representing, of all things, the role processed food plays in a healthy diet), lobbyists jockeyed for their respective products to be well placed in the new guidelines. It occurred to me, as I listened to their rationalizations, that we will never get authentic guidelines. We will never receive untainted information. Every single lobbyist in that room had a vested financial interest in getting a spot on the new symbol. The guidelines were for sale. Positions in the guidelines were going to the highest bidder.

Yes, healthy eating is promoted in the new guidelines, with plant-based eating even being endorsed and supported. I applaud the progress that has been made in the direction of solving some of the problems we face with epidemic lifestyle diseases.

Research on Vegetarian Eating Patterns

The types of vegetarian diets consumed in the United States vary widely. Vegans do not consume any animal products, while lacto-ovo vegetarians consume milk and eggs. Some individuals eat diets that are primarily vegetarian but may include small amounts of meat, poultry, or seafood.

In prospective studies of adults, compared to non-vegetarian eating patterns, vegetarian-style eating patterns have been associated with improved health outcomes—lower levels of obesity, a reduced risk of cardiovascular disease, and lower total mortality. Several clinical trials have documented that vegetarian eating patterns lower blood pressure.

On average, vegetarians consume a lower proportion of calories from fat (particularly saturated fatty acids); fewer overall calories; and more fiber, potassium, and vitamin C than do non-vegetarians. Vegetarians generally have a lower body mass index. These characteristics and other lifestyle factors associated with a vegetarian diet may contribute to the positive health outcomes that have been identified among vegetarians.

—"Dietary Guidelines for Americans," 2010

Now if only we could get the special interest groups out of the picture so this information would get as much media attention as eating animal products does.

Lobbies would have you believe that there is a place in a healthy diet for processed foods. A representative of the Grocery Manufacturers Association/Food Products Association said that it was "up to each individual American to discover how much processed and packaged foods worked for them in their lives," implying that a "nanny state" of experts telling us what to eat was not what was needed in this country. What? All you need to do is look around and see how well that's working.

Nobody likes to be told what they can and cannot eat; I just want information free from the taint of special interests, which brings me to the latest and greatest attempts by our government to attract us to healthy eating.

MY PYRAMID MEETS MYPLATE

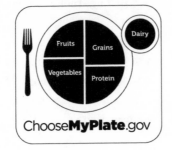

Out with the old and in with the new—guidelines, that is, for how Americans should be eating.

The decades-old food pyramid was toppled early in 2011 and replaced with a simple icon of a dinner plate to help us make healthier food choices. Divided into four primary-colored sections, representing fruits, vegetables, whole grains, and lean protein with a small side dish representing dairy, the new MyPlate is designed to show Americans, at a glance, the kinds of foods they should be filling their plates with, and in what proportions.

Considered an opportunity for Americans to understand quickly how to have a balanced and nutritious meal, the icon is promoted to be a constant reminder as you look at your own plate: whether your portion sizes are right, and whether you've got enough fruits and vegetables on that plate.

The hope is that MyPlate, as the "face" of the new guidelines issued by the USDA in 2010, will remove the confusion associated with figuring out how many servings of a food or food group create health. The accompanying new website (ChooseMyPlate.gov) includes much of the same information featured at MyPyramid.gov, as well as selected messages to help consumers focus on key behaviors: enjoy your food, but eat less; avoid oversized portions; make half your plate fruits and vegetables; switch to fat-free or low-fat (1%) milk; make at least half your grains whole grains; compare sodium in foods like soup, bread, and frozen meals—and choose foods with lower numbers; and drink water instead of sugary drinks. (These highlights are taken from the website's homepage.)

It's a step in helping people approach healthy eating but avoids hard-and-fast rules because that might, well, conjure up images of "dieting."

A lot of the advice given at ChooseMyPlate.gov is sound, to be sure. The brightly colored sections on the plate lead to suggestions like choosing whole fruit, 100 percent juice, and fresh or frozen vegetables. It even encourages shopping at local farmers' markets to get the freshest, most nutrient-dense food.

However, further click-throughs paint a slightly different picture: the whole grains section of the plate divides grains into whole and refined. The whole grain list leads with whole-wheat flour and bulgur, both refined grains. The only whole grain on the list is brown rice. In my view, this will confuse people as to what whole grains really are. Flour is not a whole grain; it is made up of refined grains, and while whole-grain flours are certainly superior to refined white flour, they are not whole grains. This is precisely the kind of deception that allows certain breakfast cereals, for instance, to claim they include whole grains. And it just ain't true. If Cheerios had whole grain oats in them, you would not have the little "O's," you would see whole oats. This is but one instance that I find misleading and that doesn't give consumers the information they need to make educated choices.

The protein suggestions are mostly all animal foods. Dry beans and peas are considered unique in that they work as both sources of protein and vegetables and are strongly recommended several times a week. And finally, the recommendations also include nuts and seeds as sources of protein. While that's excellent news, the focus is still placed on animal food as the primary source of protein. That's a big problem for me. In a culture that is suffering from so much disease as a result of the amount of animal products we consume, I would be happier to see beans, peas, nuts, and seeds as our primary recommendations for protein sources with a nod to animal food instead of the way it is presented now. A radical thought, I know, but in my opinion, we need something radical to pull us back from the edge, so to speak.

MyPlate is simpler than the pyramid and that's good. We like simple. But the results of these efforts, beginning with the first food pyramid in 1992, have been less than spectacular. As a nation we are fatter and less healthy than ever. Frankly, I think that the government campaigns for healthier eating are no match for the massive marketing budgets (and misplaced subsidies) for certain sectors in the food supply chain that, in the end, are promoting products—fast food and processed goods—that are deleterious to everyone's well-being, as well as the planet's.

When you look closely at the recommendations made by the USDA, and represented by MyPlate and its predecessor icons, you have to recognize that the USDA struggles with a dilemma: to serve the health needs of consumers and at the same time continue to pander to special interests. One striking example that is particularly telling in the MyPlate icon is the inclusion of a special side dish for dairy products. The fact that these products have been distinguished so prominently instead of including them within the protein portion is, in my opinion, a clear tip of the hat to powerful dairy lobby groups. And even though the new icon includes "foods made from milk that retain their calcium," it does not explain that the human body can only use up to 30 percent of that calcium. (I will concede that adding calcium-fortified soy milk to the dairy group is welcome.)

However, in spite of the USDA's best efforts, I believe that their approach is fundamentally flawed and only a radical shift in thinking of both the USDA and the public will result in any significant improvements.

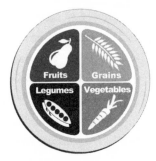

Used by permission of Physicians Committee for Responsible Medicine

Which brings me to Neal Barnard, MD, and Physicians Committee for Responsible Medicine (PCRM). In anticipation of the MyPlate launch, Dr. Barnard and PCRM created the Power Plate. To me, it's the answer. Like

MyPlate, it eliminates serving numbers, but unlike MyPlate, it does not recommend portion sizes—because all the food groups are plant based. By eliminating foods that are risky for our health, there's no need to regulate portions. With this high-fiber, nutrient-dense, vegetarian diet, people will self-regulate because eating real food will satisfy them long before the negative effects of high-calorie intake can be reached.

The message is simple. Eat from these four food groups: grains, legumes, vegetables, and fruits, and you automatically create balanced nutrition. Meat, dairy, eggs, and, of course, processed foods have been eliminated because they are not necessary for health and actually increase our risk for disease. Oils, nuts, and seeds are options and can be used as needed in each person's diet. It could not be easier.

This is the plate that I would promote if I had my way. This is how we climb out of the abyss in which we find ourselves in terms of health and wellness. If I had all the money that is being spent on subsidies, special interests, and lobbying, this is the program on which I would spend my resources, educating and marketing in the same ways that allowed processed and fast food to take over our consciousness.

In my opinion, the accessible and engaging approach that the Physicians Committee for Responsible Medicine has created is the sure path to health. The supporting website (www.pcrm.org) is simple, clean, and user-friendly. The information is easy to understand. The site contains unimpeachable research and simple ways for people to make the changes they need to prevent and even reverse disease, from shopping lists to recipes.

In my opinion, the USDA could have saved a lot of taxpayer dollars by simply listening to the voices of reason at PCRM and adopting and promoting a symbol backed by a comprehensive program that could lead Americans to healthy eating. Combined with a public relations campaign (not unlike the "Got Milk?" promotions funded by the California Milk Processor Board), we could change the health of Americans (and make a lighter footprint on the planet) in a most delicious manner.

Am I suggesting that the only way back to health for Americans is to adopt a plant-based diet and eliminate animal foods? Yes, I am. Can it be done? With education, information, and an easy-to-follow plan, just maybe . . .

PART TWO

The State of Our Food

When I came home from school every day, my Nonna would have a big pot of some kind of beans or a stew simmering away on the stove, simply prepared with olive oil, garlic, and fresh herbs from her windowsill. She served it to us as our after-school snack along with bread freshly baked by my mother. That was what we knew. If we wanted cookies, my mother baked them. If we wanted pizza, they whipped up the dough and—voilà!—we had pizza. We lived a life where food was respected and valued, where dinnertime was sacred. If you didn't make it to dinner, you'd best be dead. It was the only acceptable excuse.

They shopped for food like their lives depended on it. They would squeeze the fruit, smell the vegetables, examine the eggs, sniff the milk. They knew nothing about nutrition, but they knew that if food was fresh and whole, it cooked well and tasted right. They didn't have to spend precious time agonizing over the small print that comes on the packaged food in trying to determine what was in it and if it was any good for us. Yet the family was nourished properly and was happy and strong.

So am I asking you to head into the kitchen and bake bread? Yes . . . and no. While a lovely hobby, bread baking takes time, and I know that's at a premium for most of us. But I am asking you to return to the kitchen; dust off the pots and pans and cook dinner from scratch . . . a few times a week. And build from there.

3

What's Really Going into Our Food?

Maya Angelou famously said that when someone shows you who they are, we should believe them. The same goes with food and its labeling.

It's time to get smart about food. You need to educate yourself. There's no need to spend hours trawling the Internet reading studies. But you must begin to think differently. For instance, if a Mrs. Smith's PreBaked Apple Pie contains more than twenty total ingredients, three sugars, including high-fructose corn syrup, hydrogenated vegetable shortening, and margarine, there has to be a better choice.

THE SCOURGE OF PROCESSED FOODS

Processed foods have changed the complexion of our eating patterns. That we know for sure. Overall, their inclusion in our daily fare has left an imprint on human health that has completely changed the playing field, so to speak.

What exactly is a processed food and what's the problem?

A stroll through any supermarket reveals row after row of foods in brightly colored packages displaying food after delicious-looking food. They encourage us with catchy names and creative packaging . . . and great prices.

And while you may be thinking that you don't buy or eat these things or you think processed foods are greasy, wrapped burgers and fries, think again. Open your cabinet doors and look at what's there. I'm betting you'll find processed foods.

If the food lining your pantry shelves is jarred, canned, and/or has a list of ingredients on the package, it's processed. Any food that has been altered from its natural state for ease, convenience, and to extend its shelf life is considered a processed food.

Processed foods are most certainly more convenient. Open a box, pour in some oil and an egg and—presto!—you have a cake in minutes. Open a tube, slice frozen dough into rounds, and in minutes you have cookies, just like homemade. Add boiling water to Minute Rice and you have flavorful rice . . . in a minute.

Ease and convenience aren't the only things you get in a packaged food though. We get so much more: color to give your food that never-seen-in-nature glow; stabilizers so your gravy is never runny; emulsifiers so oil and water can mix (even though in nature, they wouldn't); bleach so your food is pristine-looking, sanitary, and disinfected; softeners so that ice cream seems as though it was churned twice (it wasn't); preservatives so you can enjoy the cupcakes in that package six months from now; artificial sweeteners so you can have your cake and eat it; artificial flavorings that give processed foods flavors more intense than anything nature could produce. Mother Nature can't compete.

The biggest problem with processed foods isn't convenience. No one wants life to be harder than it is. The problem lies with the fact that they contain a laundry list of ingredients that you probably don't want to eat. You can't pronounce or identify most of them, so you need to ask yourself if you want to eat food that contains them.

With more than six thousand different chemical additives approved to color, flavor, bind, enhance, and otherwise alter a food, it's important to note that you may not be aware of what's really in your food. Sure, you read labels and that's essential, but the FDA doesn't require that a manufacturer list approved additives (called GRAS, generally regarded as safe) individually, which is why you see phrasing like "artificial flavors," "artificial colors," or even "natural flavors."

One look at the packaged items in your pantry, freezer, and fridge tells the story. You will see "natural flavor" or "artificial flavor" on just about every ingredient list. According to Eric Schlosser, author of *Fast Food Nation*, the similarities between these two broad categories are far more significant than the differences.

Both are man-made additives that give processed food most of its taste.

WHAT'S REALLY IN THE "FOOD" YOU ARE EATING?

According to the Center for Science in the Public Interest, you will find many of the following "ingredients" in fast and processed foods—or what I call "chemical cuisine." Even with giant checkmarks, health halos, and carefully worded claims on the packages and in the advertising, there is no mistaking that processed foods are a lot less than "healthy."

Acesulfame-k: K is the symbol for potassium, so you will also see this no-calorie, artificial sweetener called "Ace K" on ingredient panels. Used mostly in carbonated beverages, it's two hundred times sweeter than sucrose. The problems, according to www.medicine.net, stem from the fact that there are no long-term studies proving the safety of this sweetener. Containing methylene chloride, a known carcinogen, excessive exposure can result in headaches, nausea, mental confusion, liver and kidney trouble, and cancer. Many experts oppose the use of acesulfame-k until more comprehensive testing is done, but the FDA does not require it, so we are the guinea pigs.

Artificial coloring (including blue 2, green 3, orange b, red 3, yellow 5, yellow 6): According to *Science News*: "Artificial food coloring ingredients (food dye) contain plenty of chemicals. Many are derived from highly toxic sources and can cause many different diseases, disorders, and mutations in humans. Although it seems unlikely that a trivial amount of food coloring in a piece of a candy you eat (like licorice) would have any harmful effect on you, you would be wrong, because it does."

Aspartame: A derivative of aspartic acid and phenylalanine, this very sweet no-calorie artificial sweetener is between 160 to 200 times sweeter than sugar, and was denied approval by the FDA for eight years because it was considered a risk to human health. Among these risks is the fact that this sweetener does not digest and enters the brain and central nervous system and can result in a number of problems, according to Dr. Janet Hull, including seizures, impaired vision, anxiety, and palpitations.

Butylated hydroxyanisole (BHA): BHA is an additive that preserves fat and oils in food and cosmetics, but its ability to preserve may also be the cause of health problems, according to Anne Marie Helmenstine, PhD, of About.com. The oxidative characteristics of BHA may contribute to carcinogenicity or tumorigenicity. Some people have difficulty assimilating this preservative, resulting in behavior changes.

Hydrogenated oil: Hydrogenation is a process by which one kind of fat is converted to another; it alters the molecular structure of fat to create a longer-lasting end product, not prone to rancidity. Also known as trans fat, it is a hydrogen-rich fat that contributes to heart disease because it is nearly impossible to digest and assimilate, accumulating in the circulatory system, blocking veins and arteries, according to the experts at www.optimal-heart -health.com.

Olestra: A synthetic cooking oil used as a calorie-free fat substitute, olestra was created by Procter & Gamble by combining sucrose and vegetable oil to create a molecule not found in nature; a molecule that cannot be digested by our bodies. It simply passes through the stomach and intestines unchanged. This can result in the depletion of fat-soluble nutrients we need to be healthy: vitamins A, D, E, and K. Because these vitamins bind to fat for digestion, they bind to this product and are excreted.

Partially hydrogenated oil: Hydrogenated oil is made by forcing hydrogen gas into oil to prolong the shelf life. The more solid the oil, the more hydrogenated it is. Partially hydrogenated oil has had less hydrogen forced into it, but it remains a rich source of trans fats.

Potassium bromate: A powerful oxidizer, this food additive is employed to improve the quality of flour but is considered carcinogenic and has actually been banned by most of Europe, Canada, and China, according to the Center for Science in the Public Interest, and has been linked to renal cancer and mesothelioma.

Propyl gallate: A food additive used to prevent the oxidation of fats in processed foods, thereby extending shelf life, it has been added to the "Dirty Dozen" of dangerous food additives by the experts at SixWise.com because of its links to cancer and food allergies.

Saccharin: This artificial sweetener, which contains no food energy, is made from benzoic sulfilimine and is much sweeter than sucrose. Found in Sweet'N Low and many other no-calorie products, saccharin was the first artificial sweetener to be mass produced. Although saccharin was thought to be carcinogenic, studies proved inconclusive, resulting in warning labels being removed, but many experts still believe there is an increased risk of cancer with continued use of this sweetener.

Sodium nitrate/sodium nitrite: Known by both names, this toxic additive also made it onto SixWise.com's list of most dangerous food additives. Used to color, preserve, and flavor bacon, ham, hot dogs, lunch meats, corned beef, and smoked fish, these additives can lead to the formation of cancer-causing chemicals called nitrosamines.

Diacetyl: A chemically produced byproduct of yeast, this additive provides a buttery taste and lends creaminess to foods. Used in everything from butter-flavored popcorn to sour cream, cottage cheese, salad dressings, icing, and even beer, it has been linked to bronchitis obliterans (a serious fixed obstruction lung disease), a condition found in employees working in factories that use it in processed food products. Although diacetyl has been deemed safe by the FDA, California is working to ban its use completely and several manufacturers have banned its use to protect workers and consumers.

Heptyl paraben: A preservative used in beer and noncarbonated soft drinks, as well as bakery products, it belongs to a family of parabens used to preserve lotions, conditioners, and shampoos. This food-grade paraben, like other parabens, has been shown to display estrogenic activity. The *European*

Journal of Cancer Prevention reported that parabens accumulate in breast tissue and do not break down, resulting in actual breast tumors.

Fructose: This monosaccharide is low on the glycemic index and can be used by the body as energy. So what's the problem? According to the American Diabetes Association, because fructose is digested in the liver, it overwhelms the function of this gland, so the body can't use it fast enough as sugar, converts it to fat, and sends it off to the bloodstream as triglycerides. Elevated levels of triglycerides increase the risk of heart disease.

High-fructose corn syrup: A Princeton University research team released results of a study in March 2010 that found that while some people (corn refiners, for example) insist that HFCS is no different from other sweeteners, it's not true. Professor Bart Hoebel found that long-term consumption of this sweetener led to abnormal increases in body fat, especially in the abdomen, and a rise in triglycerides. They say this is because, like fructose, HFCS digests through the liver, disrupting metabolism.

Hydrogenated starch hydrolysate: The result of partial hydrolysis of corn, wheat, or potato starch, HSH is one of a family of polyols that includes lactitol, maltitol, manitol, and sorbitol. These hydrogenated saccharides are used in the production of sugar-free products and are between 40 and 90 percent as sweet as sugar. And while they seem harmless, even beneficial to people in need of low or no-calorie sweeteners, these hydrogenated compounds are hard to digest and can present a problem for sufferers of celiac disease.

Invert sugar: This mixture of glucose and sucrose made by hydrolysis of sucrose and broken down into free glucose and free fructose is used to prevent and control the buildup of crystallization of sugar and extend the shelf life of processed baked goods. Like HFCS, it's another form of sugar and is a major contributor to obesity.

Lactitol: See hydrogenated starch hydrolysate.

Maltitol: See hydrogenated starch hydrolysate.

Manitol: See hydrogenated starch hydrolysate.

Polydextrose: Used to increase the nondietary fiber in processed foods, this synthetic additive is used in processed diet foods and low-calorie sweets to enhance flavor. Made from dextrose, sorbitol, and citric acid, polydextrose has been linked with bloating, severe stomach cramps, and excessive gas.

Salatrim: This manufactured, modified fat, developed by Nabisco and made from stearic acid, is used in low-fat food products. With the physical properties of fat and about half the calories, it has been subjected to very limited testing, according to the Center for Science in the Public Interest. The FDA rejected CSPI's petition to ban this product until more extensive testing was done. Consumption has been linked to severe gastrointestinal distress with no understanding of long-term effects on digestive health.

Tagatose: A low-carbohydrate, naturally occurring sweetener similar in molecular structure to fructose, produced from lactose, it is the sugar found in dairy products. Need I say more?

Monosodium glutamate: MSG, as we know this chemical additive, is used to preserve processed food and cheap restaurant food so it seems fresh. According to John Erbe, coauthor of *The Slow Poisoning of America*, MSG triples the amount of insulin secreted by the pancreas, contributing to obesity. Said to increase production of serotonin, MSG has been shown to be addictive, causing people to eat more. The National Library of Medicine has more than 115 published studies that establish the link between MSG consumption and obesity.

Benzoic acid: Benzoic acid and its salts are yet more preservatives added to processed foods and are mostly used in fruit juices and sparkling beverages to preserve the pH and as an anticorrosive agent in soda. Anticorrosive!

Sodium benzoate: Produced by the neutralization of benzoic acid with sodium hydroxide, this preservative is used in the same way as benzoic acid, for the same reasons, with better results. See benzoic acid.

Sodium bisulfate: This is an acid salt made from sodium, hydrogen, sulfur, and oxygen ions and is used to impart a sour taste and to enhance the flavor of processed foods. Used also as a preservative, sodium bisulfate has been linked to respiratory problems, including chronic cough and tracheal bronchitis. Excessive consumption has been linked to tooth corrosion, according to the National Institutes of Health.

Sodium caseinate: This derivative of casein, a milk protein, is often used in non-dairy creamers (don't ask me how, since it comes from milk protein . . .) to create a creamy flavor and texture. This presents a big problem for people with allergies to dairy products.

Sulfites: Also known as sulfur dioxide, these fruit preservatives are used in wine and include potassium metabisulfite, sodium sulfite, sodium bisulfite, and sodium metabisulfite. They are used to prevent discoloration and bacterial growth in wine and dried fruits and vegetables. The World Health Organization says that while deaths are rare, sulfating agents are linked to respiratory problems and even death in people with asthma and recommend only 42 milligrams for a 130-pound person. The problem is, a 4-ounce glass of wine can contain 40 added milligrams of sulfites; a restaurant salad, 160; and 3 ounces of dried apricots, 175.

Sulfur dioxide: See sulfites.

While some of these ingredients are considered "natural," you won't find them in a bin in the farmers' market. So, yes, I am mad as hell . . . at what food manufacturers are doing to our food and to us. Our health is suffering; disease is at epidemic numbers, and we are losing our vitality, our children, and our future.

THE COMPETITION FOR OUR FOOD DOLLARS

Most people buy a new food item because of the packaging, the appearance, or word of mouth. Taste and taste alone determines whether they will buy it again. And since about 90 percent of the money Americans spend on food now goes to buy processed foods, the competition is fierce.

The canning, drying, freezing, dehydrating, hydrogenating, and other processes used to create these foodlike substances destroy most of the food's natural flavor. So a vast and profitable industry has grown to make processed food palatable. Without this industry, processed foods would cease to exist, because they would not taste good and people wouldn't buy them. People would buy real food, like apples, and not some enhanced applelike thing that tastes sweeter and more apple-y than real apples.

And while the names of the leading fast-food chains have become a part of our day-to-day culture, with their names and products embedded in our psyches, not many of us can name the companies responsible for manufacturing the flavor of the fast food we love so much.

Which is how the companies prefer it.

This highly secretive industry will not divulge precise formulas or take interviews about their clients. The fast-food industry banks on the public thinking that the flavors in their food originate in kitchens in pots and pans simmering on the stove. Their ads show chefs slicing and dicing fresh ingredients, stirring, and tasting. Commercials show cooking schools with chefs learning to cook authentic dishes in various foreign countries. In truth, most of those flavors are manufactured in factories, like IFF (International Flavors & Fragrances), the world's largest flavor company. Off the New Jersey Turnpike, IFF is housed not far from the second-largest flavor house in the world, Givaudan, in East Hanover. And then there's Haarmann & Reimer and Takasago in Teterboro, Flavor Dynamics in South Plainfield, Frutoram in North Bergen, and Elan Chemical (yes, chemical, not food, *chemical*) in Newark. Dozens of smaller companies dot this corridor in New Jersey. Altogether, this area of the country produces about two-thirds of the flavor additives sold in the United States. It's an interesting paradox that New Jersey is known as the Garden State, conjuring images of idyllic farms and fields of fresh vegetables and fruit, when along with its gorgeous, abundant farmland, we also have these factories of fake flavors.

In the "Flavor House"

I was hired by a multinational food company to consult on a new food product it was considering. I attended brainstorming sessions, and lab and creative packaging meetings. I worked in a huge commercial kitchen creating the products from natural ingredients. Afterward, in what could only be described as the Mad Scientist Meets Willy Wonka, a team of "scientists" in lab coats (not chef coats) went about showing me how they were able to *duplicate* nature's flavors. Little bottles, filled with powerfully flavored chemicals, had long science-y names on their neat white labels. It was mystifying. These chemicals would come together like magic potions to re-create some of the most common flavors, only more intensely.

It occurred to me that flavors for potato chips, breads, crackers, juices, cereals, pet food, ice cream, cookies, candies, toothpaste, mouthwash, antacids, power drinks, beer, soda, bottled teas, wine coolers, and just about every other processed food could be—and were—created.

Although the flavors in my food came from 100 percent natural ingredients, when they were moved to the lab, they were created chemically so that the foods could be manufactured from cheaper ingredients, in larger volumes, and made to taste like real food—sort of like food "on steroids." Cookies tasted more cookielike; ice cream creamier; and chocolate more intense. Mother Nature had been hijacked... outlabbed.

A DAY IN YOUR LIFE WITH PROCESSED FOODS

It is indisputable: breakfast is the most important meal of the day. It sets the tone for how you will experience your day. After a night's sleep, our bodies and brains need energy to get going. Our blood sugar is a little low from fasting all night. We need to rebalance and begin to fuel ourselves for the day ahead. The foods we choose will give us the energy we need to get through the morning, as well as provide nutrients we need for life in general . . . or not, depending on your choices.

Not all breakfast foods are good for you. Marketers have figured out brilliant ways to ruin our day right from the beginning with high-calorie, nutrient-deficient breakfast options wrapped in brightly colored packages with health claims on them to seduce us into the trap.

According to a poll done by ABC News, one in four Americans skip breakfast altogether. More than 31 percent begin their day with cold cereal, with eggs, bacon, bagels, or pastries. Fast-food breakfasts run a distant second. (Cold pizza came up as a breakfast favorite for about 39 percent of those polled, but I don't think I need to speak to how many ways this is just so wrong.) The survey of adults showed that women were eight times more likely to eat cold cereal than men, with men choosing eggs more often. But even at that, cold cereal emerged the clear winner for both sexes.

Breakfast (and More) Cereals

Because most working people are looking for fast and easy ways to get nutrition to begin the day, we need to be vigilant with our choices of breakfast cereal. So many times, we think we are making healthier choices, when, in fact, we may not be doing so—even when the names imply health and vitality, nature and goodness, whole grain and fiber. You need to read the fine print between the screaming headlines.

A quick check of the nutritional label on most packaged cereal is all it takes to show you that most cold cereals are just boxes of candy enriched with a few vitamins and minerals. Many of them have more sugar than the average pastry! A study published in the *Journal of American College Nutrition* revealed that women who ate high-sugar breakfasts burned less sugar throughout the day than women who ate a low-sugar breakfast, which resulted in lethargy, mental fog, and weight gain.

The fact that cereal isn't marketed only as a breakfast food makes it all the more problematic for our health. It can be eaten any time of the day, with or without milk, as a snack right out of the box. Special K tells us that having a bowl of their Special K Chocolatey Delight cereal will keep your cravings at bay and your diet on track. Their commercials show a gorgeous woman chowing down on a huge bowl of this stuff (while her chocolate ice cream calls to her seductively), but the reality of their label is not so seductive. With 120 calories, 9 grams of sugar, and hydrogenated oil in a mere three-quarter-cup serving, you'd be better off with an ounce of dark chocolate, which has about 70 calories and 7 grams of sugar—and is the real thing, not some dry, manufactured, strawlike nonsense with artificially flavored chocolate bits distributed through it. You would eat a smaller volume, for sure, but think of the satisfaction of that silky smooth dark chocolate. Now think of a bowl of Special K. I rest my case.

Let's take a look at some of this toxic waste masquerading as breakfast food on our supermarket shelves. While most cereals look the same as always with similar-size boxes and designs and similar pricing, almost all of them now make health claims of some sort. Get the insulin ready, folks. You'll need it after these breakfasts.

I compiled these numbers from the actual websites of each of these cereals, so if you think they are screwy in some way, take it up with them. The commentary is completely mine; the stats are theirs.

Here are, in my view, the worst breakfast cereals you can buy today, not in any particular order. It was just about impossible to rate them in order when each one has its unique profile designed to make you fat and unhealthy.

1. **Post's Banana Nut Crunch.** Weighing in with 220 calories for a bit more than a half-cup serving, this top contender also boasts 6 grams of fat and 44 grams of carbohydrates (most of them simple) in this tiny serving.

2. **Kellogg's Smart Start, Healthy Heart Toasted Oat Cereal.** Ah, the irony! With 220 calories in a 1¼-cup serving, 17 grams of sugar, plus high-fructose corn syrup, this *healthy-sounding* cereal will do a lot more damage to your ticker by expanding your waistline than you might think from its name.

3. **General Mills' Oatmeal Crisp Crunchy Almond Cereal** delivers 220 calories in one cup, 16 grams of sugar, and high-fructose corn syrup. But it's oatmeal, right? Isn't that healthy? Not in this box. The claim that oats

can help reduce blood pressure and the risk of heart disease is true when you eat whole oats. (Even rolled oats deliver a benefit.) But when coupled with all the other ingredients in this package, well, not so much.

4. **General Mills' Basic 4**, marketed to be completely healthy, is taking us back to basics, right? One cup gives us 200 calories, 14 grams of sugar (from sugar, brown sugar, honey, corn syrup, barley malt, and brown sugar syrup), artificial colors and flavor, hydrogenated palm kernel oil, and preservatives. The Basic 4? The implication in the name is that this cereal draws from the four basic food groups. But with more than forty ingredients, including some added vitamins and minerals, it's hardly what I would call basic—or healthy.

5. **Kellogg's Frosted Mini Wheats** with 200 calories, 12 grams of sugar, and high-fructose corn syrup in a mere 24 little biscuits, is this the cereal that will keep your kids focused in school and prevent million-dollar mistakes at work because you are so on the ball? I doubt that.

6. **Kellogg's Raisin Bran Crunch** is a "healthy" cereal with 190 calories in a one-cup serving, 20 grams of sugar, and high-fructose corn syrup. Have a little fiber (4 grams) with your sugar.

7. **General Mills' Wheat Chex.** With only 6 grams of sugar, where are the 214 calories in one cup coming from? Makes you wonder if they count the molasses in the ingredient panel as sugar.

8. My personal "favorite" is **General Mills' Lucky Charms** with 110 calories and 11 grams of sugar in a three-quarter-cup serving. You might be wondering how this seemingly benign cereal got here on the list of lousy cereals. You might be thinking: only 110 calories and not too much sugar. Is that so bad? Well, this teensy three-quarter-cup serving is one that you will never see a child eat . . . a mouse, maybe, but not a hungry kid.

The label claims to be a good source of whole grains—and the package features the "Big G" checkmark. But is it? According to the Whole Grain Council, here's where information gets a little murky on labels. Lucky Charms claims to contain "whole grain oats." The U.S. standards are that a product must contain 51 percent, by weight, of whole grain to be called a "whole grain." That leaves nearly half the volume of the ingredient to be refined grains and flour, which explains why this product can say "whole-grain guaranteed" and still contain only 1 gram of fiber per serving. If this cereal gave us a serving of whole oats, it would contain nearly 12 grams of total fiber per serving. A serving of whole grain, real whole grain, according to the Council, is 1 ounce, or 28 grams. In the case of whole-grain products, a serving is a food that contains at least 16 grams of whole grains. Just so you're clear.

The rest of the ingredient panel reads like *War and Peace*: including modified corn starch, corn syrup, dextrose, gelatin, artificial flavor (yellow 5 & 6, red 40, blue 1 [all proven carcinogens]), methyl cellulose, sodium laurel sulfate, calcium carbonate, salt, and at the end, a mixed bag of some added vitamins (to ease their guilt?). You'd be better off sending the kids to school without breakfast, in my view, than with this "magically delicious" junk food.

9. How can I resist **Trix**? After all, they're for kids and part of the "Big G" whole-grain family from General Mills. When I was a kid, we could buy Trix, plain and simple; junk food to be sure, but just Trix. Now, it seems the focus is on Trix Fruitalicious Swirls, so we think our kids are getting the goodness of fruit along with their cereal.

What you're actually getting in this artificially flavored and colored poison is 120 calories (160 with a half cup of skim milk), 28 grams of carbohydrate, 10 grams of sugar, and a measly 1 gram of fiber in one cup. So much for the "whole-grain guarantee." And the calcium that's guaranteed on the box? It clocks in at a mere 10 percent of your daily need, which doesn't come close to offsetting what the sugar depletes from your blood.

So the next time you are perusing the packages in the cereal aisle of your local market, don't be fooled. Look past the claims, checkmarks, and health halos and see what's really in those brightly colored packages. Look at the number of different sugars on the ingredient list and the artificial colors and flavors. And remember just because a product has words like *heart*, *smart*, *basic*, or *whole grain* or tells you it can help lower cholesterol, it doesn't mean the product is natural or healthy. Learn to read the fine print and you'll see that most of these cereals have no place in your pantry, on your table, or in your family's tummies.

You will see this continued deception throughout packaged processed foods. Whole grains are whole grains like brown rice, barley, quinoa, millet, whole wheat, or buckwheat. Flour, flakes, or puffs can be fun to use once in a while, but make no mistake that you will not see the benefits you will from eating real whole grains. Relying on them as your sources of whole grains will not create the health that marketers are trying to sell you.

A Healthy Breakfast . . . Fast!

Froot Loops, out! Trix, out! Lucky Charms, definitely out!

What can you do to get that same silly smile on your face that you get with a bowl of crunchy cereal in the morning?

How do we satisfy our need for a quick breakfast and our love of dry cereal to start the day?

You know I want to tell you to break your fast with miso soup, a creamy whole-grain porridge, and steamed leafy green vegetables, but since I live in the real world and that ideal breakfast may need to be leaned into . . . try these healthy options and still get your day off to a great start.

Here are my top five choices, in order of preference. With almond, soy, or rice milk, these can't be beat.

1. **Erewhon Crispy Brown Rice Cereal** is gluten-free and made from whole-grain puffed brown rice. Sweetened with a wee bit of brown-rice syrup, there's nothing artificial added and no preservatives. And . . . 110 calories in a one-cup serving.
2. **Post Grape-Nuts** cereal, the butt of the twig-eating jokes of my youth, contains only four ingredients (not counting the vitamins added) and no added sugar. A great source of fiber, Grape-Nuts weigh in at 200 calories for a half-cup serving and provide 90 percent of the iron you need daily.

3. For Cheerios lovers, **Nature's Path Organic Whole O's** is a great alternative, with six ingredients, no artificial additives or preservatives, and 110 calories in a two-third-cup serving. These do contain organic cane sugar, but they sure beat anything you'll buy commercially.

4. And for the Honey Nut Cheerios fans, try **Cascadian Farms Organic Honey Nut O's**, with 110 calories in a one-cup serving and nothing artificial added. These also contain organic sugar and honey, but with only 7 grams of sugar. It's a better choice than commercial O's.

5. For the Froot Loops lovers, try **Cascadian Farms Fruitful O's**. While they contain some sugar (9 grams in a one-cup serving), there's nothing artificial added, and at 160 calories a serving, these are a great way to transition your family to healthier options.

And, finally, for breakfast cereal lovers not quite on board with miso soup and vegetables, but who want a bit more than cold cereal, try **Bob's Red Mill Organic Rolled Oats**, bulgur wheat, or unsweetened muesli, and in about five minutes, with fresh fruit and almond milk, you'll have something that sticks to your ribs.

Fast-Food Breakfast Options

Since we're talking breakfast, let's look at some options to whole grains that are not serving your health. For those of us who need more than just a bowl of cereal to begin the day, we usually turn to protein to fill the bill. Not a bad idea for us in the morning because nothing keeps us sated quite like it. It's important, again, to read the fine print before sitting down to that manly platter. It's true that with protein, you will be less likely to have a mid-morning attack of the munchies. But you are just as likely to stay sated until lunch with a breakfast of whole grains, so don't get too hung up on protein . . . and certainly not at fast-food joints.

Besides, the answer isn't at Denny's: chowing down a Grand Slam Breakfast of eggs, cheese, and bacon (and God knows what else) on a biscuit or English muffin.

An Original Grand Slam Breakfast (10-ounce meal) contains 795 calories, 450 of them from fat, 2,237 milligrams of sodium (yikes!!!), and 460 milligrams of cholesterol. One buttermilk biscuit has 190 calories alone! Denny's Belgian Waffle Slam delivers 1,030 calories (without syrup) and 1,765 milligrams of sodium. Slam, indeed.

Over at Burger King, things are just about as grim for your health: the Ultimate Breakfast Platter comprises scrambled eggs, hash browns, sausage, biscuits, and pancakes with syrup. ("Anything less and it wouldn't deserve to be called the ultimate." At least that's what their website says.) Seriously? Here's how "The Ultimate" stacks up: 1,310 calories, 26 grams of saturated fat, 455 milligrams of cholesterol, 41 grams of sugar, and 2,490 milligrams of sodium. The ultimate what? Need for a portable defibrillator?

Dunkin' Donuts serves breakfast, too. Their Maple Cheddar Breakfast Sandwich is loaded with 720 calories and 1,140 milligrams of sodium. But not to worry, the geniuses at Dunkin' also have healthy offerings, called DD Smart with a teeny sandwich dumping between 250 and 440 calories and an average of 800 milligrams of sodium into your gut. Whew! For a second there, I was worried. DD . . . stands for "double duh," perhaps?

Anthony Bourdain once said that everything tasted better with bacon. And James Beard famously said that if he was to be executed, his last meal would be bacon and eggs because few sights appealed to him more than the streaks of lean meat and fat in good bacon. Both are seductive quotes extolling the desirability of bacon, but they don't change the fact that modern bacon (and other commonly eaten breakfast meats like sausage and ham) is rich in saturated fats and high in sodium . . . both deadly for your heart. And then there are the nitrites, which have been linked to colon cancer. Nothing sexy about that.

Healthier Options?

McDonald's has, of course, plenty of unhealthy breakfast options to choose from, but in an effort to leave no demographic untouched, they have added their version of a whole-grain, healthy-breakfast option: oatmeal. Yippee, right?

Not so fast. According to Mark Bittman, *New York Times* food columnist and bestselling author, there's more to this oatmeal than meets the eye. Marketed as "a bowl full of wholesome," this simple menu item, Bittman says, is a crock full of something else.

"It's put forth as this wholesome thing when, in fact, it's sort of an amalgam of ingredients you wouldn't ordinarily have at home," he says.

Oatmeal naturally has one ingredient in it: oats. McDonald's version has twenty-one ingredients, including flavoring and coloring. Bittman says that it's misleading to imply this item is a healthy breakfast because it contains "about the same amount of sugar as a Snickers Bar" and "about the same number of calories as one of their hamburgers."

McDonald's says that about half the sugar in this healthy breakfast comes from fruit options and the rest from brown sugar, which they say is optional. But you have to ask that the sugar not be added.

No one eats plain oatmeal. We all add something to spruce it up a bit. But we don't add twenty-one ingredients . . . and since it cooks in ten minutes or less, you can see you are better off making it at home.

Other Breakfast Choices

But okay, suppose you don't eat dry cereal or fast food for breakfast. What if you start your day with fruit juice and a bagel or a whole-grain muffin? Did you do the best for your body that you could? Maybe . . . maybe not.

Fruit Versus Fruit Juice

We have all been sold on the notion that downing a glass of orange juice every morning is a great idea. While it's not the worst breakfast choice on the list, take a look at what's in it and you may rethink the prevailing wisdom here.

At 110 calories and 16 grams of carbohydrates (all in the form of simple sugar), a mere 8 ounces of orange juice packs a caloric punch. A medium orange on the other hand, gives you only 62 calories and 15 grams of carbohydrates (2.4 of which are in the form of valuable fiber). With the whole fruit, the fiber will keep you satisfied longer than the juice, which is an insulin trigger and can set your feet on the path to being hungry all day long. Whole fruit is a wiser choice, indeed.

Just look at these comparisons for yourself:

Apple juice (1 cup): 112 calories; 0.2 grams fiber
Apple (1 medium): 53 calories; 2.4 grams fiber

Grapefruit juice (1 cup): 94; trace of fiber
Grapefruit (one half): 41 calories; 1.4 grams fiber

Grape juice (1 cup): 154 calories, trace of fiber
Grapes (10): 36 calories; 0.1 grams fiber

Need I go on?

Carb Loading, Anyone?

Maybe you think you're making a better choice by swinging by Panera Bread to pick up one of their whole-grain bagels. After all, it's said to be made with spelt flour, whole-wheat flour, and flax seeds. It's got to be healthy, right?

A 4.25-ounce bagel has 340 calories and only 6 grams of dietary fiber. What about the flax seeds and all those whole-grain flours? What happened to the fiber? Well, the first ingredient in this whole-grain bagel is unbleached enriched wheat flour (translation: unbleached white flour) and the whole grains are a whole-grain blend that includes flax seeds, so the percentage of each whole grain is small. There are, however, four different sugars in these "healthy" bagels. And that 340 calories is before you put anything on it!

Their muffins are much worse, even though nothing *sounds* healthier than a Carrot Walnut Muffin. With 500 calories, 37 grams of sugar, and only 4 grams of fiber in a 5-ounce muffin, these may sound healthy, but they're anything but.

Starbucks makes an Apple Bran Muffin that even looks healthy, all crunchy and granola-ish. The reality of these little muffins is a bit more harsh: 350 calories (80 from fat), 34 grams of sugar, and 6 grams of protein—all packed in one 4.2-ounce muffin.

Each of these "healthy" breakfast choices will require at least an hour of intense physical exercise to undo the damage to your waistline, according to www.livestrong.com.

What a way to start your day.

EATING WELL ALL DAY LONG

With breakfast under our belt, we have to face the rest of our day and figure our how to navigate all the land mines that inhibit us from eating well. Most of us work outside the home and find it inconvenient or undesirable to brown-bag lunch to the office. And dinner comes at the end of a long day of tight schedules, deadlines, car pool, sports practices, part-time jobs, and other day-to-day stresses. Why can't we just pick up some takeout on the way home?

Because most of it will kill you.

Fast Food Won't Feed You Well . . . Just Fast

In previous sections of this book we discussed what has happened over the last few decades to the way we eat. The de-evolution of our diet has left us adrift in a sea of fast-food franchises that promise one thing and deliver quite another.

McDonald's, Wendy's, KFC, Burger King, Denny's, Olive Garden, Dunkin' Donuts, Subway, Red Lobster, and even Applebee's and Friday's are all leaping on the bandwagon of fresh and wholesome. They all promise you quality food at affordable prices. Some even have "under 500 calorie" menu items.

We see commercials with fit, happy people eating these foods. Subway has created a folk hero out of Jared Fogle, who lost more than two hundred pounds eating only at their restaurants. How did he do it? No breakfast; a six-inch turkey sub with baked chips for lunch; and a twelve-inch veggie sub, topped with nothing on it, for dinner, plus diet soda and water throughout the day. His under-one-thousand-calories-a-day approach worked because he cut back so dramatically on his caloric intake, not so much because he chose Subway and "ate fresh," as the ads would have you believe.

Most of the ready-to-eat food we purchase, whether in a restaurant or in a package, is compromised in quality. There is no way that superior-quality foods can be created and then sold at a cheap price. Do the math: If you bought all the ingredients to make a Big Mac at home, you would spend a lot more than the current retail price of $3.99 (even if you could get all the in-gredients). You'd need access to a chemistry lab to truly duplicate your favor-ite burger.

The Anatomy of a Big Mac

Here's what's in that burger. Now you will understand why it's so cheap. It's a lot more than "two all-beef patties, special sauce, lettuce, cheese, pickles, onions on a sesame seed bun."

Sesame seed bun: Made with enriched flour (bleached wheat flour, malted barley flour, niacin, reduced iron, thiamin, monnitrate, riboflavin, folic acid, enzymes), water, high-fructose corn syrup, sugar, soybean oil or partially hydrogenated soybean oil, plus 2 percent or less of salt, calcium sulfate, calcium carbonate, wheat gluten, ammonium sulfate, ammonium chloride, sodium stearoyl lactylate, datem, ascorbic acid, azodicarbonamide, mono- and diglycerides, ethoxylated monoglycerides, monocalcium phosphate, enzymes, guar gum, calcium peroxide, soy flour, calcium propionate, sodium propionate, soy lecithin, and sesame seed.

Special sauce: I guess the "specialness" is in the proportions of soybean oil, pickle relish (diced pickles, high-fructose corn syrup, sugar, vinegar, corn syrup, salt, calcium chloride, xantham gum, potassium sorbate, spice extractives, polysorbate 80, distilled vinegar, water), egg yolks, high-fructose corn syrup, onion powder, mustard seed, salt, spices, propylene glycol alginate, sodium benzoate, mustard bran, sugar, garlic powder, hydrolyzed corn, soy, and wheat (MSG), caramel color, extractives of paprika, soy lecithin, turmeric, and calcium disodium EDTA.

Two all-beef patties: Come complete with growth hormones, steroids, pesticides, and antibiotics.

Pasteurized process American cheese: According to our friends at Wikipedia, "Today's American cheese is generally no longer made from a blend of other cheeses, but instead is manufactured from a set of ingredients such as milk, whey, milk fat, milk protein concentrate, whey protein concentrate, and salt. In many jurisdictions, it does not meet the legal definition of cheese and must be labeled as 'cheese analogue,' 'cheese product,' processed cheese, or similar."

Pickles: It is hard to say how these are made. But there isn't much nutritional value to them to make a lot of difference.

Lettuce and onion: Perhaps not organic but these seem closest to what Mother Nature intended as we are likely to get.

Just like Mama used to make.

More to Your McNugget Than Chicken?

The Chicken McNugget is fed to our kids daily by the millions. It's a rare mother who has not given in and ordered these for her children because "they like them" and, anyhow, "they're real chicken." Well, that's what McDonald's would have you believe.

While there is, in fact, chicken in McNuggets, how much is up for debate. Their marketing says that McNuggets contain "100 percent chicken" and that's true, technically. They do contain chicken and what chicken they contain is, in fact, real chicken.

They leave out the fact that 56 percent of these little pieces of deep-fried . . . something . . . is corn. In *The Omnivore's Dilemma*, Michael Pollan cites McDonald's own brochure, "A Full Serving of Nutrition Facts: Choose the Best Meal for You," when he writes:

> The ingredients listed in the flyer suggest a lot of thought goes into a nugget, that and a lot of corn. Of the thirty-eight ingredients it takes to make a McNugget, I counted thirteen that can be derived from corn: the corn-fed chicken itself; modified cornstarch (to bind the pulverized chicken meat); mono-, tri-, and diglycerides (emulsifiers, which keep the fats and water from separating); dextrose; lecithin (another emulsifier); chicken broth (to restore some of the flavor that processing leeches out); yellow corn flour and more modified cornstarch (for the batter); cornstarch (a filler); vegetable shortening; partially hydrogenated corn oil; and citric acid as a preservative. A couple of other plants take part in the nugget: There's some wheat in the batter, and on any given day the hydrogenated oil could come from soybeans, canola, or cotton rather than corn, depending on the market price and availability.

Pollan goes on to summarize the "quasi-edible substances" in McNuggets that ultimately come not from a corn or soybean field but from a petroleum refinery or chemical plant. These chemicals are what make modern processed food possible, by keeping the organic materials in them from going bad or looking strange after months in the freezer or on the road, and include leavening agents and synthetic antioxidants to keep the various animal and vegetable fats involved in a nugget from turning rancid. Then there are antifoaming agents, like dimethylpolysiloxane, added to the cooking oil. According to the *Handbook of Food Additives*, dimethylpolysiloxane is a suspected carcinogen and an established mutagen, tumorigen, and reproductive effector; it's also flammable.

But the real kicker in a Chicken McNugget is tertiary butylhydroquinone, or TBHQ, an antioxidant derived from petroleum that is either sprayed directly on the nugget or the inside of the box it comes in to "help preserve freshness." According to *A Consumer's Dictionary of Food Additives*, TBHQ is a form of butane (i.e., lighter fluid) the FDA allows processors to use sparingly in our food: It can comprise no more than 0.02 percent of the oil in a nugget. And it's a good thing, too, since ingesting a single gram of TBHQ can cause "nausea, vomiting, ringing in the ears, delirium, a sense of suffocation, and collapse. Ingesting five grams of TBHQ can kill."

But there is 100 percent chicken in them, too. Counts for something, right?

Pizza for the Health Freak

"Health Freak, Pizza. Pizza, Health Freak" reads the headline on the Domino's Pizza website. The copy goes on to sell us the idea that "Pizza can be healthy. It's just a matter of choosing the right ingredients."

Domino's Pizza tells us that their pizza sauce is fresh from the farm to the table. Their pizza sauce is "made from the finest vine-ripened tomatoes."

It should make us wonder, then, why their sauce is made from the base of a canned, tomato paste–like food service product called Angela Mia Pizza Sauce made by Hunt's. If their sauce relies on the goodness of nature, why does it need MSG added? I guess if you go back enough steps, you'll find a fresh tomato grown on a farm in there somewhere. Hardly what I would call fresh from the farm to your front door. But I guess since fresh tomatoes are a part of the processing of their sauce for pizza, it's technically the truth.

On their website, you can build a pizza and check the calories before you order. As you'll discover, you consume 135 calories for one slice of a small (ten-inch) thin-crust pizza with onions, peppers, garlic, spinach, and mushrooms—no cheese. Now, you may think that's not so bad, right? But that's for one-quarter of a 10-inch pizza! That's a tiny serving. Most of us would devour that whole ten-inch pie and, as a result, take in 540 calories. You may say that's not bad for a meal. It's not, really. Remember that's with no cheese! Add cheese, as most Americans do, and that skimpy slice shoots up to 205 calories, with the whole pizza coming in at 820 calories! While accurate, this information can be misleading—leading us into getting fatter by the minute. People almost always miscalculate what they actually eat, and generally err on the side of fewer calories taken in.

Health freak pizza, indeed.

I could go on with examples of how you are being misled by companies that want to sell you compromised foods under the guise that they can be healthy for you. Do you think there's a chef from McDonald's at the local farm market squeezing tomatoes and checking for the freshest, crispiest lettuce? Although their commercials show glistening veggies, fresh from the farm, being washed by hand under cascades of shimmering water, nothing could be further from the truth. Do you think Old MacDonald himself is growing tomatoes for Domino's or whole grains for Stouffers? All of these images are designed to make you think there is some humanity in the food they sell; that the frozen meals and delivered pizza are homemade.

They think we are naïve enough to believe it. Let's prove them wrong. I am so weary of all this nonsense. We need to stop falling for big portions of lousy quality. It's time to get mad as hell.

Dinner from Your Microwave

So, let's say you decide that the drive-through won't cut it anymore. You swear off fast food. Wandering the supermarket frozen food aisles makes your head spin. From vegetables to dinners to pizza, there are options galore.

How do you decide what's healthy?

Frozen food companies like Lean Cuisine and Stouffers refer to their veggies as "farm-picked." Really? Farm picked? Notice that it doesn't say farm fresh, just picked. Do vegetables grow anywhere else, whether commercially, genetically modified, or organically, than on a farm? Can we get them by any other means than picking them? It's a meaningless phrase designed to make you think this frozen dinner is somehow fresh from the farm stand.

What's more important is what is actually in one of these frozen meals that you think serve your health. A study of the nutrition facts on the Lean Cuisine website doesn't exactly make me feel like these foods are made from ingredients picked at their peak of freshness. The full nutrition profile reads like a laundry list of ingredients that have little to do with nature . . . or the farm. Ingredients like modified corn starch, onion powder, whey protein concentrate, xanthan gum, mono- and diglycerides, and natural flavor aren't what my mother would have put in her Chicken Fettucine. It's not what you would put in yours if you cooked it from scratch. It would be one thing if they just called it what it is: a low-calorie frozen dinner. We would know then, that it was not natural, but low-calorie. We'd get what we get. But they go to great lengths to convince us that their food is fresh, somehow superior and so natural; the farmers are in the fields feverishly growing and picking by hand to keep the quality just like homemade.

And you didn't need to break a sweat for this homemade dinner.

That's what makes me so mad!

SOME SWEET TALK ABOUT SWEETENERS

Where do I begin with this one? Sweet is by far the flavor we want the most in our food. From breast milk to the grave, sweet taste is connected to satisfaction, comfort, fulfillment, and joy.

There's a reason we love the sweet taste so much, and it has to do with our ancestry.

The human tongue can best detect four flavors: salty, sour, bitter, and sweet, but we are drawn to sweet because we are primates, animals that evolved from eating fruit in trees. The attraction to sweet ripe fruit developed because its higher sugar content supplied energy more quickly than sour, unripe fruit and was also higher in water, so hydration was easier to come by.

Research done at Cambridge University by William McGrew revealed that primates will go through any degree of pain to get to the sweet stuff, including multiple bee stings as they rifle through the hives for honey with their fingers.

Once people figured out how to extract sugar from various foods, from beets to cane, there was no turning back. We fell in love with it in all its forms. We wanted it all the time now that there was ready access to it. The food industry cashed in big. According to Sugar Knowledge International, the industry is selling us more than 167 million tons of sugar each year, worldwide.

And just like chimps drawn to the hive at all costs, we, too, ignore the stinging consequences of excessive sugar consumption . . . from bad teeth to diabetes to high triglycerides to obesity. According to Medicine.net, we take in 165 pounds of added sugar on average, per person each year, with teenagers taking in more, to the tune of more than thirty-four teaspoons of added sugar a day. Add to that the forty-seven pounds of naturally occurring sugar in foods, and you come up with a whopping 212 pounds of sugar per person per year. Yikes, right?

The World Health Organization says that added sugar should account for no more than 10 percent of our diet each day. That's two hundred calories in a two-thousand-calorie diet or the equivalent of eight heaping teaspoons. (Consider that one full-sugar twelve-ounce soda has at least *nine* teaspoons, and it's pretty clear how we've ended up in such trouble.)

But foods with sugar taste good, so it's really easy to eat too much of them. That's the simple truth.

Discerning Sweet Taste

There is a substantial difference in the sweeteners available to us, regardless of what marketing may tell you. Fructose, sucrose, and glucose all behave differently in the body and cause specific reactions. It's time we make all this clear so you can choose the sweet flavor that best suits your needs and health.

Sucrose

By definition, sucrose is what we know as table sugar, a disaccharide that's derived from glucose and fructose. White, crystalline, and odorless, sucrose is formed by plants and cyanobacteria and is found in many plant sources along with fructose. In many fruits, like pineapple and apricot, sucrose is the main sugar, but the most common sources are sugarcane and beets.

Originally a luxury food, sucrose became a commodity after a refining process was invented by Raymond Lemieux, beginning the evolution that would make it a cheap and commonly used ingredient. A major ingredient in desserts, pastries, cookies, pies, and cakes, sucrose has become synonymous with junk food because of the role it plays in it.

Sucrose is digested in the stomach by a process known as acidic hydrolysis and is an easily absorbed macronutrient that provides a quick source of energy, by provoking a rapid rise in blood glucose almost immediately upon ingestion. Eaten in excess, sucrose can contribute to adverse health effects like metabolic syndrome, insulin resistance, high triglycerides, and hyperglycemia.

Glucose

Glucose is a monosaccharide, an important simple sugar in human biology. Our cells use it as a source of energy and a metabolic intermediate, meaning it is a precursor for important biological molecules. It is a byproduct of photosynthesis, and scientists can only speculate as to why glucose is the sugar so readily used by the body. What they do know is that glucose is critical to the production of proteins and in the metabolism of fats.

A precursor to the making of vitamin C, glucose is found in most dietary carbohydrates, like whole grains, beans, and vegetables. Broken down by the small intestine and lumen of the duodenum, much of the glucose we consume is used directly as energy by the brain, intestines, and red blood cells. The rest is stored in the liver, fatty tissue, and muscle cells as glycogen. The liver cell glycogen can be converted back into glucose and returned to the blood for use when insulin is low or absent.

It is the source of fuel that we can use most efficiently and, as a result, is the most essential to the human body.

Fructose

Fructose is simply fruit sugar and is one of the three important dietary sugars, along with glucose and galactose (a monosaccharide that combines with glucose). It is also one of the components of sucrose.

Dr. George Bray, MD, from Louisiana State University, who wrote what is considered the definitive paper on the role of high-fructose corn syrup in obesity and obesity-related illnesses, says the biology of natural fructose is different from other sugars.

More chemically reactive than glucose, it circulates in the blood at much lower concentrations. Fructose is absorbed into the liver, where it is converted to the precursor of triglyceride synthesis.

Human milk contains no fructose, so our bodies are not naturally used to assimilating it. The primary source of it in traditional diets came from fruit, honey, and to some extent, nuts and some vegetables. In our modern diet, the main sources of it are in its refined form, high-fructose corn syrup and purified cane sugar.

There is naturally occurring fructose in some foods, like apples, pears, and their juices, but fructose differs from glucose in our bodies in other ways. It is absorbed from the intestines by a different mechanism than glucose. It's why apple and pear juice is of some concern to pediatricians. The way the fructose must be absorbed can cause diarrhea in small children.

When glucose is present with fructose, it eases the absorption of it by the liver, its primary organ (gland, really) for metabolism. Glucose directly stimulates the insulin release from the pancreas; fructose does not. Fructose enters the muscles without insulin; glucose enters in an insulin-dependent manner.

Dr. William J. Wheelan, a biochemist at the University of Miami School of Medicine, says, "When fructose reaches the liver, the liver goes bananas and stops everything else to metabolize the fructose." He also says that eating fructose instead of glucose results in lower circulating levels of insulin and leptin, both of which decrease appetite, and higher levels of ghrelin, which increases appetite, making the connection between obesity and excessive fructose consumption.

Outside of its natural state in fruit, commercially produced fructose was developed to be used in commercially produced foods. It is, without question, the sweetest of all naturally occurring carbohydrates.

High-Fructose Corn Syrup

Farmers in the United States have managed to produce 500 additional calories per person every day; each of us is, heroically, managing to pack away about 200 of those extra calories per day.

—Michael Pollan, "The (Agri)Cultural Contradictions of Obesity," *The New York Times Magazine*

If fructose is the sweetest of all naturally occurring carbohydrates, then high-fructose corn syrup is off the charts in that department.

High-fructose corn syrup got its name because the processing of the corn into this sweetener increases the fructose levels. Corn, as a grain, is a glucose-based carbohydrate. To make it sweeter, manufacturers needed to up the ante on the fructose. They do that in the process. The corn's starch is separated from other parts of the kernels, and enzymes are added to convert some of the glucose to fructose. After filtering, some of the resulting syrup is filtered again to create a very high-fructose base. The two syrups are mixed to create a corn syrup that is 55 percent fructose . . . high-fructose corn syrup.

Crystalline corn syrup was developed in the 1950s and proved it could compete with sugar on every level, from flavor to versatility. In 1967, the Japanese figured out how to convert dextrose to fructose and created high-fructose corn syrup from corn starch, so a corn sugar could be produced in mass quantities. With corn a heavily subsidized crop (for animal feed), this new sweetener unlocked a way for food manufacturers to sweeten their products for a mere fraction of what it had been costing, resulting in lower manufacturing prices. But rather than pass those lower costs on to the consumer, they increased the portion sizes for the same prices and—voilà!—we became a culture of big food and big people.

The Corn Refiners Association has several websites it uses to put forth the message that corn sugar, as they prefer to call high-fructose corn syrup, behaves no differently in the body than any other sugar. They have paid experts, corn farmers, and dieticians to appear in videos to convince Americans that it's not high-fructose corn syrup that has made us an obese nation, but all added sugars.

They are not entirely wrong. Americans do eat entirely too much added sugar in their diets. The "acceptable" amount of added sugar is nine tea-spoons for men and six teaspoons for women, which is a lot of added sugar in and of itself. The average American eats twenty-two teaspoons of added sugar (with our teenagers taking in thirty-four teaspoons daily), according to the American Heart Association. And that doesn't include the naturally occurring sugars in foods like fruit and vegetables.

Where they stretch the facts is in saying that glucose and fructose digest in the body in the same way. We have seen here that these two sugars digest quite differently in the body, so while calorically similar, it's a bit off the mark to say there is no difference between them.

No matter how you use semantics or how many American-as-apple-pie farmers you have telling us about corn and nature, there's no escaping the facts: high-fructose corn syrup, while originally from a natural source, is anything but good for us.

Faux Sweeteners

Artificial sweeteners are in a class all by themselves to be sure. We have come to use them on what seems to be a never-ending quest to lose weight. They are just one of the many tricks we use to try to circumvent the misery of that process. But studies reveal that artificial sweeteners may not be all they are cracked up to be, explaining why, with all the sugar-free foods out there, we continue to get heavier and heavier.

According to studies done at Purdue University and published in *Behavioral Neuroscience* (February 2008), we are trained to begin to salivate when we taste something sweet, in anticipation of calories. So when that sweet taste hits the tongue with no calories attached, we go on a quest for the calories we expect. The study also revealed that when animals ate naturally sweetened foods, their core temperature rose, as their metabolism revved up in antici-pation of calories to burn. The animals eating artificially sweetened foods showed no temperature increase, meaning that their metabolism didn't in-crease in anticipation of burning calories and would, instead, store them, re-sulting in weight gain.

John Yudkin, professor of nutrition at the University of London and one of our earliest proponents of a low-carbohydrate diet, wrote extensively on the subject of refined sugar and its effect on health. His books include *Sweet and Dangerous*, published in 1974, which built on his book *Pure, White and Deadly*, published in 1972. In it, Professor Yudkin said, "I suppose it is natural for the vast and powerful sugar interests to seek to protect themselves, since in the wealthier countries, sugar makes a greater contribution to our diets, measured in calories, than does meat or bread or any other single commodity."

Sugar may not be as sweet as we think.

100 PERCENT BEEF (OR CHICKEN OR THE OTHER WHITE MEAT): WHAT'S REALLY IN THAT STUFF?

Since we're talking here about the foods that don't serve our health, you wouldn't expect me to skip over meat, would you? It is a big part of our food culture—and an important ingredient in the compromised quality of food being sold to you.

This isn't the part where I go all radical vegan on you, either. Living a vegan life is my choice, and I would love it if more people lived healthy, compassionate lives, but I know that some people are just not there yet. And it's okay. I live by a different philosophy from the ladies behind the *Skinny Bitch* books in that I believe people will be more willing to try out my lifestyle through education about what's in the food they are eating. We all turn off to those awful political attack ads during campaigns; why would I use those tactics to attract people to compassionate living? Wouldn't compassion get me further?

There is a prevailing belief in our culture that we're American, descendents of chest-thumping cowboys. We're made of cheeseburgers and steaks! We need our meat! We need it more than Neolithic hunters, more than lions and tigers. If we can't have meat, what will happen to civilization as we know it? Would we all become vegan hippie socialist terrorists?

Well, no.

But you could become unhealthy . . . and not so much from eating meat as by what's in the meat you're eating. So before you buy another burger, another chicken (in a bucket or not), or another carton of milk, another block of cheese or carton of eggs, there are some things you should know. And then you can decide for yourself if you want to continue eating meat . . . or any other animal protein for that matter.

When we think of meat, we think of a lot of things: the beach, baseball, tennis, boating, golf, picnics, barbecue; burgers sizzling on grills all over the country fill the air with the scent of charred animal parts. And for many people, there is no more seductive perfume. We have seen complete ad campaigns showing men standing over their grills, euphoric with joy, yelling out "meat!"

But what about all the saturated fat, growth hormones, steroids, and other nasty stuff that causes heart disease, stroke, cancer, and diabetes lurking in that juicy flesh we love so much? Can we have our burgers and eat them, too?

It seems that we have parallel universes existing in America. There is a hyperconscientiousness that has taken over the American psyche when it comes to food awareness. Organic food sales have taken off like a rocket; films like *Food, Inc.* enjoy Hollywood premieres. The collective awareness of the effects of food on health has risen dramatically. At the same time, the majority of Americans still hit the Golden Arches regularly, drink high-calorie Coolattas from Dunkin' Donuts, and think KFC's dinner in a bucket is a good idea.

More and more people want to know what's in the food they choose, so we might as well begin with those burgers sizzling on the grill. What, exactly, is in the meat you are eating? Is there more to your burger than meets the eye? Sadly, the answer is yes, but happily, there is a solution. And no, I am not referring to organic lentil burgers with sprouts (although they are delicious and much more heart-healthy than even the healthiest organic meat-based burger).

When it comes to meat, the idyllic images we have of cows, pigs, and chickens lazily grazing in sun-dappled pastures is far from the truth, even if the pictures on the labels imply otherwise; even if Mr. Perdue would have you believe he wanders through the henhouse and speaks to his chickens by name.

The majority of meat production is now completely dominated by factory farms: 95 percent of pigs, 78 percent of cattle, 99.9 percent of chickens to be precise, and 70 percent of eggs. *Food, Inc.* showed us, in graphic detail, the none-too-pretty journey from farm to table for most animals. In the majority of instances, animals are fed completely unnatural diets, which is part of the problem with conventional burgers. When cows are grass-fed and eating a diet natural to them (they are vegans, ironically . . .), their meat contains less than 2 grams of saturated fat per ounce, while grain-fed, factory-farmed cattle contain just under 10 grams of saturated fat per ounce. That's an astonishing difference and one of the reasons heart disease is associated with consumption of red meat. It's no small thing to consider the ramifications of about 12 grams of saturated fat in a 6-ounce burger versus almost 60 grams.

But it doesn't end there.

Since the 1940s, factory farms have employed the use of nontherapeutic antibiotics for healthy animals to help ensure they do not get sick. The animals live in unnaturally tight quarters; a sick one can infect the whole herd. So we dose them up before they become diseased rather than change the conditions in which they live . . . because that would cost money. These preventive drugs have another benefit, but again, hardly for the animal. It turns out that these antibiotics also make the animals fatter faster, which maximizes profits! So it's a win-win for the factory farm ranchers. They fatten animals quickly and offset the disgusting unsanitary conditions in which these creatures are forced to subsist until slaughter, packed into feedlots and confined enclosures where an enormous amount of feces serves as the perfect breeding ground for bacteria and disease to spread from one animal to another. Sound delicious yet?

The Union of Concerned Scientists says that about 70 percent of all antibiotics used in the United States are not distributed by doctors, but by livestock producers. When a farmer can walk into a feed store and purchase a hundred-pound bag of tetracycline, we need to worry about the quality of meat they are producing. As Jonathan Safran Foer points out in *Eating Animals*, the factory farm system is dysfunctional, broken, unethical, and destructive to the environment and human health.

We try ball players in open court for the use of performance-enhancing steroids, yet we eat them on a daily basis in our burgers, steaks, and ribs. Yup, steroids—similar to the ones athletes use.

According to Cornell University researchers, hormones added in meat and dairy production "make young animals gain weight faster. They help reduce the waiting time and the amount of feed taken by an animal before slaughter in meat industries. In dairy cows, hormones can be used to increase milk production. Thus, hormones can increase the profitability of the meat and dairy industries."

Now, there are a variety of hormones produced by our bodies that are essential for normal development of healthy tissue, but synthetic steroid hormones used as pharmaceutical drugs have been found to affect cancer risk. For instance, lifetime exposure to the natural steroid hormone estrogen is associated with an increased risk for breast cancer. We should be concerned about the hormones being added to our foods.

As early as the 1930s, farmers realized that cows injected with compounds drawn from cows' pituitary glands produced more milk. However, it was not until the 1980s that it became possible to harvest enough of this compound for large-scale use in animal production. In 1993, the FDA approved the use of rbGH (recombinant bovine growth hormone, also known as bovine somatotropin, rbST) in dairy cattle. Current estimates by manufacturers of this hormone indicate that 30 percent of the cows in the United States may be treated with these hormones.

The female sex hormone estrogen was also shown to affect the growth rates in cattle and poultry as early as the 1930s, and once manufacturers understood the chemistry of it, it became possible to make the hormone synthetically in large amounts. In the early 1950s, synthetic estrogen was used regularly to increase the size of cattle and chickens. Be clear . . . estrogen.

DES was one of the first synthetic estrogens made and used commercially in the United States to fatten chickens, but when it was discovered that it caused cancer and miscarriage in women, its use in food production was phased out in the late 1970s. Scary stuff; it's like we're the subjects of a mad scientist's experiments.

In modern animal production, there are six different kinds of steroid hormones currently approved by the FDA for use in food production: estradiol, progesterone, testosterone, zeranol, trenbolone acetate, and melengesterol acetate. Estradiol and progesterone are natural female sex hormones; testosterone is a natural male sex hormone. Zeranol, trenbolone acetate, and melengesterol acetate are synthetic growth promoters, which are hormone-like chemicals that cause animals to grow faster. Currently, federal regulations allow these hormones to be used on cattle and sheep, but not on poultry or pigs.

But only because they have not been shown to work on poultry or pigs. Not because they are worried for our health.

Here's how clever these guys are. They give the steroids to the animals in the form of a pellet planted just under the skin of the ear. The ears are thrown away at slaughter, so there is less likelihood of hormone residue left in the animal in the edible meat because federal regulations prohibit the use of the hormones in this manner. They can hide the use of hormones this way and be able to say on their labels that no hormones were added to the meat. And some of the steroids are available in a form that can be added to animal feed so, again, they can legally say on labels that no hormones were added to the meat.

Dairy cattle may be injected under the skin with rbGH, which is available in single-dose packages to reduce the chances of accidental overdose. How nice.

Estradiol, progesterone, and testosterone are natural sex hormones produced by the animals' bodies. So there is no regulatory monitoring of these hormones because the regulators tell us that they can't separate or tell the difference between the hormones used for treatment, those produced naturally by the animal, and those administered by the farmers for growth. But a tolerance level has been set up for the synthetic hormones, which is the maximum amount of a particular residue that may be permitted in or on food. They don't monitor the hormones that can do us the most harm, just the synthetic ones.

The levels of naturally produced hormones vary from animal to animal to be sure, but there is a range that is known to be normal. They say it's not possible to differentiate between the hormones produced naturally by the animal and those used to force growth, but that isn't true by their own logic. If we know the range of normal hormone levels, wouldn't it stand to reason that levels that exceed normal ranges should come into question?

To add insult to injury, the FDA also tells us that since they can't regulate these natural hormones, they can't tell how much of the hormones remaining in the meat is from the treatments. Scientists are working on creating a better system to measure steroid hormones, but for now it's a crap shoot.

You may be asking how harmful these steroid hormones really are. Things get a little murky here, so the conclusion is ours to draw . . . and the risk is also ours to take.

Early puberty in girls has been associated with a higher risk for breast cancer. Family history, height, weight, diet, and exercise are also known risk factors to be considered. Steroid hormones have long been suspected to cause early puberty in both sexes.

We are bombarded with results, statistics, and specifics with countless studies, but the results have been routinely inconclusive. Look at just two of them and see if you won't be scratching your head as I was.

In the 1980s, the Centers for Disease Control and Prevention (CDC) conducted a study in Puerto Rico when it was discovered that girls were reaching puberty as early as the age of eight. Samples of meat and poultry showed higher than normal levels of estrogen. Residues of zeranol were also found in the blood of some of the girls in question. But because these results were not verified by another laboratory, they were said to be inconclusive.

A study in Italy was conducted on beef and poultry because of breast enlargement in very young boys and girls. However, samples of the suspect meat and poultry were not made available for testing, thereby negating the theory, since the suspicions could not be proven.

I'm not sayin' there's something fishy here; I'm just sayin'.

I am not sure what it will take for us to be more concerned about eating animal foods. How many beef recalls, egg recalls, salmonella outbreaks, e-coli contaminations, undercover exposés of unsanitary practices in meat packing plants will it take before we realize that factory farming is polluting the planet, destroying our health, and contributing to unspeakable cruelty? Have our brains gone to mush? Are we immune to suffering in ourselves and in others? Do we not care about our own health and the health of the planet? Do we just talk a good story and carry our little canvas bags to the store and breathe easier because we have done our part for "greening"?

What do we do? What if you're not ready to hit vegan eating full-on?

In my view, organic meat is not the answer and never will be, but it's a baby step in the right direction (that direction being a plant-based diet with veggie and bean burgers sizzling on the fire). But for now, as you transition to a healthier way of eating, look for USDA-certified organic meat that is grass-fed. It will cost you a pretty penny, but if you choose to eat meat, what is your health worth? You are guaranteed that certified organic meat is free of hormones, antibiotics, pesticides, and other toxins. However, you will need to look even harder to find certified organic, grass-fed meat. Grass-fed doesn't mean organic; organic doesn't mean grass-fed.

The same goes for your eggs, dairy, and cheese. Look for organic, grass-fed products, and in the case of eggs, cage-free. These will not be that easy to find, but they are worth the search because they will give you what you want . . . animal food without the things you don't want . . . additives, pesticides, hormones, steroids, and other toxins.

How an animal was raised and what it was eating before it was slaughtered will become more and more important issues as we strive to make healthier choices for ourselves and the planet. Simply stated, if you're not ready to be vegan, you're not ready . . . yet. I can wait for you to get here. I pray every day that you find your way to a plant-based diet. But until you do, if you aren't sure where your burger comes from, you might want to think twice about eating it.

As you watch the happy families in the Norman Rockwell–esque settings of Boston Market commercials and drool over the chicken, skin glistening and surrounded by starchy side dishes, what you are really seeing is a hormone-laced toxic animal that was raised and slaughtered under the most un-Rockwell-esque conditions.

THE TRUTH ABOUT DAIRY

In his *New York Times* exposé in 2010, Michael Moss wrote about the USDA's efforts to encourage cheese consumption to satisfy their obligations to the dairy industry. The USDA also has the task of tackling the obesity epidemic that threatens to shorten the lives of an entire generation and break the back of the health-care industry.

How does this government agency serve two masters? How does it promote agriculture and health when the two are in conflict?

Sadly, it doesn't. We, the consumers, lose. The powerful forces and financial clout that are the backbone of the dairy industry trump our health each and every time.

According to Dr. Marion Nestle, nutrition expert, activist, and author of *Food Politics* and *What to Eat*, dairy lobbying groups "aided and abetted by the USDA convinced nutritionists that dairy foods were equivalent to essential nutrients and the only reliable source of dietary calcium, when they are really just another food group and one high in saturated fat at that."

That was some time ago. We all grew up hearing that milk builds strong bones. It is a myth still held to this day. It is just one of the many myths put forth as truth in order to sell more or less of a certain food to us.

And the USDA is still at it.

With all we know about dairy (in particular cheese), from the perils of saturated fat to growth hormones to the simple fact that cheese doubles the calories in any dish, they still try to shove it down our throats. The USDA acknowledges that cheese is high in saturated fat, but says it's still an important source of calcium. "When eaten in moderation and with attention to portion size, cheese can fit into a low-fat, healthy diet," the department said.

There are two major points to be made here, both of which blow this thinking out of the water.

First, to call dairy food an important source of calcium is misleading on a good day. Have you ever wondered about the populations of the world that consume little or no dairy? They also have the lowest incidence of osteoporosis. In addition to regular physical activity, these populations consume a largely plant-based diet and, therefore, require less calcium (since they are not losing as much calcium to the high concentrations of amino acids in animal food that cause the depletion of calcium from blood and bones).

And how much of the calcium in dairy can we actually absorb and use? We hear in all the ads about building strong bones and milk being nature's perfect food and all the calcium we get. So let's look at the math, shall we?

In one cup of cow's milk, there are 300 milligrams of calcium, which is a lot. Here's where it gets sticky. Your body can only absorb and use up to 32 percent, about 96 milligrams. Broccoli, on the other hand, has 178 milligrams of calcium in one cup, but your body can use 53 percent or 94 milligrams. Pretty comparable in the calcium department and with broccoli, you also get truly essential vitamins and minerals, no growth hormones or saturated fat or excessive calories like you do with milk.

It was pure marketing and lobbying that sold us the idea that dairy was and is the best source of calcium for the human body.

Second is the USDA's use of the word *moderation*. If you look at the average fast-food pizza from Papa John's (you know, "Better ingredients, better pizza"), a slice (one-eighth of the whole pie) of a medium cheese pizza offers up 210 calories, 70 from fat, 18 percent of it saturated fat, and 530 milligrams of sodium and 1 measly gram of fiber. Pretty hefty, right? Now think about how many of us eat one slice of a medium pizza? No one I know. Most people are downing the entire twelve-inch pizza on their own, because it just isn't that big, is it? So that means you are eating more than 1,680 calories, 560 of them from fat and 4,440 milligrams of sodium.

Moderation? Is this what the USDA had in mind?

So why, you may ask, is the USDA so cozy with the lobbying groups? It is the job of the agency. From its beginning in the 1860s, the USDA was charged with the task of promoting American agriculture and sales, with the full support of Congress (which was largely agricultural at the time). It was not until the 1970s that the agency took on the additional responsibility of governing food assistance programs and became the lead federal agency in providing dietary advice to the public.

Much of Marion Nestle's work and a good chunk of *Food Politics* is devoted to talking about the USDA's conflict of interest in working to develop dietary advice that includes eating less of certain agricultural commodities. The interest with the most money on the table wins.

WHAT MAKES YOUR SODA SO "SPECIAL"

In my view, soda is one of the most subversive and destructive forces in the loss of our health. While not actually a food, for those people who drink soda, it can be its own food group.

As far back as the 1500s, Spanish colonists took note that Indians of South America overcame fatigue by chewing on the leaves of the coca shrub. But it wasn't until 1860 that the first pure crystals of cocaine were extracted from coca by German biochemists. It was used in very small quantities as a stimulant in beverages. In the 1880s, Angelo Mariani's incredibly popular wine beverage, which was laced with cocaine, won him praise from the likes of Thomas Edison, who called the drink "brilliant," and he was even honored as a benefactor of humanity by Pope Leo XIII.

In the late 1880s, a new nonalcoholic beverage was born in Atlanta to quench the thirst of America and provide a little boost of energy. Originally sold as a syrup to be mixed with cold soda water at local drugstore soda fountain counters, Coca-Cola contained cocaine from the coca plant and lots of caffeine from the kola bean. This brew also included lots of sugar, along with caramel color, lime juice, citric acid, phosphoric acid, nutmeg, coriander, orange flavor, and cinnamon. (Coca-Cola did once contain an estimated nine milligrams of cocaine per glass, but in 1903 it was removed.)

In 1906, the Pure Food and Drug Act was passed, and one of the officials in charge of its enforcement made it his mission to prove that the "Coca Cola habit" America was forming was harmful to health. By 1922, this same persistent official told *Good Housekeeping* magazine that if a child drank three or four six-ounce colas a day, he or she would ruin his or her health for life.

Today, most soft drinks contain phosphoric acid, caffeine, sugar or an artificial sweetener and/or high-fructose corn syrup, caramel coloring, carbon dioxide, and aluminum. While we don't experience acute reactions to these ingredients, like stomach cramps, vomiting, or diarrhea that one would expect when normally ingesting poisons, we do feel temporarily energized by the caffeine and the sugar.

The truth is, however, that these ingredients cause the body to experience imbalances that result in many of the diseases that plague us today.

Phosphoric acid is used in soda to create an acid medium that enhances the absorption of the carbon dioxide. The sour flavor is overcome by adding lots of sugar, so it's palatable—and calorically dense. Our bodies maintain a concentration of phosphorus, calcium, and potassium to provide the right balance in the bloodstream to build new bones and strengthen existing bone tissue. The influx of excess phosphorus causes calcium to decline as well as accelerating the excretion of calcium through the urine. As a result, in the body's effort to create balance, calcium is leeched from our bones, and especially from the teeth, spine, and pelvis. You can dissolve a tooth in it. This process continues over a lifetime, resulting in osteoporosis, which we are beginning to see earlier and earlier in life. It is no longer the disease of old people.

Phosphoric acid is the same compound that is one of the ingredients that cleans scum from your shower walls. Phosphoric acid causes the body to use its alkalizing minerals to attempt to neutralize this intense acid. So we lose valuable minerals like magnesium and potassium as well as our calcium. This throws off our sodium-potassium balance, which increases the production of bile, forms a plaquelike substance in the intestines, and can result in colitis.

Excess phosphoric acid also contributes to heart disease because it reduces the secretion of hydrochloric acid, which is necessary for the digestion of protein and fats and the absorption of minerals, leading to anemia and the overgrowth of harmful bacteria in the stomach and bowels.

Caffeine is an addictive chemical that acts by blocking the neurotransmitter receptor sites in the central nervous system, which means it has a depressing action in the brain, heart, and kidneys. The resulting stimulation of caffeine constricts cerebral arteries, increases heartbeat, raises blood pressure, and dehydrates the body.

With the release of adrenaline and an accompanying increase in blood sugar, the pancreas reacts by secreting insulin to keep blood sugar stable. Insulin drives blood sugar levels down by forcing it into cells for oxidation and energy production. Excess sugar is stored as fat. This bizarre cycle places incredible stress on both the adrenal glands and the pancreas.

So what? Adrenal exhaustion and the resulting cortisol deficiency cause the release of arachidonic acid, forming prostaglandin-2, which can lead to arthritis. And a deficiency of cortisol leads to overcompensation and overproduction of cortisol, which results in belly fat.

In spite of the kick of energy, caffeine addiction actually leads to mental sluggishness and an exhausted body when we are deprived of the "hit." While caffeine and sugar make for a seductive combo to sell soda, these ingredients are destructive to health.

But if you think a dark color means more caffeine (like coffee), note that Mountain Dew contains 50 percent more caffeine than colas.

The ill effects of *sugar* and *high-fructose corn syrup* have been well-documented in these pages and elsewhere. A twelve-ounce can of soda delivers about eleven teaspoons. In the United States, about 50 percent of the carbohydrates we consume are in the form of sugar, and that trend continues to rise. Since our bodies convert excess sugar to fat, you can see how soda is problematic for our health.

But what if you are drinking artificially sweetened sodas to avoid all those calories? Just check out the facts about these chemical toxins in the section Faux Sweeteners. You'll see you're getting more than you bargained for with these, too.

Carbon dioxide is another offensive ingredient. The waste product of metabolism when we exhale, we are now ingesting the very compound that it is the body's nature to eliminate. Does that make sense to you?

Meanwhile, the phosphoric acid in the soda eats away enough *aluminum* from the can itself to be harmful to health. Soda companies stepped right up and plastic-coated the interiors of the cans, but the phosphoric acid leaches toxic amounts of aluminum into the soda despite this coating. Aluminum is deposited in brain and bone tissue, resulting in inflammation of neurofibrillary tissue in the brain, and an increase in the risk of bone breakage (along with calcium leeching).

Still not convinced? Here are some uses for soda, especially colas, that might surprise you:

■ A lot of state highway patrols carry two gallons of cola in their trunks to remove bloodstains from the roadway after a car accident.

■ Soaking a steak in a bowl of cola will result in its total disintegration in two days.

■ Pour a can of cola into a toilet bowl and let it stand for one hour. Flush and reveal a sparkling clean bowl.

■ Cola's citric acid can clean stains from vitreous china.

■ You can remove rust from car bumpers by rubbing them with crumpled up aluminum foil dipped in cola.

■ Car battery terminals can be cleaned of corrosion by pouring a can of cola over them.

- You can loosen a rusted-tight bolt by holding a cloth soaked in cola on the bolt for a few minutes.

- You can remove grease stains from clothes by adding a can of cola to a load of greasy laundry with your detergent.

- Cola can clean road haze from your windshield.

- Because the active ingredient in most colas is phosphoric acid, its pH is 2.8. It will dissolve a nail in about four days.

- Soda distributors of cola have been using it to clean the engines of their trucks for the last twenty years.

Still think soda is "the pause that refreshes"?

4

The Politics of Food

THE SCIENCE OF NUTRITION

How did we come to be in such a mess? If you ask me, we are simply in information overload: We know a lot about food, just not much about what to eat.

And the reason for that? Nutrition science.

Much of the confusion stems from a desire for ease and convenience at all costs, combined with a lack of common sense. The fact is that most of us are not scientists, but the simple truth is that nutrition science is for sale. The bulk of the research being done in nutrition isn't on actual food, but on the micronutrients that make up food, funded by the people who manufacture the food being studied. It's important to understand the distinction here.

Nutrition science is based on the premise that there is something missing from our food, something deficient with food in its natural state and that finding out the biological function of specific nutrients will magically resolve the diet-disease connection for us.

The science of nutrition was, in fact, developed to discover the cause of specific nutritional deficiencies. And at first, it was great. Wonderful things were discovered. A vitamin C deficiency was found to cause scurvy; a calcium deficiency creates bone density loss.

These important discoveries became the domain of industry and business, which turned this exciting information into advertising bonanzas! Processed foods were developed that were enriched; supplements were touted as the latest, greatest creations; natural food, in all its nutrient-dense glory, was ignored.

Creating fear of nutritional deficiency has become the driving force in nutrition science, making it the official handmaiden of the processed food industry. Every single function of every single micronutrient discovered is heralded as the key, the missing link, the one factor that will lead us to a life of health and happiness, the cure to what ails us, the second coming of food; the epiphany to end all epiphanies . . . until the next discovery.

Study after study is conducted on human nutrition, but an important point has been overlooked. Humans have diverse constitutions and diets. We live vastly different lives with differing levels of activity and environments. We come from different cultures and traditions. All these factors come together to create a confounding set of circumstances in which to attempt to study human eating habits and health. That's why the results of so many studies are conflicting and confusing. How do we study people's habits without changing their habits? And how do we compile all these differences into one result? We don't, which is why the study results rarely come to a consensus and so are reported as "inconclusive" and the beat goes on with no one getting the information they really need to make healthy choices.

The primary function of nutrition science is to study nutrients, not food; it dissects food, deconstructs it, and removes it from reality. So what does it have to do with us and our health?

The exception here is nutritional epidemiology, the study of the causes of disease in large populations. Epidemiology has shown us a hard truth. Read *The China Study* by T. Colin Campbell, PhD, for some pretty eye-opening information on how food affects health. In this vast work, Dr. Campbell and company studied the eating habits of more than 6,500 Chinese living in sixty-five mostly rural counties in China. This site was chosen because nowhere else could they find a population of this size with such genetic similarities that tended to live in the same place, in the same way, and eat the same foods for entire lifetimes. As I said, studies are often inconclusive because people's habits and lives are so diverse. The similarities of the population in *The China Study* allowed for a study that revealed clear patterns. In a population of similar genetics and lifestyle habits, they compared the health consequences of diets rich in animal foods with those of a plant-based, whole-foods diet and concluded that eating a plant-based diet, steeped in whole, unprocessed foods, naturally low in fat, resulted in substantially reduced risk of disease and an increased chance of actually reversing disease.

Dr. Campbell argues that "most, but not all of the confusion about nutrition is created in legal, fully disclosed ways and is disseminated by unsuspecting, well-intentioned people, whether they are researchers, politicians or journalists." In his view—and I agree—there are powerful commercial interests that stand to lose a lot if America was to switch to a plant-based diet, so information is given out in ways that keep us reeling with confusion.

In reading books by experts like Dr. Campbell, Marion Nestle, and Michael Pollan, I have come to some conclusions. There are three truths that need to be emphasized (which I included in my introduction but repeat here because I feel they are so vital to our future health and well-being):

1. People who eat a modern, Western diet are killing themselves in record numbers from all manner of "lifestyle diseases": heart disease, cancer, stroke, diabetes, obesity.

2. People who eat traditional diets of their culture, no matter what that tradition may hold, do not experience the same levels of disease as cultures "enjoying" our modern diet of convenience.

3. People who abandon a modern diet and adopt a diet of whole, unprocessed foods, cooked in the ways of their ancestors, get healthier and even reverse disease. (I am one of those people. I was unconvinced of the power that food held in our lives until I saw it for myself in my own life, in my own return to health from cancer. So trust me on this one.)

I find it more than a little interesting that no one is talking about these truths.

In current marketing, nutrition science is used to distract us from the fact that eating fast-food, drive-through dinner in a bucket; drinking chemical brews fizzy with bubbles and loaded with sugar is making us unhealthy and obese. It is the manipulation of science in the service of big business and bigger profit. This manipulation results in massive profits, massive amounts of money being made; which feeds a sort of collective amnesia, which fuels the cowardice of government and even credible science.

Think about it. Whenever the media presents bad news about the way we eat—a recall for example—the first response is from some government talking head assuring us that this or that study is being reviewed and we should carry on as usual, eat as usual; that our food supply is the safest in the world. We really know the outcome before it's announced: The government review will be inconclusive and the offending product will be defended by the industry in question's nutrition expert. The study is questioned. More experts testify. The whole circus is designed to slow the flow of information so that we forget there was a problem or are so confused that we can't follow the facts.

Look at what happened in 2008 when roughly 143 million pounds of beef was recalled by the USDA because Westland/Hallmark Meat Packing Company in California had allowed "downed cows" (an indication of mad cow disease) to get into the food supply. The largest meat recall prior to that was in 1999, when 35 million pounds of beef were pulled off shelves for listeria contamination. Almost immediately upon recalling the product, then undersecretary of agriculture Richard Raymond said, "We do not feel this product presents a health risk of any significance. But the product was in noncompliance with our regulations."

That's why they recalled the beef? Not because of the risk of having potentially diseased animal meat in our food supply?

And the meat sizzled on.

Instead of presenting the consumer with the simple facts, we are subjected to complicated reports, studies, statistics . . . semantic tap-dancing. Instead of advising our overweight population to eat real, whole, unprocessed foods, we pick food apart, looking for the magic bullet that will cure all our ills . . . and still allow us to indulge our passions for fast food.

It's this search for the single cause, the single ingredient . . . the one evil-doer in food that is keeping the status quo. Nutrition science, pharmaceutical companies, and even medicine perpetuate this promise of a new discovery that holds the key to perfect health. And we just behave as we like, waiting for that bright, shiny day when someone else makes it all right again . . . without any painful change.

WHY ARE WE SO EASILY MANIPULATED?

People have been making movies, writing books, speaking out, telling the truth about our food. People are trying to teach humanity how to respect food again, how to treat it . . . how to use it to create health and make a lighter footprint.

What is the answer? Can we separate the issues of public health and special interests so we can have access to advice that is without influence and potential profit-making? Can we start to recognize the ways in which corporate lobbyists corrupt our food systems and do something about it . . . in the ballot box, at the supermarket, demanding better from the people and agencies charged with the nation's and the planet's well-being?

And the most important question: do consumers want healthy products?

We say we are tired of junk food; we are tired of the lies and deceit in advertising; we blame corporate America for making us overweight and sick with the products they create and market to our families and to us.

But we continue to buy processed foods, and the more of it that we can get for our dollar, the happier we are. We have stopped considering quality and look for the biggest sizes. We choose for price and size alone. I am not out of touch or elitist. I know that we can buy more calories of processed foods than of fresh whole foods, and in some cases that is an absolute necessity if we are to feed our families. Or so we have been led to believe. In my view, we need to begin to see the price tag attached to that processed food and find a way, as a society, to make fresh food accessible to all of us, not the privileged few. How? Demand feeds supply. If we demand better and stop buying junk food, they will make what we want . . . so they can sell us something.

It's up to us now, regardless of the economy. We must grow up . . . just a little. We must stop living our lives like petulant children who want what we want, when we want it without a care about the consequences. We party on, like drunks with lamp shades on our heads. We think that someone else, some hippie, liberal tree hugger will clean up our mess. We have highly evolved brains and are very good at figuring things out. We build cities; we created math, invented cell phones and computers. We are capable of things like the Sistine Chapel and the David. We can make Twinkies that last for years in plastic packages.

With our great ability to create, we should be able to make decisions that serve and support life.

With all our studies, seminars, self-help books, and government committees investigating the problems, we still say that there's no solution . . . maybe we do not want to see one.

If we were serious about solving the ills of the world, we would begin to live life as though it mattered . . . every minute of every day. This may sound simplistic in the face of the complicated issues we face, but simple is good and action is essential if we are to survive what we have created.

Imagine how the world could change if we just ate (as Michael Pollan says) real food, not too much, mostly plants; if we showed compassion to all beings; if we stopped buying worthless junk we didn't need and realized that without clean air and water we are lost. I have a strong feeling that everything would change . . . fast.

This is our problem. We have created it. That's the bad news.

The good news is that we can change it. In fact, that's the best news. In a world where everyone is out to brainwash you and steal your power, you must remember you have the ultimate say. You decide if you will live a healthy life or not. You decide if the planet will be healthy or not.

So what's it going to be?

PART THREE

What Do We Do?

There is a lot of confusion about what's healthy and what's not. In some cases, I wonder whether some product on the supermarket shelf is actually food. But there's little doubt that by listening to misleading advertising that focuses on individual ingredients or nutrients rather than the food as a whole will only lead us further astray. Labels like "gluten-free," "great source of calcium," or "can help lower cholesterol" distract us from the truth of what's in the package.

While it seems there's more bad news about our food supply than there is good news, in reality, there's a lot we can do as consumers to change the course we are on.

It's time to get back in touch with real food so we can enjoy real health.

5

You and Your Food

In a nutshell, the easiest way to health and wellness is to focus on whole, unprocessed foods as much as possible. These would be foods that are as close to their original state as possible. These are foods grown and nurtured the way Mother Nature intended, without the use of chemical enhancements.

Whole, unprocessed foods contain such a concentration of nutrients that work together synergistically; they are superior to anything food science and chemistry can come up with.

In our modern life, a lot of us have lost touch with "as nature intended" and may find even that simple phrase confusing with all the bells and whistles on packages. Marketing tells us grain-fed meat is "natural," but there's nothing natural about a cow eating grain. It is not and never has been a natural part of a cow's natural diet. You will never see a cow grazing on corn when out to pasture. They eat grass. So "natural" has become fairly bastardized in terms of its meaning.

As a result, a lot of us are going through life, eating a modern diet of processed foods, but popping vitamins and supplements, thinking it's natural and healthy . . . and still not enjoying robust vitality because we have lost our relationship with real food. We need to rekindle that love affair.

Natural food is elegant in its simplicity, delicious in its flavor, and completely nurturing to us as humans. It's what we are meant to consume. It doesn't need disguises or dancing fairies to "sell" us the idea of it.

Consider this: When you walk down the street and see a vegetable garden, lush with life, does it need a dancing clown to take your breath away? Or are you instinctively drawn into the natural beauty and life before your eyes? Think of how you feel in a farm market surrounded by bins of fresh food. Happy Meals could never make you this happy.

Natural foods are kissed by the sun; nourished by the rain, wind, and soil; and are rich, concentrated sources of the nutrients we need to thrive as humans . . . all wrapped in delicious flavors and textures. But broccoli tastes like broccoli, not ranch dressing, so natural foods may take a bit of getting used to because we have waded so deeply into the sea of artificially enhanced flavors.

Whole grains, vegetables, beans, nuts, seeds, fruit, herbs, and spices come together to create the perfect nourishment for humanity.

Marketing has changed our relationship with food and works hard to seduce us into believing that every day is a reason to indulge. We work hard; we deserve this; we're worth it and it would be s-o-o-o-o-o-o-o-o easy to just pick up the phone, call Domino's, and go comatose in front of the television again. The way we eat in our modern world is like an out-of-control party where everyone is passed out on the floor. We're not having any fun anymore, but we are so used to the party now that to return to sensible, normal eating seems grim and deprived when it's anything but; natural foods make eating special in a new way.

The cause of most of our ills is simple. We want more than we can have and marketing has promised we can have it. But reality and marketing are at opposite ends of the spectrum. The rise in degenerative disease, the degradation of the planet, and the increase in obesity come down to the fact that we have developed bad habits that are taking their toll.

AND NOW IT'S UP TO YOU

Day to day, you choose, shop, and buy the food that your family and you will consume. You decide at any given moment, from any number of viewpoints—economic, cultural, environmental, whatever—what you will buy and use. It's entirely up to you. What you choose to eat is the only decision over which you have complete control . . . even if you think you don't. Only you can make the changes needed to ensure health, a clean planet, and a safe food supply. You do it by demanding better. You demand better by "voting" with your dollar. Big business tracks trends; they track shopping; they track the interests of their customers. By telling them what you want, you can effect change and begin to see products on the shelves that you actually want to eat . . . and are good for you. Just take a look at how far the accessibility of natural, fresh, and organic foods has come over the last decade or two. They have become as familiar to us as any other kinds of foods. Our awareness of food has already begun to change. Now our actions have to change.

YOU ARE WHAT YOU EAT

And you thought it was a joke. It turns out that we are, in fact, what we eat. And what we eat drives how we feel and how we behave. New research being done at the Mayo Clinic has revealed some telling information that may help answer the age-old question: "Why can't we just make healthy choices?" Finally!

"Different foods signal pleasure both through the substances they contain and the chemicals they cause the brain to release," says Gianrico Farrugia, director of the Enteric Neuroscience Program at the Mayo Clinic.

Dr. David Kessler, former commissioner of the Food and Drug Administration under Presidents George H. W. Bush and Bill Clinton, is a pediatrician and served as the dean of the medical schools at both Yale and the University of California, San Francisco. His book, *The End of Overeating: Taking Control of the Insatiable American Appetite*, speaks to this new brain-gut connection and the insidious way in which products are marketed to us.

"Fat and sugar, fat and salt, fat, sugar, and salt stimulate us to eat more and more," Kessler writes. "Does the food industry understand the inputs? Absolutely! They understand that fat, sugar, and salt stimulate us and they understand the outputs. They understand we keep on coming back for more and more.

"Have they understood the neuroscience? Have they understood how fat and sugar work? I don't think so. But we now have that science. But what's important is the fact that they have figured out—they've learned it experientially—what works and they construct food to stimulate us to eat more."

This brain-gut connection has necessitated a new field of science: neurogastroenterology. I know; I know; more studies with more confusing scientific statistics, right? Maybe not this time. Calling our digestive system a "second brain," this seemingly unglamorous science has revealed the gut as both a physical and emotional powerhouse with more than two hundred million neurons, which is more than contained in our spinal cord. Oh, and remember the digestive system does its work independently of the brain.

Dr. Kessler uses a great example in an article he published, called "Deconstructing the Vanilla Milkshake." In the article he asks what it is about the milkshake that you love? The fat? The sugar? The flavor? What stimulates you to come back for more?

"It's the sugar," says Kessler. "The sugar is the main driver. But when you add fat to the sugar, it's synergistic." Kessler explains that sugar and fat, in combination, elevate the brain's dopamine circuitry (like when you ingest an amphetamine or cocaine). And here's the scary thing: this elevation doesn't habituate; it doesn't go down time after time. Fat and sugar create a potent, multisensory food that stimulates the brain's neural circuitry and needs more and more stimulation, leading to the conclusion that the more fat and sugar you eat, the more you need to feel sated.

Is he saying that food manufacturers are manipulating addiction?

It sure sounds that way.

The food industry certainly understands what works. Based on past history, memory, and experience, our brains take cues and stimulate thoughts of wanting what creates arousal. The food industry has taken fat, sugar, and salt and put it on every street corner, on every shelf, available to us 24/7. They have made it socially desirable to eat it at anytime. "Eat great, even late," screams Wendy's ads. The emotional gloss of advertising is icing on the cake (pun intended) for their seduction. You look at an ad and fall in love. You want it. Food has become entertainment. We live in a food carnival.

Look at how they do it. They take some animal, like a chicken. Before it gets to the fast-food joint where you will buy it and eat it, it's fried in the manufacturing plant, loading, according to Dr. Kessler, about 30 percent of fat on top of the animal's original fat content. It's then fried again in the restaurant (and I use the term loosely). Often it's coated in a spicy red sauce made of . . . wait for it . . . fat, sugar, and salt. In the end, what you really just ate in your box of wings was fat on fat on fat on sugar on fat and salt. It sounds gross in these terms, but in terms of making you want it, it's brilliant.

Dr. Kessler believes that the food industry, advertising, and marketing have created a conditioned behavior in Americans that he calls "hyper-eating." Through conditioning, our brain's reward circuits are in constant activation, so the anticipation of food, the smell of food, the sight of food makes food hard to resist. Marketing has staked a big claim in that fact. They don't show fat, juicy burgers or glistening pizzas, dripping with cheese, in their ads for kicks.

Regular exposure to foods rich in fat, sugar, and salt can literally change the way your brain works, contends Dr. Kessler. He thinks humans are wired to focus on the strongest stimulus in our surroundings. When it comes to food, the greatest stimuli are fat, sugar, and salt. The mere thought of such foods travels to the reward center of the brain, releases dopamine (the chemical associated with pleasure), and we want to eat . . . which releases more chemicals, "opiods," which provide emotional satisfaction. Over time and repeated behavior, these neuro pathways are strengthened so that the mere mention, a slight whiff of a favorite food, sets the cycle of desire in motion.

You have just created a habit.

More and more of these foods are needed to keep the level of satisfaction high and the pleasure strong. Just like the bag of chips says: "Bet you can't eat just one."

The new scientific evidence we have connecting our food and our gut, our hunger with our mood, shows that our behavior is becoming seriously conditioned and driven. And we are passing this behavior on to our children. This is learned behavior and it can stick with us for life. In essence, our brains are being activated, hijacked, and manipulated . . . but it doesn't mean we can't fight back. We have been conditioned over the last decades to eat as reward or as comfort . . . as the cure for whatever ails us at the moment. We have a bad day; we eat. We have a good day; we eat. That "bastard" leaves us; we eat. It's our anniversary, graduation, birthday, christening, bris; we eat. We celebrate, commiserate, comfort, and control with food.

There is good news in all this. According to Dr. Kessler, now that we know our brains are being purposefully stimulated in an attempt to manipulate us, we can do something about it.

Imagine your favorite food in front of you right now. It's perfect, exactly what you like and how you like it. What are you thinking? Are you still focused on the information in this book? Are you still with me? Or are you thinking of the taste of that food on your tongue, the aroma of that food in your nose? Are you salivating, distracted? You begin a dialogue with yourself. "I really should continue reading." "Oh, that smells so good." "But it has so much fat and so many calories. I really shouldn't."

According to Dr. Kessler, you just lost the fight. When you have that little dialogue in your head, especially about why you shouldn't eat something, the obsession begins and you amplify the experience and reward of the food. You only want it more.

So what do we do?

To break the cycle of addiction to foods that are literally stealing our future, we have to change how we think.

Look what happened with cigarettes. When I was a kid, there was nothing sexier than someone smoking. I remember my mother, sitting at the head of the dinner table, with a cigarette in a black holder and thinking how positively gorgeous and sophisticated she looked. Glamorous movie stars, suave lovers, and rebellious youth were the images we held in our heads of smoking.

But then reality changed our view of tobacco and smoking and now, well, it ain't so cool anymore, is it? Now we feel sad for those poor huddled masses in front of office buildings puffing away, their yellowed fingertips pushing cigarettes into their pursed lips, the misery of their addiction obvious to us and maybe even to them.

It's time to change the image we have of junk food; change the image we have of the foodlike substances dancing in our heads. We have to see past the dancing clowns, delicate fairies, kindly old colonels, freckle-faced kids to the truth.

We have to decide that there is more to life; that there is something more important to us than fat, sugar, and salt. Then we can change our behavior. Something must motivate us to change. For some of us, a light goes on in our heads watching a documentary or Dr. Oz or reading a book. For me, it took fear; it wasn't until I was diagnosed with cancer and facing my own untimely death at twenty-six years of age, that I was able to give up the deadly combo of foods that had created my situation. My life was more important to me than frozen Snickers bars.

In a word, that is how we must learn to think. The food industry will not change on its own. Yes, they will continue to roll out "low-fat," "light," "healthy" fare to market because it allows them to capitalize on current headlines and trends. By creating all these pseudo-healthy products, they create a constant stream of something to talk about in the media. So they are never far from your consciousness. In truth, they don't care if you ever order the salad with grilled chicken. They don't care if you take the free pedometer with your Happy Meal and they don't care if you buy one fresh apple instead of apple pie. They care that you come into their stores, take in the aroma of the familiar fatty foods they are known for, and buy.

And so they will create fake healthy product after fake healthy product so they never lose that special place in your heart.

The change needed is in our minds as well as our bodies.

Not so long ago, food was simpler. There were three flavors of ice cream: chocolate, strawberry, and vanilla. We had a few cereals to choose from and pizza was, well, pizza with cheese, along with anchovies (for some) and pepperoni if you were splurging. M&M's came in only primary colors.

Now we have countless varieties of ice cream, cereal, bread, salad dressing, candy, toppings for pizza and burgers, fried, grilled, and barbecued chicken options, and don't even get me started on the options for sides. We have a billion (or so it seems) flavors of coffee, tea, and other beverages. There seem to be hundreds of flavors of yogurt . . . frozen and not.

Studies now show that when complexity of flavor is built into food, the effects of desire become more powerful. "The complexity of the stimulus increases its association to a reward," says Gaetano Di Chiara, an expert in neuroscience and pharmacology at the University of Cagliari in Italy. He goes on to say that experience plays a role in this stimulation for reward. When you see a bowl of M&M's, you know what to expect because you have eaten them in the past. You know the reward that is coming. The more potent and complex a food, the greater the reward it may offer, so we become more stimulated. Think of ice cream topped with M&M's or cookies with M&M's in them. You know the M&M's are good, but how cool might they taste in cookies? Wow!

While there's still a lot to be discovered in this new field of neurogastroenterology, we do know that foods high in fat, sugar, and salt are literally altering the biological circuitry of our brains. Science has seen them change the connections between our neural circuits and our response patterns. We know these foods are rewiring us, so to speak.

And with an industry that knows exactly what it's doing, we must be wide awake and see the truth for what it is. Maya Angelou famously said that when someone tells you who they are (in deeds, words, actions), believe them.

Nothing could be truer for the food industry we must navigate.

Let me tell you a little story about Starbucks. A venture capitalist (who requests anonymity) familiar with the business cited them as a company that has recognized and responded "brilliantly" to cultural need. Caffeine and sugar in coffee has an energizing effect, but Starbucks has taken it to another level. They offer something far more primal than a cup of joe. They made their goal to offer "warm milk and a bottle."

Wanting more customers during the afternoon hours led to the creative thinking that gave us the Frappuccino. The creation of a rich, sweet, and comforting milkshake-like product transformed their business. And our waistlines.

A Starbucks Strawberries & Crème Frappuccino with whipped cream comes with 18 teaspoons of sugar. The Double Chocolatey Chip Frappuccino with whipped cream weighs in at 640 calories, 22 grams of fat, and 100 grams of carbohydrates (almost all sugar . . .). Of course without the whipped cream, it slims down to a mere 500 calories. For a coffee drink?

Did the product and its strategy work? Yes, it did. Starbucks discovered that by making enticing foods constantly available and keeping them novel with cool-sounding names, people will come back for more and more.

By encouraging us to consider any occasion for food an opportunity for reward, the industry invites us to indulge more often. "The number of cues, the number of opportunities to eat have increased, while the barriers to consumption have fallen," says David Mela, senior scientist of weight management at the Unilever Health Institute. He goes on to say that few of us are immune to the omnipresence of food, especially foods that are readily available, seemingly decadent (read: reward), and cheap. "There is constant, constant opportunity."

Now what?

YOU CAN'T CREATE CHANGE
WITHOUT CHANGE

There are lots of ways you can break this cycle of fast food and the addiction to fat, sugar, and salt. They all require discipline and a bit of work, but all will pay off in freeing you.

1. You can plan when and what you will eat and not deviate from that plan as much as possible. This can be a bit exhausting to be so constantly vigilant, but it works.

2. You can practice control. I know: what a grown-up concept! If you eat less and eat more slowly, consuming foods that are nutrient dense and high in fiber, your hunger will be kept at bay for about four hours. This way you can begin to discern if you are really hungry or if you are just grabbing that donut because it's there and it's habit.

3. Avoid fast-food joints altogether. Seriously. This may sound easier than it is in practice, but to change the quality of our food; to break the cycle of this addiction to fat, sugar, and salt; to take back our health, we must avoid these greasy spoons like the plague.

These steps are a bit of tough self-love and require a good bit of discipline. On a kinder and gentler note, taking control of what you choose to eat is as simple as paying attention, or as world-renowned Buddhist master Thick Nhat Hanh calls it, "eating mindfully."

To get to the root of the problem—any problem—is to change how you think and how you act.

Simple, right?

It really is. When we slow down and enjoy our food, we take on a different quality in our life. When we can sit and enjoy each bite of food, we develop an awareness of our surroundings, the flavors and nuances of the foods, the way we feel as we eat. Now I know what you're thinking. You have three kids fighting at the table; your husband is grouching about his day; soccer practice is looming; the PTA meeting is in half an hour; and I am asking you to eat in peace.

Yes, I am. You can't change your life without changing your life; it's really that simple. Even within the chaos that is modern life, we need to find a small bit of peace in the day to eat and be aware. We must make our health a priority if we are going to get out of this life alive.

The way we eat influences every single aspect of our day. When we respond to certain stimuli, certain feelings or emotions will manifest in us. Think about how you feel when you eat a meal under stress. Now think about how you feel when you eat a relaxed meal. Obvious, right? Think about when you eat and why. Think about how you feel after eating when you have eaten because you are stressed or sad or depressed. Do you feel bloated, puffy, maybe even guilty? Finally, think about how you feel when you eat under happy circumstances. Relaxed? Sated? Fulfilled? Maybe even happy? Being mindful allows you to control how you eat, and when you control how you eat, it's easy to control what you eat. Fat, sugar, and salt addictions are broken. You are free.

In our house, eating is a ritual that we observe with sanctity akin to religion. It's how I was raised. I set the table each night, with cloth napkins, real dishes, and silverware. Please, please get rid of paper plates and plastic microwave dishes and use real china. Please! Your experience of your meal will change . . . your view of food will change . . . and the planet will have less trash. A win/win/win! I serve the food I cook in beautiful serving bowls, having cooked what we will need for this meal with perhaps a little left over to give me a start for my next meal preparation. We sit for each meal. It's a celebration of the blessings we have in life; we reconnect at each meal; we talk about our day; we relax. We take the time to experience the meal.

Now before you roll your eyes, let me say that I, too, live a wild-and-crazy life filled with travel, work, seminars, classes, community obligations, impossible demands on my time and family . . . just like you. I don't have help in the house. I cook, clean, work out regularly, and take care of the family. I work full-time. But I decided long ago that this is how it would be in our house. I grew up with mealtime as the time of day when we stepped off the carousel of life and decompressed at the table. I work hard to maintain this time in our modern life of distractions and connectedness, but we are the better for it. You will be, too.

Being mindful takes no more effort than it takes to be unconscious. It's not extra work. Mindful living makes everything a bit more meaningful, like being just a little more awake. When we are mindful, we are conscious of every breath and thrilled to be alive. We become truly present within ourselves and, as a result, for each other. Wouldn't it be nice to lose that desperate distracted quality that always has you just a wee bit lost: looking for your keys, your wallet, your briefcase; exhausted like a hamster on a wheel?

There are experts who will tell you that being mindful is too much work to maintain and that we should develop healthy habits that then become mindless and robotic. But in order to develop those healthy habits, we need to be mindful, at least for a period, right? So why not just move to a more mindful place of being and see where that carries you in life?

It's not about obsessing over every single bite you take or thinking about food all the time. Mindful eating is a way of thinking that allows you to eat freely with respect for your body and all living things because you have become a feeling, thinking person, not a zombie stuffing his or her face with fast food.

It's not all airy-fairy esoteric, this mindfulness. There are tangible steps you can take to create an awareness of what and how we eat. I have found these few steps work wonders for waking me up to what I choose to eat. These simple steps will turn you into a mindful eater in no time:

1. Never eat unless you are sitting down. But eating in your car doesn't count. Or at your desk while you work. I mean sitting down in a spot or in a setting where you can create a spirit of awareness of what you're consuming. When we eat while we walk, drive, talk on the phone, watch television, work at our desks, text, surf the Internet, or stand over the sink, we lose touch with what we are eating, how it tastes and feels in our mouths. We just consume mindlessly, eating much more than we intend or need.

2. Take food out of the pots and pans, transferring it to serving dishes. Just this act elevates the experience of your food. Even commercials for frozen meals show the food tumbling from the pan to a serving plate. Just this simple act makes eating more sacred, a little more special. It makes you more aware of the food: the colors, aromas, textures.

3. Chew your food. This seemingly natural act is a bit of a lost art. Most of us wolf down our food, swallowing it practically whole. Chewing allows you to really taste the food and slows us down just a wee bit. Slowing down helps us to eat less. Remember the old adage: it takes twenty full minutes for your brain to signal your stomach that you are full. If you're really honest with yourself, by the time twenty minutes have passed, most of us have had three helpings, the dishes are done, and we're back in front of *Dancing with the Stars*, if we ever left the glow of our TV screen at all.

Mindfulness creates a respect in us for all living things, beginning with our own bodies. Once mindfulness becomes a way of life for us, we can no longer disrespect our bodies or those we love with artificial foodlike substances. We will no longer be enslaved to what they market to us. Our vision for our lives and our world becomes bigger than the ninety-nine-cent bargain meals in colorful packages.

Once we know who we are, what we are, the value of our bodies and our lives, we will know what to eat. Our humanity and intuition will guide us, not marketing. Eating mindfully is a practice that will help us understand who we are and our connection with nature.

In the end, we are all connected. What we touch, do, and say affects each and every single living thing around us. We are an integral part of the web of life, and what we do has an impact on all things around us. When you harm your body with food unfit for human consumption, you harm your family, your friends, your community, your city, your world. Think about that the next time a kindly old colonel invites you to have your dinner from a bucket.

Changing the way we live and eat is the single most important ingredient in creating a healthy society and a future in which we thrive. We can no longer live in denial of the implications of our actions, divorced from the source of our amusements and indulgences. We must step into the light and take back our health and our future.

SATISFACTION GUARANTEED

When faced with the idea of changing from a diet of Golden Arches and dinner in a bucket, washed down with gallons of sugary drinks, to simple fare like whole grains, beans, and vegetables, many people have a knee-jerk response. The food will be awful, tasteless, and boring . . . and they will be hungry all the time. It won't be any fun. It will be grim and deprived. We hardly think it will be an exciting new culinary adventure.

That thinking (and you know it's true) signals one of the biggest differences between our American eating culture and just about everyone else in the world. The perception of satisfaction with a meal differs greatly in other cultures. We were all raised to clean our plates, not waste food. After all, think of the starving children of the world. It's what our parents told us to get us to eat . . . and it stuck. As immigrants came here and discovered abundance like they had never seen, having more food to eat was a sign of affluence. That, too, stuck. And finally, as transport made it easier to get more food, and supermarkets grew in size and convenience, we had access to more food . . . and that really stuck. Supermarkets today are like Disneyland—huge, colorful festivals of packaged foods.

In countries like Italy and France, more often children are raised to appreciate a feeling of "longing," anticipation of the next course of the meal. They are taught to savor each bite, enjoy the textures and flavors. They still take the majority of their meals at the table, with friends and family. They are encouraged to experience the meal, not wolf it down between television shows or activities. Eating is still somewhat sacred in other countries.

In 2006, a study published in the journal *Obesity* was done on how Parisians and Chicagoans ate. While the French paid attention to their internal cues of satiety, the Americans took their fullness cues from their plates. When it was empty, they were full. This tells us something very important about how we eat and how we listen or do not listen to our body's cues.

Most of us ignore the body's subtle signals of hunger and fullness. We are either "starving" or "stuffed." We rarely pause at or even recognize the pleasant midpoint . . . satisfied. But reacquainting ourselves with that middle ground of satiety could be the key to managing our weight, maintaining our health, and making a lighter footprint on the planet. It will help us to eat more like humans.

According to food psychologist and one of the authors of the *Obesity* study, Brian Wansink, PhD, of Cornell University, overweight people have a harder time recognizing when they are full. The study also concluded that overweight people are more susceptible to the messages in ads, on signage, and from other sources like television and radio, urging them to eat more. And in my view, the food industry knows exactly what it is saying and to whom it is saying it. It's not the fit, slim triathlete succumbing to its food seduction. It knows full well it's the schlub who hasn't seen his feet in years and who has lost hope who will seek solace, satisfaction, and fullness in the fat, sugar, and salt it sells.

This should make you mad as hell. It's an affront to humanity by big business, in my view. This study tells us that we are being consciously manipulated by food marketers to sell us more and more processed food. It's another link to how easily we can lose ourselves in the seduction of food and stop listening to our instincts.

We need to understand that there's more to satiety than being stuffed like a Thanksgiving turkey. We have lost sight of simple satisfaction. In our lust for more bang for our buck, we have placed a higher value on being stuffed than on feeling great.

When you are aware of satisfaction, it allows you to enjoy your food more and to anticipate flavors to come. Imagine finishing a meal and not having the discomfort of a bloated belly and guilty conscience after eating. Imagine being content, not having to loosen your pants.

Hunger is not a bad thing. It's an alarm that tells us we need calories to function. It's a response by the hypothalamus region of the brain in answer to signals like glucose or fatty acid levels in our blood, hormones like ghrelin from our stomach, leptin from our fat cells, and nerve signals from our intestines. We know hunger signals us to take in food for energy to keep going. The latest theories suggest that "fullness" releases bursts of dopamine (our feel-good hormone), and when we're hungry, these little bursts of joy stop. It makes sense; think how cranky you get when you're hungry.

Here's where it gets tricky. Our modern diet, rich in saturated fats, seems to throw our satiety/hunger equilibrium off balance. According to a study published by the *Journal of Clinical Investigation*, bingeing on treats high in saturated fats caused an impaired sensitivity to leptin and insulin, which causes us to ignore signals of being full. And this effect can last for days. This tells us that a weekend binge could be the reason we find it so hard to get back on the bandwagon on Monday morning. It's why the advice to eat well for six days of the week and eat all you like of whatever you like on the seventh day is some of the worst advice ever. It sets you up for the thinking that eating well, treating your body well, is a drag, a deprivation, and you only have to hold on for a few days and then it's party time again. More important, it will make Monday seem all the more grim as the party ends and you face six days of broccoli and sprouts. I know this to be true. It was not until I broke this thinking for myself that I was able to fully enjoy and appreciate the deliciousness of real, healthy food.

When you begin to eat a healthier diet, when you begin to feed your body with food that can fuel your activity and leave you feeling alive and vital, you actually begin to crave those foods. Your body wants that fuel. One of the reasons we feel so awful all the time is that we eat food that makes our body work so hard to digest it, leaving us exhausted and miserable. It's true. When you eat food that is fit for human consumption, designed by nature to nourish us well, we want that food. It's our instinct to feel well; it's our instinct to be strong and vital.

Because we have chosen to eat poorly for so long, many of us don't even realize we don't feel well and vital. We don't know how awful we feel until it changes. We think all the little aches and pains and other chronic problems are just a part of life or aging. But it's not true.

When I changed my diet to whole, unprocessed foods, I was young and athletic. But after a few weeks of eating appropriate food for me, it was like a fog lifted. I had none of the aches and pains that I had associated with aging (at twenty-six!). I felt renewed with more energy than I could have imagined. My morning fog was gone; my late-afternoon lethargy was gone, too. I wasn't cranky. My knees stopped aching. My lower back didn't ache.

Eating a plant-based diet will give you gifts far beyond the delicious flavors and textures you will come to enjoy. You will see changes and feel energy you thought long gone. I can't imagine not wanting that for your life. And if all it means is giving up Big Macs (knowing what they are now), isn't that worth it?

6

Get Smart About What You're Eating

Now that you have become more than just peripherally aware of the compromised quality of our food supply, it's time to get smart so you know what you're getting when you shop for food. You can only make wise choices when you know what you're seeing on labels . . . and what might not be on the label.

The smart shopper has the best shot at avoiding the kinds of ingredients you don't want to eat . . . or support with your dollar.

HOW TO READ A LABEL

I know; duh, right? Don't you just pick up the package, turn it over, and read? Sure, but you may not know what exactly you're seeing.

It's complicated. We are confused by all the conflicting information, buzzwords, and claims being made on packages, so we just chug along, heads in the sand, and keep eating what they sell us. But we have to take some responsibility here and make the changes we know we need to make in our diets.

One of the reasons we have seen such dramatic imbalances in human health is because we have radically changed our patterns of eating over a very short period of time. We have created dietary chaos. Much of what we call food in our modern world is actually unfit for human consumption. The literally thousands of chemically processed colors and flavors created to enhance and preserve our foods are absolutely alien to who we are as human beings. Our biological history has no way to deal with this stuff. And I'm not talking about the basic constituent nutrients that remain in many modern foods; that is not in dispute. The quality of nutrients seems to have lost its place of importance in the world of food.

Our human form has evolved over millions of years and has, for lack of a better description, an organic familiarity with foods in their natural form. The fine balance of nutrients that Mother Nature placed within whole, unprocessed foods maximizes the nutritional impact of said foods like nothing science can dream up. It's impossible for nutrition science to improve on foods in their natural state. Outside of natural processes, like cooking, drying, pickling, sautéing, slicing, and dicing, modern food science has done nothing to improve on the natural goodness of food. It has improved profit margins, but not human health. It has created false and stimulating flavors, but done nothing to enhance the actual food in a way that benefits humanity.

The appeal of convenience, low price, added flavor, and enriched nutrients is all an illusion to cover up the compromised quality of food. With fat, sugar, and salt, you can make cardboard taste exciting to the palate. These are the dominant flavors in all junk food and the basis for their appeal. Food companies, along with nutrition science, have figured out ways to make any substance taste like any food. And we are helpless, lost in a sea of enhanced flavors, confusing labels, and seductive marketing. In the hands of the food industry, rubber can take on the texture, smell, and flavor of strawberry jam . . . and they can make anything taste like chicken. The food industry is counting on your losing your sense of taste (on so many levels), as well as your good judgment, so they can continue churning out new and ever more exciting junk food to line their pockets.

Since 1994, the FDA has required that packaged foods carry a nutrition label along with ingredients so that, in theory, consumers know what's in the food they are buying and can choose accordingly.

Nutrition labels are usually vertical boxes with lots of information on them to inform you. At the top of the label you will see the serving size or the number of servings that the nutrition information is based on. This is one of the most important parts of the label because all the other information in the nutrition panel is based on the serving size.

The next part of the label includes information concerning fat content and type, amount and type of carbohydrates, protein, sodium, fiber, and sugar. It's important to note that the FDA now requires the amount of trans fats in products be listed. They will be listed with fats and cholesterol amounts. Each will be shown in grams or milligrams and the percentage of the daily value (the amount needed daily) of the nutrient. This can be a bit misleading because these percentages are based on a 2,000-calorie-a-day diet, but it gives you an idea of how the food in question can fit into your daily needs.

The next part of the label reveals the vitamin and mineral content of the food item you are considering. The FDA requires listings on calcium, iron, and vitamins A and C, but not others. Manufacturers often add other listings of percentages, like folic acid, potassium, or magnesium if the product contains significant amounts of the nutrients in question.

The bottom part of the label is not always there, but when it is, it is significant. Suggested Daily Requirements serve as a reminder of general dietary needs based on 2,000-calorie and 2,500-calorie daily diets.

We need to begin to use these little panels to guide us in the quality and quantity we should be eating.

The ingredient list on a packaged food is not so easy to decipher as the nutrition panel. As you know, ingredients are listed from greatest quantity to least. Some common buzzwords on packages won't hold up under the scrutiny of label reading if you know what you are looking at.

When a package makes claims like "immune boosting" or a "good source of antioxidants," what is the label really saying to us? Unless the food is fresh, you might be getting more than you want. A packaged food is fortified with nutrients that allow them to make these claims, but before putting it into your shopping cart, check out the nutrition panel for calories, fat, sugar, and sodium. Just because a product is fortified doesn't make it healthy.

"Made with whole grains" is a phrase we see a lot, but as we have seen, it simply means there is some form of whole grains somewhere in the product. The order that the whole grain appears on the ingredient panel is the indicator of just how much whole grain is present. The nearer to the beginning of the list, the more of any ingredient.

Trans fats are now listed on the nutrition panels and that's a good thing. Here's the rub, though. When a label makes the claim that a product is "trans fat free," it may not be entirely true. The FDA allows for the "free" claim if a product has 0.5 grams of trans fat per serving. So you may be seeing partially hydrogenated oil in a "trans fat free" product and wonder. No need. The product has trans fats. It's a loophole. Avoid these products.

Often products say that they are lightly sweetened or low in sugar, but since the FDA has no requirement or guidelines for this, who's to say what that means? Sugar is listed on labels under many names, including sucrose, glucose, fructose, corn syrup, maltose, dextrose, brown sugar, organic cane juice, raw sugar, turbinado sugar, high-fructose corn syrup, date sugar, and fruit sugar. If you see a bunch of these, this product is anything but lightly sweetened.

A new buzzword is that a product is made with real fruit. Best to head right to the ingredient panel and see if you see fresh fruit as an ingredient. Often, just a touch of real fruit is in the product, but the bulk of the sweetness comes from some form of sugar.

Natural and artificial flavors are seen in just about all packaged and processed foods. As you will see, the differences in them are minimal and the fact that manufacturers are not required to list these ingredients separately should worry you when you see them on an ingredient panel.

Many people get discouraged by reading labels because it seems you need a chemistry degree to decipher the list of additives. Let me make it easy for you: if you can't pronounce it, don't know what it is, skip the product. And if Michael Pollan has his way, labels will become easier to understand. He is currently working with experts to create a universal label designed to show ingredients and nutrition more clearly.

NATURAL VERSUS ARTIFICIAL

Scientists have come to the conclusion that humans acquired the sense of taste to avoid being poisoned. Edible plants, nuts, seeds, and berries generally had a sweet taste while toxic ones were bitter. And while our taste buds can detect subtle nuances in food, the basic tastes—sweet, bitter, salty, sour, astringent, and umami (discovered by the Japanese in research and translates into the detection of richness and deliciousness triggered by amino acids)—they offer a limited detection compared to the human olfactory system, which can take in and decipher thousands of chemical aromas. Research suggests that flavor is primarily the smell of gases being released by the chemicals you have just put in your mouth. They now believe that as much as 90 percent of the taste of a food comes from the aroma.

I know this is getting more like Mr. Wizard than a cookbook. Stay with me. You'll see why this is important to know when you are choosing food.

The act of drinking, sucking, or chewing releases foods' volatile gases, which flow from your mouth, up your nostrils, and up the passageway in the back of your mouth to the thin layer of nerve cells called the olfactory epithelium, located right between your eyes at the base of your nose. Your brain steps in, deciphers the smells, combines them with taste signals from your tongue, and decides if this is something you want to eat.

People's preferences are formed in the first few years of life, through how we are socialized. Babies naturally prefer sweet tastes, like mothers' milk, and reject bitter flavors. But as we grow, we learn to appreciate other foods by what we are fed.

With all we know about the body, the human sense of smell is largely confounding to science. More than other senses, our sense of smell is greatly affected by psychological factors and surroundings. People can grow used to bad or good smells. We can stop noticing a smell that at first was overwhelming. Aroma and memory are inexplicably linked. An aroma can trigger long-forgotten moments of our past. Flavors of childhood seem to leave an indelible mark and we often return to them as adults for comfort and reassurance. The perfumes of our youth take us back to what we remember as better times, simpler times . . . a fact that is not lost on fast-food chains and their flavor houses.

Think about it. Cinnamon smells like Christmas; tomatoes and basil evoke memories of summer.

Childhood memories of Happy Meals will translate into frequent visits to McDonald's as adults. Especially in hard times, these fast-food masterminds are counting on your childhood memories and your search for comfort in uncertainty so they can steal your future by stealing your health.

According to author Eric Schlosser, the flavor industry has its beginnings in the mid-nineteenth century, as processed foods began to be manufactured on a larger scale. Early food processors turned to perfume companies to help them create flavorful additives for food. Originally working with essential oils, the industry quickly changed when a German scientist discovered methyl anthranilate, one of the first artificial flavorings ever created. With the sweet smell of grapes as its signature, this chemical became the chief flavor compound in grape Kool-Aid.

After World War II, the flavor industry shifted to the United States, first in the garment district in New York and eventually to New Jersey for larger plant capacity. Man-made flavors were used mostly in baked goods, candies, and sodas until the 1950s when the sales of processed foods exploded. Inventions and technology kept up; until by the mid-1960s companies were creating the flavors for Pop-Tarts, Bac-O's, Tang, and Tab, along with thousands of other products.

The American flavor industry now sees revenues of about $1.4 billion annually, with about ten thousand new processed food products being introduced each year. Nearly all of them require flavor additives to be palatable. Flavor innovations keep creating new ways to entice you to eat more junk food.

And food additives are cheap because they are so potent. They appear at the end of the ingredient list for this reason, but yet, they are why we love junk food so much.

The FDA does not require companies to disclose the ingredients of their flavor or color additives as long as the chemicals in them are considered by this same agency to be GRAS (generally regarded as safe). This allows companies to maintain the secrecy of their formulas and hides the fact that flavor compounds often contain more ingredients than the food they are flavoring. "Artificial flavoring" gives us little insight into the chemical magic and skill that makes processed food taste just like strawberries . . . or chocolate . . . or blueberries.

Check this out. Schlosser says a typical artificial strawberry-flavored milkshake, like those sold in popular fast-food chains, can contain the following ingredients: amyl acetate, amyl butyrate, amyl valerate, anethol, anisyl formate, benzyl acetate, benzyl isobutyrate, butyric acid, cinnamyl isobutyrate, cinnamyl valerate, cognac essential oil, diacetyl, dipropyl ketone, ethyl acetate, ethyl amyl ketone, ethyl butyrate, ethyl cinnamate, ethyl heptanoate, ethyl heptylate, ethyl valerate, ethyl lactate, ethyl methylphenylglycidate, ethyl nitrate, ethyl propionate, ethyl valerate, heliotropin, hydroxyphenyl-2-butanone (10 percent solution in alcohol), a-ionone, isobutyl anthranilate, isobutyl butyrate, lemon essential oil, maltol, 4-methylacetophenone, methyl anthranilate, methyl benzoate, methyl cinnamate, methyl heptine carbonate, methyl naphthyl ketone, methyl salicylate, mint essential oil, neroli essential oil, nerolin, neryl isobutyrate, orrise butter, phenethyl alcohol, rose, rum ether, gamma-undecalactone, vanillin, and solvent.

I am exhausted just typing that. And people drink these every day. Kids drink these toxic brews. Oh, my God.

Many of the processed foods today are like blank canvases and whatever chemicals are added will give the food the desired flavor. Ethyl-2-methyl butyrate smells just like an apple. Methyl-2 pyridyl ketone makes something taste like popcorn; ethyl-3 hydroxybutanoate, like marshmallow. The possibilities are nearly endless. The most foul of processed food can be made unbelievably desirable through the miracle of chemistry.

But do we want to eat it?

What about natural flavors you ask? We see those words on labels all the time. According to the FDA, natural flavors must be derived from natural sources . . . herbs, spices, fruits, vegetables, beef, chicken, yeast, bark, roots, and so on. Consumers love seeing natural flavors on a label, believing that they are more healthful products. But the distinctions between artificial and natural flavors are arbitrary and absurd, based more on how the flavor is made, not on what it contains. Make sense? It will.

Terry Acree, professor of food science at Cornell University, says that a natural flavor has been derived with out-of-date technology. Natural and artificial flavors often contain the same chemicals but are produced through different methods, making them "natural." Amyl acetate provides the flavor of banana. When distilled from banana with a chemical solvent, it is considered natural. But when it's produced by mixing vinegar with amyl alcohol, with sulfuric acid as a catalyst, amyl acetate is an artificial flavor. Not much difference, right? As a result, natural flavor is now listed among the ingredients in everything from granola bars to hot sauce and is not necessarily healthier or purer than an artificial one.

Natural and artificial flavors are now manufactured at the same chemical flavor plants, places where few people would find Mother Nature's influence.

The Vegetarian Legal Action Network has petitioned the FDA for full disclosure on labels for foods containing natural flavors. The thinking behind the petition was to have food processors list the origins of their flavors on their labels. Right now, vegetarians have no way of knowing whether a flavor has roots in beef, pork, or other animal products, none of which we want to eat.

Ray Kroc, who bought McDonald's and grew it to what we know, once said that the french fry was sacrosanct and the preparation of said fries was sacrosanct. In that spirit, at the beginning, french fries were hand-washed, peeled, cut, and fried at McDonald's. But as they exploded in growth, this was no longer feasible. The business demanded that they streamline labor and save money, so McDonald's switched to frozen fries. Customers did not notice, but this one change had a profound effect on our diet and system of agriculture. This familiar food became an industrialized, highly processed commodity and hardly the food we knew. It changed everything.

McDonald's fries now come from huge manufacturing plants that peel, slice, cook, and freeze two million pounds of potatoes each and every day. This capability, along with McDonald's rapid expansion, literally changed the way we eat. In 1960, Americans ate about four pounds of french fries per person per year. By 2000, that was up to thirty pounds, and today, McDonald's is the largest purchaser of potatoes in the United States.

And of course, it's the flavor of these famous fries that stoked this success and growth. As a hallmark of McDonald's, the fries have been praised by people far and wide, including James Beard (makes me wonder, really, what all the fuss is about him and his influence on the food world . . . bacon and fries . . . oy). But the taste doesn't stem from the kind of potatoes or the technology that processes them or the equipment that is used to fry them. Other chains, stores, and businesses use the same potatoes and technology. So what's the secret?

The cooking oil.

For decades, McDonald's cooked its fries in a mixture of about 7 percent cottonseed oil and 93 percent beef tallow, so the fries tasted a little like burgers—and had even more saturated fat per ounce.

By the 1990s they were taking a lot of heat about the level of saturated fat and cholesterol in their fries and so, amid great fanfare, they switched to vegetable oil. But how would they keep that unique flavor (and your dollars) flowing? A look at the ingredient list shows us how. Toward the end of the list (yes, list . . . twelve items to be exact) of ingredients is the seemingly benign phrase "natural flavor."

Those two words tell us a lot about the fast-food industry, not just the fries at McDonald's. They tell us why most fast food, not just fries, tastes the way it does . . . and why, being the food that most Americans eat regularly today, natural foods are having such a hard time competing.

And "natural color" is not much better, considering that it comes from what could be considered an unusual source. Cochineal extract (also known as carmine or carminic acid) is made from the dessicated bodies of a female insect (*Dactylopius coccus costa*) from Peru and the Canary Islands. The bug eats red cactus berries, which accumulate in the females and their unhatched larvae. So companies collect, dry, and grind them into pigment. It takes about seventy thousand of these little bugs to produce a pound of carmine, which is used to make processed foods look pink, red, or purple. Dannon yogurt gets its color from carmine, as do many frozen fruit bars, candy, fruit filling, and Ocean Spray pink grapefruit fruit juice drink. Yuck.

But it's all natural, right? Boy, have we been duped.

TO DYE FOR

One more thing on label reading. This one is big, so I thought it deserved some attention. When my younger brother was found to be allergic to artificial colorings in food, not the foods themselves, just the colors, it changed the way my mother read labels. It has been decades since that time, but food dyes and colors have become big business.

A fact that should make you blistering mad: Americans now eat five times as much food dye as we did fifty years ago. That may not sound like a lot, so let me put it in more concrete terms. Manufacturers put about fifteen million pounds of synthetic dyes into our food each year, and that number continues to grow with each new processed food product put on the market.

While natural colorants like beets are available, most manufacturers opt for synthetic dyes to make our food more colorful and exciting to the eyes. It will come as no surprise that they do it because . . . it's cheaper.

And here's the kicker. Three of the eight main dyes used have been linked to cancer, according to the Center for Science in the Public Interest. New research shows that Yellow 5, Yellow 6, and Red 40 contain compounds including benzidine and 4-aminobiphenyl and have been directly linked to cancer. Lucky Charms, anyone? Containing all three of these potentially carcinogenic compounds, this brightly colored cereal doesn't seem so "magically delicious," does it?

From cereals to ice creams, our exposure to these synthetic dyes could come at a high price, according to the CSPI, especially for our kids. Study after study has shown that synthetic food dyes are linked with hyperactivity, ADHD, and an inability to focus. A British study conducted in 2007 revealed that children eating foods or drinks with the most commonly used dyes displayed hyperactive behavior within an hour of consumption! That was back in 2007, with the results published in the esteemed medical journal the *Lancet*, but it hasn't stopped us from the use of such toxins in our foods and it sure hasn't stopped the sales of Lucky Charms. What's it going to take?

GMOS (GENETICALLY MODIFIED ORGANISMS)

G-M-what's? GMOs are genetically modified organisms that are engineered in a lab, in petri dishes, without any influence from Mother Nature, and then used to create new breeds of foods (and other living things). DNA and other compounds, like pesticides, are incorporated into organisms for an end purpose. We know little about the long-term effects of these foods on us and the planet.

"Round-Up Ready" is the name given to soy and corn that was developed by Monsanto and involves the pesticide Round Up being integrated right into the seeds before they are planted. The theory they are trying to sell is that this will require less pesticides to be sprayed, but according to experts at Cornell University, this practice has ended up requiring a more intense use of pesticides as the plants around the corn and soy (and the corn and soy themselves) grow resistant to the *Round Up*. Mistake? Coincidence?

Don't be naïve.

And these are just two of the thousands of genetically modified foods being mixed into the ingredients in many foods today.

Genetic modification also allows for cross-breeding that is far removed from natural hybridization, although manufacturers of these products would have you believe otherwise with their propaganda. The theory behind GMOs is simple. Scientists select specific genes from one organism and introduce them into another to confer a specific trait. This technology can be used to create new varieties of plants and animals more quickly than conventional methods and produce traits not possible through traditional, natural techniques. The mad scientists behind GMOs would have you believe that their process is just like mixing red and yellow peppers' DNA to create an orange pepper, but it isn't. For example, genetic material from salmon can be injected into strawberries to make them more resistant to cold weather. That's messing with Mother Nature in the most unnatural way.

Look at it this way. Two peppers, even of different colors, would hit on each other in a bar, date, and mate. But a strawberry and a salmon, well, not so much. The consequences of this work are alarming, with ramifications we cannot begin to imagine.

While marketers try to sell us on the concept of GMOs as foods that improve yields, are more nourishing for developing countries struggling with famine, and require less use of toxins to grow them, nothing could be further from the truth. While Monsanto and other chemical giants continue to promote these false ideas, there has been no independent proof to support their claims. Only studies conducted within their companies have shown the results they market in their public relations campaigns.

There is, however, increasing concern among independent scientists about the safety of these crops and the resulting foods. The spread of pesticide-resistant plants, the possible toxicity to natural habitats and the species who thrive there, and the impact on human health all remain unanswered questions and are of paramount concern to experts.

So why do these companies do this? Why take such risks with the collective health of humanity and the planet?

GMO crops and foods would give companies like Monsanto and DuPont the ultimate control over human life . . . the control of food. They have already changed the way commercial farmers farm; this is just the next step to world domination, in the sense of food.

Do you think that the chemical executives sitting in their high-rise glass-walled offices with spectacular views care for one moment about the health of populations in developing countries? Or in the industrialized world, for that matter?

With more than 167 million acres of GMO crops planted in the United States, making our farmers the largest producers of these crops, there is solid reason for concern. The United States accounts for more than all GMO crops grown around the rest of the world. And if you are thinking it's just about corn and soybeans, here is the laundry list of crops now grown using GMO technology (and don't you think it's weird to even use the word "technology" when talking about growing food?): corn, cotton, soybeans, canola, squash, sugar beets, rice, dairy products, farm-raised salmon, papaya, and alfalfa, to name a few. GMO ingredients play a role in more than 70 percent of our food overall.

How can this be? How did these potentially disastrous organisms get into our food in such a high concentration? Public relations would have you believe that the FDA approved GMOs after rigorous testing and long-term studies. Nope. In fact, there are no safety testing requirements, according to their own website. The only testing done on GMOs is done by the companies themselves and is meticulously designed to avoid problems, according to Dr. Arpad Pusztai, the leading researcher in this field.

The FDA, under the first President George Bush, was specifically directed to promote the research of biotechnology, and not ironically, the person in charge of developing the policy was the former attorney to the biotech giant Monsanto, who later became their vice president. The results of his policy showed that GMO crops were not different from traditional crops in "any meaningful or uniform way." Therefore, testing was not required.

It didn't stop there. The latest outrage perpetrated on Mother Nature came under the Obama administration. In one week, this administration deregulated two very important crops that can affect our future: alfalfa and sugar beets. Deregulation of alfalfa, the nation's fourth-largest crop and a prodigious pollinator, could spell disaster for natural crops. Used mainly in animal feed, GMO alfalfa would contaminate not only soil and crops, but the meat you eat as well. In January of 2011, this important crop was completely deregulated, meaning that there are no restrictions on the growing of GMO, Round-Up Ready alfalfa by Monsanto and no labeling is required . . . so you, the consumer will have no idea. This deregulation also removed what are known as "buffer zones," specific distances designed to prevent the contamination of organic alfalfa crops by GMO crops, making it virtually impossible to produce organic alfalfa. Indirectly, this means that it could become impossible to produce organic meat and dairy products, since alfalfa is such a big part of their feed.

In a further outrage, in February 2011, sugar beets were deregulated, allowing for GMO sugar beet crops to be grown without restriction or labeling requirements to avoid "a sugar shortage," according to Tom Vilsack, secretary of agriculture for the Obama administration. God forbid we should consider using a wee bit less sugar. We'd rather screw up the natural order to feed the hungry mouths of business and lobby groups!

This is significant for a lot of reasons. Vilsack says that to regulate GMO crops would be "burdensome" to business, but whose business? The deregulation of these crops and the resulting contamination puts an unreasonable burden on all those dedicated farmers and businesspeople working hard to produce and create organic foods. The deregulation of these crops significantly threatens the ability to produce certified organic products, according to Senator Patrick Leahy (author of the original Organic Foods Production Act). The biotechnology industry has declared war on the organic food industry and through shrewd lobbying has won a decisive victory . . . and will continue unopposed with the onslaught of genetically modified foods that are controlled by only a handful of multinational corporations.

Are you mad as hell yet?

It gets better. Scientists who worked for the FDA came to the overwhelming consensus that GMOs were distinctly different from other crops and could lead to unpredictable and hard-to-detect toxins, allergens, new diseases, and nutritional problems. They urged their superiors to conduct long-term studies.

They were ignored.

As a result, only one in four Americans knows that they have eaten or are eating GMO foods. The Campaign for Healthier Eating is committed to educating Americans about what is really in their food. One of the goals is to change the regulations so that GMO ingredients in food must be listed as such. The labeling is voluntary now.

So what do we do?

Read labels, when you can find them, and work to understand them. Begin with your produce. You know those pesky little stickers that are so hard to remove from everything we buy? They could turn out to be your best pals.

If produce is grown with GMO influence, the little stickers will show a 5-digit number beginning with "8." If the produce is organically produced, the stickers will show a 5-digit number beginning with "9," and conventionally produced veggies and fruits will have stickers with a 4-digit number. But don't get your hopes too high that you'll beat them at their own game. With voluntary labeling, you have no idea what you are getting most of the time unless it's certified organic.

With processed foods, there is no way to tell what GMOs may be lurking in your food, well, foodlike substances. GMO ingredients are widespread and well hidden. Even some so-called natural food companies employ GMO ingredients so you really have to know the players to win at this game . . . unless you are buying certified organic foods. And with all of the deregulation going on around us, certified organic could become a moot point. At this time, there is only one organization dedicated to rooting out GMOs and letting the consumer know if the products they are using contain GMOs, whether the product is organic or not. The Non-GMO Project's mission is simple: they are "committed to preserving and building sources of non-GMO products, educating consumers, and providing verified non-GMO sources."

Genetically modified foods and other toxic additives in our foods should scare us witless and have us all mad as hell.

ORGANIC OR NON-ORGANIC, THAT IS THE QUESTION

I turned to my friend and colleague David Steinman to help me explain the importance of organic foods. David is a journalist, environmentalist, and consumer advocate. His book *Diet for a Poisoned Planet* grew out of his own personal concern for the amount of toxins present in the food he was eating. What began as an investigation into contaminants found in the fish in the

Caveat Emptor

According to the Campaign for Healthier Eating, knowing which companies use these questionable ingredients can help you avoid them. Not surprisingly, most large food corporations routinely use these ingredients because they are cheaper. And since so many smaller companies are being swallowed up by bigger corporate giants, you will not always know what you are getting. Here are some of the biggest players so you can keep their products out of your shopping cart. This is a really long list and not even close to complete. That would be another book! Look in your pantry and fridge and see how many of these brands are in your home already.

Aunt Jemima	Heinz	Nature Valley
Beech-Nut	Hershey's	Nestlé
Betty Crocker	Hormel	Ocean Spray
Blue Sky	Hostess	Pepperidge Farm
Boca	Isomil	Peter Pan
Campbell's	Keebler	Pillsbury
Coca-Cola	Kellogg's	Procter & Gamble
Crisco	Kraft	Progresso
Dannon	Land O'Lakes	Quaker
Duncan Hines	Libby's	Similac
Eggo	Life Savers	Skippy
Enfamil	Marie Callender	Smucker's
Frito-Lay	Morningstar Farms	Stouffers
Good Start	Nabisco	Yoplait
Hansen		

Santa Monica Bay has grown into a lifelong mission to educate consumers and fight for cleaner, less toxic foods.

In this world of chemically grown crops, there are big differences in the way our favorite fruits and vegetables are grown. Some crops are sprayed with far more pesticides than others, and some absorb more pesticides than others into their edible parts. These differences in pesticide saturation are very significant. The bottom line for predicting health risks associated with any particular toxic chemical exposure is that the more frequently one is exposed and the higher the level of exposure, the greater the risk. Conversely, the less frequently one is exposed and the lower the concentration, the lower the risk. It is that simple.

Vegetable and Fruit Survival Guide

In order to determine which vegetables and fruits are safest, I examined detailed government food inspectors' reports and private studies of chemical residues in more than 150 fruits, vegetables, beans, nuts, and seeds. The study I found most useful was a huge research effort called the Total Diet Study, an ongoing study conducted by the Food and Drug Administration. It is the most accurate assessment ever made of pesticide contamination of our food supply.

The most recent Total Diet Study measured the total number of residues found in some thirty-six market basket samples, including fresh and canned fruits and vegetables. Most canned produce has far fewer pesticide residues than fresh—although that should never dissuade you from eating fresh fruits and vegetables. Organic fruits and vegetables are the safest, lowest-toxin fruits and vegetables available, and I strongly recommend that you seek out organic produce, especially as a substitute for the most pesticide-saturated foods. Organic farming is booming in this country as consumers demand safe, purer foods.

Organic foods are not readily available in many places, though, and for many people their higher cost is a burden. My goal in writing this book has been to show people which foods are safe and which foods are so high in toxins that organic or other substitutes are advisable.

I've divided foods into "green light," "yellow light," and "red light" categories. I trust that what this means is obvious. Green light foods are your safest choices. Yellow light foods are more saturated; cut down on them and, when possible, buy organic. And red light foods are dangerous.

This division of foods into green light, yellow light, and red light groupings is a simplification of a huge amount of data. My goal in dividing food this way has been to make it clear that there are significant differences in the toxicity of different foods.

Within each green light, yellow light, and red light section, I sometimes list foods without giving an exact number of residues. These foods have been analyzed in ways that tell me how safe they are, but they were not covered by the Total Diet Study, so I don't have an exact number of residues to report.

Fruits

Green Light	Number of Residues
fruit cocktail (canned in heavy syrup)	55
grapefruit (raw)	53
peaches (canned in light/medium syrup)	42
pears (canned in light/medium syrup)	6
watermelon (raw)	33

Other Green Light Fruits		
bitter melon	dates	guavas
limes	passion fruit	plantains
coconut	figs	lemons
papayas	pineapples	tangerines

Yellow Light	Number of Residues
applesauce	97
bananas	71
cantaloupe	131
oranges	116
prunes	126

Other Yellow Light Fruits		
feiojas	casaba	persimmons
blackberries	kumquats	currants
honeydew	cranberries	pomegranates
blueberries	nectarines	
kiwifruit	crenshaw melons	

Red Light	Number of Residues
apples	342
apricots	157
cherries (sweet, raw)	215
grapes	172
peaches	266
pears	176
plums	171
raisins (dried)	200

Vegetables

Green Light	Number of Residues
asparagus	22
black-eyed peas (cowpeas)	18
cabbage	28
cauliflower (fresh/frozen, boiled)	12
corn (canned)	1
corn (cream-style, canned)	14
corn (fresh/frozen, boiled)	3
eggplant (fresh, boiled)	36
green peas (fresh/frozen, boiled)	22
lima beans (mature)	19
mixed vegetables (frozen, boiled)	65
okra (fresh/frozen, boiled)	29
onions	2
peas (mature, dry, boiled)	15
pinto beans	1
radishes	32
red beans	7

Green Light	Number of Residues
sauerkraut (canned)	18
snap green beans	34
sweet potatoes (fresh, baked)	50

Other Green Light Vegetables

alfalfa sprouts	fava beans	radicchio
adzuki beans	fennel root	rapini
bamboo shoots (canned)	garlic	red chard
bean sprouts	jicama	rhubarb
beets (fresh)	kidney beans	shallots
cassava	leeks	snow peas
chives	lentils	watercress
cilantro	mushrooms (fresh)	yams
daikon	navy beans	

Yellow Light	Number of Residues
avocados	67
beets (fresh/frozen, boiled)	56
broccoli (fresh/frozen, boiled)	91
brussels sprouts	127
carrots (fresh, boiled)	63
coleslaw (with dressing, homemade)	121
green beans (fresh/frozen, boiled)	153
iceberg lettuce (raw)	132
lima beans (immature)	87
potatoes (scalloped)	81
potatoes (white, boiled without skin)	93
radishes (raw)	101
spinach (canned)	35
tomato sauce (plain, bottled)	80
tomato (stewed, canned)	49
turnips (fresh/frozen, boiled)	83

Yellow Light		*Number of Residues*
winter squash (fresh/frozen, baked, mashed)		118

Other Yellow Light Vegetables		
artichokes	jalapeño peppers	red peppers
bok choy	kale	rutabagas
cherry tomatoes	kohlrabi	serrano chilis
chili peppers	mung beans	soybeans
choysum	mustard greens	string beans
dandelion greens	okra	swiss chard
dill	parsley	tomatillos
eggplant	parsnips	turnip greens
endive	poblano peppers	turnips
escarole	pumpkin	
green peppers	purslane	

Red Light	*Number of Residues*
celery	240
collard green (fresh/frozen, boiled)	260
cucumbers (raw)	189
green peppers (raw)	256
potatoes (white, baked with skin)	205
summer squash (fresh/frozen, boiled)	185
tomatoes (red, raw)	214

Nuts and Seeds

Green Light	*Number of Residues*
pecans	14

Other Green Light Nuts and Seeds	
almonds	sesame seeds
Chinese pine nuts	sunflower seeds

Other Green Light Nuts and Seeds	
flax	walnuts
hazelnuts	water chestnuts
pistachios	watermelon seeds
pumpkin seeds	

Yellow Light	Number of Residues
lychee nuts	
radish seed	

Red Light	Number of Residues
nuts (mixed, no peanuts, dry roasted)	246
peanuts (dry roasted)	282

Juices

Green Light	Number of Residues
lemonade	10
pineapple (canned)	6

Other Green Light Juices	
apricot nectar	lime
carrot	mixed vegetable
cranberry	prune

Yellow Light	Number of Residues
apple (bottled)	71
grape (bottled)	49
grapefruit	42
tomato	35
orange	77

Other Yellow Light Juices	
boysenberry	

EATING WITH THE SEASONS

We live in a country where we can get any fruit or vegetable any time of the year. That's good news and bad news for us. It's good because it's a sign of abundance. It's not so good because in all that abundance, we have lost touch with what's in season, how foods change and shift from cold to warm weather. We eat strawberries at Christmas and beef stew in the summer and wonder why our bodies are uncomfortable in the weather of any particular season. Mother Nature has blessed us with the greatest variety of foods that are constantly changing, constantly providing us with new excitement, with the particular nutrients and level of moisture we need in any particular weather.

If we eat in season.

Fresh produce is at the heart of eating well . . . and the main reason you will decide that this is the life for you. The true glory of a plant-based diet comes from the freshest ingredients. Now hang on, I am not going all Alice Waters on you (although I love and respect her) and tell you that it's heirloom tomatoes or nothing. But think about it. When your ingredients are fresh and seasonal, your recipes are delicious.

Personally, I come alive when the farm markets in my community are in season. Winter is long and dreary for me once they close down. There is nothing like connecting with the person who grew my food and nothing at all like the flavor of vegetables and fruit freshly harvested or picked that morning. The produce at a farm market travels less distance and did not ripen under lights on a truck so the food is fresher, the flavors more authentic. They are kissed by fresh breezes, warm sunshine, gentle raindrops.

It's important to me that I buy locally as much as possible. When I buy locally produced foods, I know that less fossil fuel was burned to transport it; I can look into the eyes of the farmer who grew it and ask questions, like what, if any, pesticides are being used. I am supporting the rural economy of a small family farm. It's a win-win-win-win for me.

Never in modern history has there been such an interest in food and at the same time, such a lack of confidence in the basic quality of the food we are buying, which makes eating local more relevant to us. According to Paul Ray and Sherry Anderson, authors of *The Cultural Creatives,* a new way of thinking is springing up in America, a culture of relationships, community, social justice, and the belief that nature is sacred. These new "creatives" are more altruistic, less materialistic, and more spiritual and they are driving a new food culture with the focus on local food because of its many benefits.

Sustainable agriculture has grown from a chic chef phenomenon to a part of our everyday culture. Concern for the impact of commercial farming on the environment is no longer the province of hippies and elitists. It is growing into the accepted mainstream consciousness.

The benefits of eating locally produced food when you can are almost too numerous to mention, but here are my top reasons to go local as much as you can:

1. Eating local eliminates the middle man of distribution and can eliminate the wasteful spending on packaging and marketing that accounts for about 20 percent of food costs and drives prices through the roof.

2. Eating local saves fuel because food is not being transported so far before sale. The food is fresher and in season.

3. Eating local makes for improved food quality because the food is grown more sustainably, in smaller crops by family farms that can pay attention to how they grow and harvest. And fresher food is more flavorful and nutrient dense.

4. Eating local makes you want to cook. The food is so fresh and alive; the air at a farm market is perfumed with the aromas of fresh fruits and vegetables. It's completely inspiring. And fresh foods don't need a lot of fussy enhancement to be delicious.

5. Eating local makes food shopping more meaningful because we are getting great quality for our money. We are supporting local farms and we are not just accepting industrially produced foods like those sold in many supermarkets.

6. Eating local supports the local rural economy. By purchasing food from a local family farm, we ensure that they continue to exist and are not

swallowed up by commercial enterprises or developers. You get great food and help to save precious farmland.

7. Eating local helps us reconnect to our food by connecting with the people who produce it.

8. Eating local helps you play a part in restoring the quality of our food supply. A new, more sustainable system is thriving because farmers are working with their customers and producing food in a more traditional way. Caring for the land and the food becomes second nature. When we care for the farmers who care for the land that produces the food we eat, we thrive as a society. It's also important to me to buy organic produce as much as possible, as you have seen. I shop for local and organic first, and work my way down the list to commercially produced food when I have no other option.

Organic is more than just for the health of us and the planet. I have discovered in my own research that organic food is, in fact, more nutrient dense than commercially produced varieties. According to Organic Info, an online clearinghouse for all sorts of information on organic foods, organic produce contains 50 percent more vitamin C than commercially produced veggies and fruit. That's worth a few extra cents to me. And since the demand for organic produce has risen so dramatically, more farmers are growing it and the prices are becoming much more competitive. See? Your demand for better food yielded results.

However, circumstances and availability may drive the way you buy fresh fruit and vegetables. I am very blessed to live in a region where farm markets and CSAs are abundant, so in season, I have access to the most delicious food at the most delicious prices . . . you will never see produce more reasonably priced than at a farm market . . . organic or not. Not everyone enjoys such abundance, so listen . . . and I mean this. Wherever it is that you must buy your vegetables, whether it's a farm stand, a CSA, a supermarket, or a corner bodega; whether those veggies are organic, local, or commercially produced . . . buy and eat fresh veggies.

In the end, armed with information, you can make the best choices for your health. With marketing and subsidies, corruption and greed, special interests and bottom lines, we must do the best we can. We can make informed choices, eschewing products we know do not serve our health, and demand better from the people growing, producing, and manufacturing the food we eat.

So, here's a little primer on eating what's freshest at any time of the year. Want to learn to love your veggies? Eat them in season and you will see the difference.

Spring

During those first warm days of spring, is there anything better than letting the sun kiss your skin as you munch on freshly picked strawberries? Spring is that time of year when we trade sweaters for sundresses and T-shirts; boots get packed away and the sandals free our feet to be caressed by warm breezes. We walk around with silly smiles on our faces, drunk with the new life that surrounds us. At first, I want to just bask in the newly rediscovered warmth of the days, but soon enough, my thoughts turn to the foods of the season and my excitement takes on new depths.

The delicacy of spring foods lends a sweetness to the cuisine that is unmatched at any other time of year. The sheer nature of the foods themselves gives all your meals an air of romance and fancy. Shyly blushing apricots, graceful asparagus, earthy mushrooms, the first tender leaves of herbs, and delicate bitter greens like arugula and dandelion wake us from our winter slumber and freshen us for the warm weather. . . . And strawberries, whose gorgeous time is excruciatingly short, but when in their prime, still warm from the sun, have a tangy sweetness that screams, "It's spring!"

Fruits and vegetables, while largely available to us all year are at their peak of flavor and nutrient density when they are in season. Chinese medicine holds that various organ functions and emotions are governed by various seasons and nourished by the foods of that season. In the spring, we say that our livers and gall bladders require some refreshing after a long winter so we are comfortable in the warmer weather on the way. By eating the foods of spring during the spring, you provide your body with the nutrients it needs to feel refreshed for summer.

The stars of spring cooking and health are:

apricots	chives	rhubarb
arugula	dandelion	rosemary
asparagus	fennel	scallions
beets	leeks	spinach
broccoli	mushrooms	strawberries
carrots	new potatoes	Vidalia onions
cauliflower	parsley	

Summer

Now we're talking. Summer. It's my season. Sure, I love Christmas and all that goes along with the festivities; I love the delicacy of spring; I love the freshness of autumn and the crisp chill in the air. I love roasted squash and pumpkin pie. But give me a pair of strappy sandals and a sundress, corn on the cob and a fresh salad, and I am all set. Hot sun, fresh foods, light cooking, and time outdoors are all signatures of the season, and Mother Nature has provided us with the perfect foods to keep us as cool as . . . well, cucumbers.

I could spend hours picking berries and tomatoes. I love the moisture I get from summer squash. I love standing over a hot grill, veggie burgers and delicately seasoned veggies sizzling over the fire. Served with a crisp cold salad, lettuce and basil leaves fresh from my garden, and all is right in my world.

Eating the foods of hot summer ensure that our circulation stays stimulated, keeping our bodies cool and energized, because in Chinese medicine, we say that our hearts and circulatory systems are enlivened and vitalized at this time of year.

One caution: buy only organic corn, as most of our commercial corn has been genetically modified and is an environmental nightmare waiting to happen. Sorry to rain on your corn-on-the-cob parade, but reality is what it is, and I think we need to send a loud message to growers that we will not support and eat genetically modified corn.

Summer beauties include:

basil	garlic	peppers
blackberries	lettuce	plums

blueberries
cherries
collard greens
corn
cucumbers
figs
melons
mint
mustard greens
nectarines
peaches
radicchio
raspberries
tomatoes
yellow squash
zucchini

Autumn

The end of summer makes me sad, but I am consoled by the crisp, fresh air that tells us autumn has arrived. The farmers' market's bins of corn are replaced by barrels of apples, the air scented with their perfume.

As we move indoors after an active summer, we turn on the ovens and seek warmth and comfort as we face the long cold days of winter that we know are on the heels of this beautiful season. And Mother Nature is more than happy to accommodate us with her bountiful harvest of veggies and fruits just right to get us ready for winter.

The produce of fall is less moist, less cooling, and more inclined, through longer cooking and nutrient density, to keep us warm and cozy, comforted and sated. According to Chinese medicine, this is the time of year when we turn more inward and nourish the body with warmth for the cold days ahead. The sweet fruits and vegetables of the harvest help to balance and nourish the spleen, pancreas, and stomach, helping us to feel calm, centered, and warmer.

almonds
apples
butternut squash
cranberries
endive
escarole
figs
garlic
ginger
grapes
greens (kale, collards, bok choy)
mushrooms
onions
pears
pecans
persimmons
pumpkin
spinach
sweet potatoes
walnuts
watercress
winter squash

Winter

I love to bake. I don't even mind baking a batch of cookies on a hot summer Sunday afternoon. No kidding. I think baking opens the heart of a home and invites the love of the world inside. No one is in a bad mood when they smell chocolate chip cookies baking. Consternation is forgotten when the perfume of apple pie fills the air.

Winter cooking is a symphony of hearty soups, whole-grain pilafs, veggie and bean stews, hot casseroles that go steaming from oven to table, and pasta dishes smothered in hearty sauces. Vegetable dishes are simpler, as the fare is more limited. There are no fresh berries and tender lettuce leaves to freshen our meals, so we rely on heartier veggies that we cook in a variety of ways to keep our diets balanced and our bodies flexible.

According to Chinese medicine, winter is a time of dormant energy. We tend to stay indoors more, curled up on the couch under a cozy blanket. Our kidneys and bladder are influenced strongly in this season, so we cook and use foods in ways that keep the body warm and densely nourished with nutrients to keep our kidneys strong. When the kidneys are working well, we are not so chilled come those long winter days.

You will see some tropical choices in this list because they are really in season in the winter months. They serve to keep our cooking—and our energy—fresh with all the heavy foods we are eating for warmth.

banana	dates	pomegranates
cauliflower	dried fruit	raisins
citrus fruits	mushrooms	rutabaga
chocolate	hazelnuts	seeds
coconut	onions	spices
cranberries	parsnips	turnip

PRESERVING FRESHNESS

Moving through the seasons, eating the food of a particular time of year, is a delicious way to eat. There is nothing better than the flavor of something picked fresh and eaten immediately. Preserving food yourself, though, can be rewarding and delicious and a great way to keep your commitment to use the best-quality ingredients. When you preserve food, it's quite different from commercially preserved foods.

Sadly, that fresh-from-the-farm experience is not always available to us for whatever reason. Happily, we can work to preserve that experience in a natural way.

Yes, it's a wee bit of work, but the first time you crack open a can of tomatoes that you preserved in August for a marinara sauce on the coldest night in February, the scent of fresh basil and tomatoes fills you with memories of summer and you have hope that the sun will kiss your skin again. When you open a jar of fruit preserves that you made from local berries in season, it's heaven.

The most natural ways to preserve food at home are canning, freezing, and dehydrating. Various fruits and vegetables lend themselves to specific methods, but some of them can work in a variety of the methods. Natural forms of preserving food preserve the nutrients as well, so you win in all ways.

There are rules of thumb to follow, though, when it comes to preserving food. Delicate or young produce is best preserved through freezing. I take the last of my summer basil, lightly blanch and towel-dry it, and then freeze for use in the colder weather. (If you don't blanch the basil . . . or parsley or thyme or sage or oregano . . . before you freeze it, it will turn black. The light blanching preserves the color.)

Ripe, mature fruit and vegetables, like tomatoes, cucumbers, cauliflower, zucchini, yellow squash, peppers, peaches, apples, and pears, are best preserved by canning in mason jars. It's a bit of work, but so-o-o-o worth it when you enjoy the results.

Drying foods is a method I use mostly for fruit, so that I know what's in my food and there are no chemicals or sugar added. I also dry mushrooms and tomatoes for the same reason. I am not much for drying foods, but there are occasions where it works great for a recipe, so I do a little bit of it each season.

Fresh or preserved by you, local, seasonal, organic food is the key to health and wellness.

7

The Chemistry of Food and How It Affects You

ACID AND ALKALINE BALANCE

I was having a cup of green tea with chef Chris Koch, who manages the back-stage cooking for my television show and is a great chef in his own right. We were talking about his own journey back to health through changing his food. Over the years I have known him, he has gone from rolling his eyes at my "weird" ideas to almost completely vegan in his own cooking. He has lost thirty-eight pounds and looks ten years younger than when I met him fifteen years ago.

I asked him what connected the dots for him, and he said that when he discovered and understood the acid/alkaline balance in the body, everything he had heard me say over the years made sense. It made me think.

This will get a little Mr. Wizard-ish, but understanding acid and alkaline balance and the role food plays will change the way you think about the food you choose . . . just like it did for Chris. So stay with me. And then we'll cook; I promise. See, if you understand the physical impact of your choices and how those choices are literally blocking your body from health, I think you'll connect the dots for yourself and go for it.

We hear a lot of statistics, but have you ever wondered if (and how) most of the common diseases raging through modern society have a common cause? Many experts in the field of alternative health think this can be explained in two words: pH imbalance.

As babies, we are full of alkaline reserves and our metabolism moves along smoothly. When we die, we rapidly turn to acidic waste.

Understanding pH is easy. Finding balance in our modern world, well, not so much. The symbol pH, or "potential of hydrogen," stands the amount of acidity or alkalinity of any solution. A pH of 7.0 is completely neutral; 0–7.0 indicates acidity; 7.0–14.0 indicates alkalinity. A pH of 7.4 is considered most healthy and the goal number we should seek.

The human body struggles to maintain a healthy pH balance. Why? The natural by-product of cellular energy production and the utilization of nutrients within the cells is acidic by nature. So there must be sufficient buffering or neutralizing effects to keep the body from becoming too acidic.

Water, the most abundant compound in the human body, composes 70 percent of what we are. Our pH is a balance between positively charged ions (acid-forming) and negatively charged ions (alkaline-forming). Our body continually strives for a balance between these two forces, and when this delicate balance is compromised, problems begin.

An overly acidic condition, meaning a pH balance below 7.0, is a dangerous condition that can weaken the body and compromise all of our systems' functions. A continued acidic condition gives rise to creating an internal environment that is perfect for the growth of disease. A balanced pH environment allows for normal body functions necessary for the body to stay strong and resist disease.

A healthy body maintains adequate alkaline reserves to handle any emergency that might arise, but excess acids must be neutralized by those stores, and if the acidity continues, the body is weakened and becomes a great host for disease. Experts say that if an acidic condition is left unchecked, an imbalanced pH can interrupt all cellular activities and organ functions, from the beating of your heart to the neuron firings of your brain.

Not a new concept, and experts have been examining and studying the acid/alkaline balance for decades. But lately, it has been getting more attention because of the role it plays in weight loss. A habitually acidic pH contributes to weight gain by triggering a condition called "insulin sensitivity," which causes erratic production of insulin. See, when the body is flooded with insulin, it converts every calorie it can into fat. So the more insulin we produce, the more fat we store. This increased pressure to produce more insulin literally burns out the beta cells that cannot then function so well. As the body floods with insulin on a continual basis, our body converts calories to fat to store for the impending famine it thinks is coming. So unless you balance your pH, your attempts at dieting will be thwarted by your own body's response to starvation, the result of a chronically acidic condition.

You may be wondering what this has to do with why you should ditch junk food and adopt a diet rich in plant foods. Most pH imbalances are to the acidic side of the scale, causing the body to "borrow" minerals from organs and bones to neutralize, buffer, and remove the acid; minerals like calcium, sodium, potassium, and magnesium. This continued strain results in conditions such as:

- Cardiovascular damage like constricted blood vessels and the reduction of oxygen

- Weight gain and obesity

- Bladder and kidney conditions, including kidney stones

- Immune deficiency

- Acceleration of free-radical damage, including cancer cell growth

- Hormonal imbalances

- Premature aging

- Osteoporosis

- Joint pain, aching muscles, lactic acid buildup (not from exercise)

- Low energy/chronic fatigue

- Sluggish digestion/elimination

- Yeast overgrowth

Still think pH balance has nothing to do with you?

So what throws our pH off? Bet by now you have guessed that our diets play a key role. The more junk you eat, the more chronically acidic your pH, the sicker and heavier you get.

Every single processed food you eat contributes to your pH being off-kilter. Our typical modern diet, rich in meat, poultry, eggs, and dairy foods, is a big contributor, but junk food takes the prize as the main cause of acidosis. White flour and sugar, soda, caffeine, chemicals (both pharmaceutical and as additives in our food), and artificial sweeteners are all acid-forming and play a major role in throwing our pH into chaos.

There are several ways to test your pH to see whether or not you are in balance, from saliva to urine, but in the end, your dietary choices can ensure that your pH stays slightly alkaline, keeping you robustly healthy.

Check out this sampling of typical foods to see where they fall on the pH scale. This will help you to make choices that support your health as well as show you what needs to be eliminated.

SWEETENERS
Most alkaline: stevia
Alkaline: maple syrup, rice syrup
Least alkaline: raw honey, raw sugar

Least acidic: processed honey, molasses
Acidic: white sugar, brown sugar
Most acidic: NutraSweet, Equal, Splenda, Sweet'N Low

FRUIT
Most alkaline: lemon, watermelon, lime, grapefruit, mango, papaya
Alkaline: dates, figs, melons, grapes, kiwifruit, berries, pears, apples, raisins
Least alkaline: oranges, bananas, cherries, pineapple, peaches, avocados

Least acidic: plums, processed fruit juice
Acidic: sour cherries, rhubarb
Most acidic: cranberries, prunes

VEGETABLES AND BEANS

Most alkaline: asparagus, onion, parsley, raw spinach, broccoli, cauliflower, garlic

Alkaline: okra, squash, green beans, beets, celery, lettuce, zucchini, sweet potato, eggplant

Least alkaline: carrots, fresh tomatoes, corn, mushrooms, cabbage, peas, potato skins, olives, soybeans, tofu

Least acidic: cooked spinach, kidney beans

Acidic: potatoes without skin, pinto beans, navy beans, lima beans

Most acidic: chocolate

NUTS/SEEDS

Most alkaline: none

Alkaline: almonds

Least alkaline: chestnuts

Least acidic: pumpkin seeds, sunflower seeds

Acidic: pecans, cashews

Most acidic: peanuts, walnuts

WHOLE GRAINS

Most alkaline: none

Alkaline: none

Least alkaline: amaranth, wild rice, quinoa, millet

Least acidic: sprouted wheat bread, spelt, brown rice

Acidic: white rice, buckwheat, oats, rye

Most acidic: white flour, pastry, pasta, packaged cereals

MEATS

Most alkaline: none

Alkaline: none

Least alkaline: none

Least acidic: venison, cold-water fish
Acidic: turkey, chicken, lamb
Most acidic: beef, pork, shellfish

EGGS/DAIRY
Most alkaline: none
Alkaline: breast milk
Least alkaline: soy milk, goat cheese, goat milk, whey

Least acidic: eggs, butter, yogurt, buttermilk, cottage cheese
Acidic: raw milk
Most acidic: homogenized milk, ice cream

BEVERAGES
Most alkaline: herbal teas, water
Alkaline: green tea
Least alkaline: ginger tea

Least acidic: commercial tea
Acidic: coffee
Most acidic: alcohol, beer, soda

It's important to note that the placement of foods in categories has noth-ing to do with the actual pH of the food, but rather with its tendency to cre-ate an acid or alkaline condition in the body. For example, lemons are highly acidic by nature, but after digestion and assimilation, they are quite alkaline. Meat will test as most alkaline (like us), but after digestion, it leaves a very acidic residue in the intestines, making it acid-forming.

In general, foods are categorized as acid or alkaline based on the residue they leave in the body after digestion. Most animal foods, for example, tend to be more acidic, while cooked vegetables tend to be more alkaline than raw. Most experts in holistic medicine believe that Western diets are generally too acidic because of too many processed foods with too few veggies and fruits to make balance. We keep piling acid on top of acid and wondering why we are acidic.

Many of us live in an acidic state most of the time. When we metabolize foods, acids are produced. Our body keeps balance and control by eliminating excess acids through the lungs, kidneys, intestines, and skin. However, a constant and consistent bombardment of our body with acid-forming foods will overwhelm the body and leave you with fatigue, headaches, colds, allergies, and malaise. Do you think it's a coincidence that people with migraines are advised to eliminate acid-forming foods like white sugar, caffeine, and chocolate from their diets? This dysfunction of the body is a sign that it's trying to balance this chaotic state.

If you are eating a diet rich in animal protein and processed foods, you can rest assured you are living in a more acidic pH state than is healthy. While some acid-producing foods are necessary to keep the pH balance in line, it's good advice to eat more alkaline-type foods, with acid-producing foods eaten at a much lower percentage of your diet. A good rule of thumb is to consume 80 percent alkaline foods and 20 percent acid-producing foods for health.

The coolest thing about this very science-y concept is how easy it is to make it work for you. Simply stated, if foods are highly processed, from an animal, chemically enhanced, artificial, sugary, or take the form of a drug, then it's likely to be acid producing. If foods are natural, minimally or not processed, whole, high in fiber, nutrient-dense . . . and plant-based . . . live foods, you can rest easy that they are more alkaline.

Now does some of this make sense to you? Can you see what your modern diet is creating?

THE GLYCEMIC INDEX

Human hormones and metabolism have remained virtually unchanged over the last 100,000 years or so, much of which we spent as hunter-gatherers. Grains (and eventually their by-products) were not plentiful until the establishment of agriculture. With the advent of farming, human health actually declined, according to anthropological experts. Now hang on, don't panic.

Let me explain. Farming is such hard work and it allowed for populations to live in closer proximity to each other, so infectious disease spread more easily. Cultivation of crops also allowed for families to set down roots and space the births of their children more closely. Tribes had longer intervals in between children because they did not wean until the age of four or five when their teeth were ready to chew hard food. But with the advent of soft grain porridges, which did not require much chewing, children were weaned earlier and families grew in size. This changed the human situation in countless ways. Humans evolved and adapted to this way of life and eating and grew to thrive.

But while people have eaten grains for about a hundred centuries now, it wasn't until the last half-century that we began eating most of our grains in highly processed forms. And that's the point of this whole anatomy and anthropology lesson. The extent of the processing of our foods, in particular grains, is terrifying. Most prepared breakfast cereals, even those without added sugar, act exactly as sugar does in the body. As far as our bodies are concerned, there is no difference between a bowl of processed grain and a bowl of sugar. We are not equipped to handle this load of fast-acting carbohydrates, either. As we saw earlier, glucose is the gold standard of energy that we need to metabolize to keep our bodies and minds functioning optimally. Our brains are exquisitely dependent on a continuous supply of glucose, ensuring survival. And while too much of this good thing can cause tissue damage, as with diabetes, the body is designed to keep blood glucose levels within a tight range, and it does it against all odds. Never before has the body had to assimilate such heavy doses of simple, high-glycemic carbohydrates as it has in the last fifty years, since the advent of highly processed foods.

In an attempt to get a handle on the effects our modern, processed diet has had on health, in particular, diabetes, David Jenkins, professor of nutrition at the University of Toronto, tested various foods to determine which best served this rapidly growing epidemic. It was 1981 and the "glycemic index" was born. By ranking foods from 1 through 100, depending on how rapidly the body converted them to glucose, this work overturned some established theories about simple and complex carbohydrates and created a new set of standards. For instance, prior to glycemic-index rankings, a baked potato was considered a complex carbohydrate, but with its exorbitantly high rating of 85, it was quickly reclassified.

It works like this: high-glycemic foods dump large amounts of glucose suddenly and dramatically into the bloodstream, triggering the pancreas to secrete insulin, the hormone that allows glucose to enter the body's cells for metabolism (energy) or storage. When glucose levels in the blood spike, the pancreas overresponds and secretes lots of insulin. The foods that cause blood sugar to spike leave the gastrointestinal tract quickly, basically pulling the rug out from under you. With so much insulin circulating, blood sugar levels plummet, triggering a second wave of hormones, including stress hormones like epinephrine, since the body is now under stress with sugar levels all over the place and the brain unsure of its energy source. Sure, the sugar levels normalize but at a cost to the body.

And while you may think that cost is only diabetes (bad enough . . .), you would be wrong. Putting the body through consistent and constant physiological stress multiple times a day can double the risk of a heart attack. Double! So each candy bar, each white flour bagel, each donut increases your risk for a heart attack not only from the high concentration of sugar, but because of the literal stress you place on your poor heart with each ingestion of simple sugar.

And then there's hunger. When your pancreas overresponds and secretes a lot of insulin, and blood sugar levels drop like a rock, your brain thinks your body is starving because there's no sugar available. It doesn't recognize the fifty pounds of extra weight you tote around; it only knows you need sugar, so it sends you waddling to the fridge to get a quick sugar fix, like soda or fruit juice. Experts are beginning to think that each serving of sugar-sweetened drinks in particular multiplies the risk of obesity by as much as 1.6. Why beverages in particular? A meal has to go through your digestive tract, where the brain gets the satiety signals that slow down your consumption. When you drink, it's quick. You can slam back sixty-four ounces of Coke before you know what hits you, and the roller-coaster ride of blood sugar spikes and spins out of control. With this routine of extreme glucose-insulin cycles that characterize today's modern diet loaded with refined sugars and carbohydrates, our bodies are constantly buffeted by these insulin surges and glucose drops, creating a decreased response to insulin's signal to take in glucose, commonly known as insulin resistance. The cells slam their doors shut, figuratively speaking, leaving high levels of glucose circulating in the bloodstream, prompting the pancreas to secrete even more insulin to attempt to regulate sugar levels. This ongoing cycle sets the perfect stage for type II diabetes. How sweet do those soda, candy, and snack breaks sound now?

Robert Lustig, MD, professor of Clinical Pediatrics at the University of California at San Francisco, says that nutrition science made a wrong turn more than thirty years ago when it decided that the path to improving the collective health of Americans and reining in the rising tide of obesity was to encourage people to eat less fat and more carbohydrates. Ironically, this well-intended attempt to help Americans get healthier may have actually exacerbated the problem by encouraging more carbohydrate consumption. The junk-food-producing pirates at food conglomerates everywhere responded by creating product after product that was reduced-fat, low-fat, or no-fat, but loaded with sugar and other refined carbohydrates to feed this need to indulge without guilt.

A quick look around any airport, mall, amusement park, or movie theater will show you the results of this direction. In 2008, only one state out of fifty showed less than 20 percent of its population as obese or overweight. One state! And for the first time, we saw six states showing more than 30 percent of its populations as overweight or obese. In 2009, not one state qualified as healthy, meaning that 15 percent or less of the population was overweight.

That's how well the whole low-fat, no-fat thing worked (she said, her voice dripping with sarcasm). They took out the fat, loaded products up with simple sugars, refined carbohydrates, artificial flavors, and colors (since all these low-fat products lacked the taste that comes with . . . fat). They overloaded our livers with fructose and other sugars, disrupting metabolism and expanding our waistlines, which continue to grow unchecked.

Yikes!

8

Your First Steps

You are now armed with information about what's really going on with our food. The problem is that information can do one of two things: inspire you to make changes and become healthier or paralyze you because you do not know where to begin. Even armed with all your new knowledge, it can be daunting to change so radically in our society of fast and processed foods.

Well, to ensure that your response to reading this book is the former, let me help guide you on your first steps so the transition is smooth and painless . . . and delicious. Consider it your blueprint for success.

WHO'S CHANGING?

Even the most committed and inspired of us need a little help from our friends, as the saying goes. So as you begin the process of change, I think it's important to have support so that you stay motivated until living and eating well and naturally is your new habit.

When I began my own journey, I met my husband, who had been eating a macrobiotic diet for many years. He served as my coach and cheerleader as I made my way down that then-unfamiliar path to natural health. He likes to say that the only person you can change is yourself, and he's right in a lot of ways. You can influence others, as he did me, especially by example, but in the end you can only change what you are doing and take others along for the ride.

You have to begin somewhere. Take a look at how you and your family are eating now. Breaking unhealthy habits and replacing them with healthy ones can be challenging, and incorporating new ones a bit daunting at best.

My advice is to remember that you did not develop unhealthy eating habits overnight and you won't break them overnight either. Becoming the Gestapo of food in your house won't win you fans or make converts of your husband (or wife or partner) and kids. Gradual change, with consistently achieved goals, will result in change you love and can all embrace.

If you have read this far, you know the consequences of not changing your food, but it's important not to lecture your loved ones or they will run for the hills every time they see you walk to the kitchen. Instead, let them know that the new foods you will be trying will be a sort of culinary adventure and one of the side benefits will be better health.

Involve your loved ones in the change. If they are invested in the idea, it will go easier. If your kids are athletic, encourage them to examine how they feel when they eat healthy foods. Was their athletic performance better? Did they have better endurance? If appearance is more their appeal, encourage them to try healthy options for a few weeks and see how their skin, hair, and weight look after just a few weeks of eating well. You know their hot buttons more than anyone. Use them to encourage the change to begin. Once they are onboard, it will be a breeze.

Yes, there will be the one in the household who digs in his or her heels and will not, no matter what you say, do, or try, will not come along on the change easily.

Debbie, a mother of four and a student and friend of mine, told me how her family worked to change together. Diagnosed with breast cancer, Debbie had quite the impetus to change . . . and did, with the full support of her husband. With a combination of diet and surgery, Debbie survived her battle with cancer and is enjoying robust health today.

She wanted her whole family to change to healthier ways so they could have a chance at avoiding disease, if possible. Her husband was already onboard, had lost weight, and felt great. Her teenage daughter loved how her skin and hair looked and never even thought about her weight anymore; she loved the food and was sold. Her teenage son, an athlete, with his mother's encouragement, decided to see how his performance was affected by the food he ate. His sport was everything to him. He discovered that he was stronger and had more stamina when he ate well. Another one sold.

Her little ones were a bit more challenging. Her youngest liked cooking and being with Debbie in the kitchen. When she began studying cooking with me, he wanted to know who I was, so Debbie pulled out one of my cookbooks so he could relate. He wanted to make a recipe from the book right away. He loved it and now loves eating healthy foods.

But her third child said he did not and would not eat vegetables. Debbie tried everything, but when he saw her cooking with his young brother, he began to allow her to put some vegetables on his dinner plate. Then he tried small bites. She began to notice that he would stand at the kitchen door and cautiously watch as she cooked with his brother. In a matter of time, with her continued gentle encouragement, he joined in, and now the whole family enjoys healthy foods.

It can be done. You just have to commit, be gentle, and make it a fun adventure.

WHERE DO I BEGIN?

The question I am most often asked is: "If you could give people one piece of advice to begin to make the change to healthier eating, what would it be?" Here you go . . . wait for it . . .

Eat vegetables.

It's that simple really. Eat vegetables. They change everything about your health.

Seriously, you can do a web search of "health benefits of eating vegetables" and come up with 1,240,000 results with articles. None of them are bad news. None of them tell you to eat fewer veggies.

So whether you like it or not, eating your veggies is the key . . . and the good news is they will change your life.

Eating vegetables is the easiest way to change a poor diet into a healthier one. Adding freshly prepared veggies to your current diet of fast food will improve that diet.

According to the CDC, very few of us eat the vegetables and fruit we need to live healthy lives. In fact, only 27 percent of Americans are eating vegetables more than twice a day, with the obese among us eating the least, with fewer than 10 percent eating what we really need for health (five to nine servings a day, or about four and half cups). Twenty-five percent of Americans eat only one serving of vegetables each day, and of them, 40 percent eat only potatoes. Ay, ay, ay . . .

Vegetables contain essential vitamins, minerals, and fiber that can help protect you from chronic disease. The CDC goes on to say that people who eat sufficient amounts of vegetables and fruit during their day are more likely to have a reduced risk of the lifestyle diseases that plague us.

According to the Harvard School of Public Health, it's impossible to argue with a diet rich in veggies and fruit . . . lower blood pressure, reduced risk of heart disease and stroke, type 2 diabetes, obesity, and some cancers. They also have a mellowing effect on blood sugar and can keep us sated longer.

It's old news, but we need to start listening . . . seriously.

Going for nine servings a day isn't as hard as it sounds. It's less than five cups and there are so many veggies to choose from, you will find yourself meeting the goal easily and deliciously without breaking a sweat (although you should get to the gym at some point in the day to break an actual sweat).

Just try these simple tips to get you going. Before you know it, you'll be making healthy choices, munching away on delicious veggies and fruits without thinking much about it.

1. Keep fruit out where you can see it. Keeping a bowl of fresh fruit where you can see it will increase the chances of your making it a choice when you are looking for a snack. Keep the Snickers Bars out of sight, please . . . out of reach, too, in my view.

2. Make vegetables part of every meal, every day. Fill half your plate with vegetables at each meal. Fresh, crisp salads, stir-fried vegetables, roasted vegetables, vegetable stews and soups: a plate half-filled with brightly col-

ored antioxidant-rich fare will make it so easy to reach this goal . . . deliciously.

3. Be adventurous. Variety is the key to getting all the nutrients you need from your veggies. Each one has its own unique balance of essential nutrients. So each week, explore the produce section and try something new. What's the worst thing that can happen? You won't like something, but it's more likely, you will open your palate to a new world of tastes and textures.

4. Bag potatoes. Seriously. There are so many veggies to choose from, and while I know you love your spuds, they are among the least nutrient-dense of all the choices you have available to you. And I am not saying to give up potatoes entirely, I am saying that there's more to life, if you get my drift.

5. Make a meal out of your veggies. As you make the transition to healthier eating, try creating one meal a week where fresh veggies take center stage. And then pay attention to how you feel the next day. Soon, you'll be wondering why it took you so long to give up meat, dairy, poultry, and junk food. You will love all the delicious ways to prepare vegetables . . . and your body will love you for eating them.

Once you're on the bandwagon of veggies and have revamped your pantry, you're well on your way to never hitting the drive-through window in desperation again.

SMALL CHANGES, BIG RESULTS

As you munch your veggies, try these strategies. You'll love how easy they make your transition to a healthy lifestyle and how well they work.

1. Each week, as you add a new veggie or other healthy food to your diet, take away one food that you know isn't serving your health. It will create consistent change, a constant stream of inspiration, and new foods to

experience, and in just a few months, your transition to healthy eating will be complete.

2. Don't eat "white" foods at dinner (and then work to move them out of the rest of your life, too). White foods include: white flour, white sugar, white rice, white pasta, white bread, etc. The only "white" foods to consider? Tofu and daikon.

3. Drink a glass of water before you snack. This will tell you if you are really hungry or just thirsty, which is often the case. Have a drink and then give yourself a couple of minutes. If you're still hungry, then have your snack. Chances are you'll find you are actually hungry a lot less than you think.

4. Never eat in front of the television. Seriously, it's tempting, but it makes you completely mindless about what you are eating because you're involved in what you're watching. Next thing you know, you look down and the bowl, bag, or platter is empty.

You can also come up with your own mind tricks. Dennis, a father of two, who works at home and does all the cooking for the family, has his own strategies for cutting back on junk. He has switched up from potato chips to baked multigrain chips and only allows himself that indulgence if he has worked out hard at the gym that day. If french fries call his name, he throws half of them away before he even starts eating, so he's not tempted to polish them off.

You don't need to be a rocket scientist to change the way you eat; to change from the standard American junk-food fare that is robbing us of our future. You just have to understand what our modern diet is doing to our bodies. Once you know, you can't un-know it, and change will come and come easily.

HELP ME MAKE IT THROUGH THE NIGHT (AND THE DAYS TO COME)

There are tips and tricks to get you through the transition. They will help you over the hump until your body begins to recognize its nature, read its signals, and feel authentically human.

1. Add high-fiber foods to your daily diet to keep you full longer.

2. Ensure that you get an appropriate balance of protein, fat, and carbohydrates in your diet so you are sated more easily. This is a big one. When I changed my way of eating so many years ago, I was plagued by sweet cravings. Apple pies chased me down the turnpike in my dreams! My trainer told me that when I found the appropriate balance of fat, protein, and carbohydrates for me and my activity, the cravings would end. I played and tweaked my diet until I found the right balance for me. And while I still love dessert, I am no longer enslaved to it.

3. Chew well so your body can digest efficiently. Chewing also helps you eat slowly. Remember that it takes twenty minutes for your body to recognize that it's full (usually in that time, we have had four helpings, washed the dishes, and are back in front of CNN).

In the end, though, the experts all agree. It's a change in mindset that will get you where you want to go. We can read all the studies published; we can buy books, surf websites, and listen to lectures by people we respect. But if we do not change how we look at food; if we do not change the purpose of food in our lives; if we do not put our health before indulgence, we are lost.

It comes back to mindfulness. It comes back to choosing for life instead of choosing for a few seconds of mindless pleasure. As you shift your food choices and your thinking, you will begin to feel a vitality, an "aliveness" that cannot be described. It must be experienced.

So before you set this book aside and say, "She's nice, but she's nuts," think about how you think. Consider how you have been duped, dulled, and manipulated by the food industry. Think about how weak, tired, and lethargic you feel most of the time.

PART FOUR

Health Care Begins in the Kitchen

I t's easy to see how we got into the mess we're in once you trace a bit of our food history. It's time to break the cycle and change the way we think about feeding ourselves.

Society seems to be of the belief—a belief that food marketers foster—that there is simply no time to cook in our modern world. We all lead such busy lives and have such important extracurricular activities that we just can't seem to find our way to the kitchen. We're told by the good people at Lean Cuisine that slicing and dicing ingredients for a fresh dinner is anything but relaxing. So just pop one of their frozen entrees into the microwave, and it will taste just as fresh without the work. After all, their veggies are "farm picked."

What nonsense! Perhaps you don't like cooking. Maybe you'd rather watch television, garden, go for a run, chill out in between jobs. I don't know. I'm not even sure I care what you would rather be doing. Just don't delude yourself. We all have the same twenty-four hours in a day. We choose how we spend them.

I don't think I have ever heard anyone say "I was so busy today that I forgot to shower and brush my teeth." We wouldn't consider blowing off something so essential to our lives, would we?

But we'll blow off cooking and eating well, the very foundation of our health.

And the food industry has made it s-o-o-o-o-o-o-o easy to do just that. Just because a meal can be ready in just three minutes instead of seven doesn't mean it will satisfy us.

Look, I don't want to sit in judgment of anyone. If your life is happy as it is, with your frozen dinners and fast-food breakfast sandwiches, then bully for you. I can only ask you to take a private, personal inventory and just between you and . . . you, are you happy with how you feel? Could you feel better? Are you willing to do what it takes? Are you sick and tired of feeling sick and tired?

Since food became an industry, business has been selling us on the idea that our meals have to be ready faster, with less mess and even less work. We are bombarded with quick, easy meal ideas in magazines and newspapers and on cooking shows. Rachael Ray has built an empire on meals ready in thirty minutes or less made from a myriad of packaged pre-prepped products with a few fresh ingredients thrown in.

The question to ask is simple. Are we happier, healthier, or more satisfied as a result? Do we have more time to do whatever it is we do, since we are not cooking? What are we in such a hurry to do that we can't enjoy the process of cooking and eating?

What has been lost in the process of selling us on fast meals? Our health; our love of food. We believe that we are a food culture because we are obsessed with food and chefs. We have entire networks devoted to food. We have magazines, newspapers, websites, and blogs all dedicated to food. But in truth, America is an eating culture. A food culture cares about quality, flavor, the process of getting the food on the table, and the purely sexy joy of that process. An eating culture . . . well, it just consumes. It's like our society has become that old joke about the "see food" diet . . . we see food and we eat it.

This cultural problem sends an awful message. It tells us that fresh, natural meals prepared and enjoyed at home are not worth the work. And the chefs that help promote this fast-and-easy, slick-as-a-Persian-bazaar style of cooking are walking advertisements for the processed food industry.

Wholesome, natural, and delicious is the answer. I am not asking that you spend three hours a day at the stove; grind your own flour; bake your own bread, as nice as that is. I am saying to take an hour of your day and cook a meal. I am suggesting that your life will change if you do.

Make the time to sit and eat together with your loved ones (or alone . . . you are worth it). Quick-and-easy won't get you anywhere. Quick-and-easy will leave you frustrated because you will always want for more. Quick-and-easy will make you feel like a failure whose health and loved ones are an afterthought.

I know for a fact that spending time in the kitchen each day preparing food is one of the most beautiful, fulfilling, satisfying, and nourishing things in life . . . period. It's what makes us human at the most primal level. It will make you happy in ways that are deep, rooted in life, and good for you.

If you want to make the most of your health and your life, you simply must, must, must return to the basics of healthy food choices and cooking. In the end, try as they might, industry lobbyists, slick salesmen, and glossy ads cannot force you to buy the poison they sell. That choice is yours.

9

The Cook's Brain

If you're like most people I know, when you finished reading the text part of this book, you thought "now what?" Every time I read a book by experts like Michael Pollan or Marion Nestle, I am left with the same question.

Welcome to "now what?" Change begins with our choices; how we move through the world; the footprint we leave; the products we consume. But nothing, nothing will create as dramatic a change as what we choose to eat and drink.

And while I am not asking you to bake bread from scratch (lovely though it is . . .) or grow your own food (you should learn how, though; it could be necessary in the coming times . . .), I am asking you to cook. Simple, elegant, natural foods that will nourish the body, mind, and spirit. Food that will become the catalyst for real change in your life.

See, I think we have lost our way when it comes to food. People are so confused. Each day we hear statistics that are scarier than anything that Stephen King could imagine. So now we're not only confused, we're scared witless! So we do nothing; change nothing, and robust health eludes us. I hear it all the time; people are literally paralyzed with fear and confusion, so they do nothing.

Well, what if I told you that it's simple, delicious, and totally relaxing to eat foods that will nourish your body and soul, help you achieve your ideal weight, live peacefully and compassionately, and slip right past all the obstacles that keep you from making healthy choices? Yeah, right, you say?

It begins in the kitchen. You need to learn to cook. And while cooking classes are fun, entertaining, and helpful and cookbooks are thrilling, fun, and gorgeous, you can cook without any of it. You just have to understand what you are doing. You have to discover the "how" in how to cook.

It all starts with your brain. Positive thinking can change everything for you, but it is not so easy to achieve and maintain. We live in a culture that sets us up for failure and cashes in on our insecurities. Every television ad we see is telling us that we are losers, but if we buy their pills, perfume, lotion, burger, drink, mouthwash, clothes, or car, we will be sane, sexy, smart, funny, healthy, fit, and thin. These messages reinforce the notion that we cannot be whole, complete humans without the stuff they are selling.

I'm suggesting we use that kind of thinking to gain confidence to dust off the pots and pans and get back to the kitchen, back to nourishing our bodies with food that serves the purpose of our lives.

But change is hard, especially when it comes to breaking a lifetime of bad habits.

Habits form in the brain. (I told you . . .) When we do something repetitively, our brains and bodies go into autopilot, functioning without much thought. Mindless eating and unconscious living means we eat too much—and too much of all the wrong things—exercise too little, depend on pharmaceuticals to keep us up and keep us down. We get into a rut. Our life becomes routine, replete with habits that are not contributing to our health and wellness, so we have to give ourselves a good shaking up or we'll continue in this downward spiral that is typical of our culture of indulgence and convenience that is eating us alive.

Letting old habits fade and new ones take their place starts with developing a positive vision of the outcome you want. If you think that you can't do something, then you probably can't do it.

I remember something very valuable that a swim coach said to me when we were training hard and doing fast-interval drills. He said, "Stop telling yourself that you can't do this."

To move forward, you must ask yourself what your life will be like as you change. How will your life be enhanced? Your mind is a powerful tool. Use it to your advantage.

New habits, healthy habits can be created by reprogramming yourself and taking your brain off autopilot. The key to lasting weight loss and health is to simply reinforce a new practice. But here is the cool thing: Whatever actions you take—and repeat—will become automatic in a mere twenty-one days. Just as your present lifestyle may be killing you now, it can quickly be turned around to become your source of strength, health, and fitness.

If you have never cooked before, it can be a daunting idea. You are heading into unfamiliar territory, like a ninety-nine-pound weakling, walking through a sea of muscles and tattoos for his first gym workout. But, with understanding and some basic skills, in a few short sessions in the kitchen, you will be whipping up meals as though you have been cooking all your life.

10

Stocking a Healthy Kitchen

When I changed how I ate more than twenty-five years ago, I was on the clock, so to speak. I had been diagnosed with cancer and given only months to live. If I was going to affect my condition with my food choices and regain my health, I had to change and change completely . . . fast.

I cleaned out my cupboards, donating all my processed and gourmet foods to a local food shelter. I restocked completely with whole grains, beans, and condiments needed for my health. I was miserable, food-wise. It was unfamiliar and overwhelming. I didn't know where to begin; how to progress; how to move forward. I felt paralyzed. I hated the food. I never looked forward to a meal. I missed my frozen Snickers Bars (I kept a bunch of these candy bars in my freezer at all times), pizza, and Tab.

I knew I had to make this change, but I was lost in a sea of doubt and fear . . . and flat-tasting food.

It took about thirty days of cooking, struggling, and praying for strength before I discovered how delicious natural foods can be. It was like a veil being lifted off my eyes. But it was hard. I was a complete and total slave to sugar, fat, and salt. The most challenging thing in my life was giving up my devotion to sugar. I was an addict; there is no way to clean it up. I could go no more than an hour or two without a "fix." For that first month, when I first made the change in my diet, I wanted to slap every person I saw enjoying something sweet.

Now, I admit I had incentive. My choices were sugar or death. It made the commitment a bit easier emotionally, but not physically. The withdrawal symptoms were not unlike withdrawing from drugs. I struggled and fought for my life every day those first few weeks.

But once I broke the stranglehold that processed food, in particular sugar, had on me, it was like life began. It wasn't until I changed that I could see how enslaved I was to sugar. It wasn't until I changed that I could see how awful I had been feeling and how my cancer did not come "from out of the blue."

Changing your cupboard is the best place to begin. It was the thing that made the difference for me. If the food in your pantry is designed for health, then you are more likely to use what's on hand and eat well. You need to do what I did. You need to make it completely inconvenient to eat poorly.

It's along the line of the thinking of the Dalai Lama when he said that people often find it difficult to do charity for charity's sake. So he advises them to do it for their own good karma, to plant karmic seeds for their own redemption. In time, they see charity for its own beauty and they do it because it's the right thing to do. He calls it "selfish charity," charity being done for one's own good, not the good of others. But it leads to true virtue.

You may not like the food at first, so eat well for other reasons: your daughter's wedding; your family's future; so you can play catch with your son; to avoid a heart attack; to fit into a little black dress for your high school reunion; to avoid cancer or diabetes. Choose a reason that will motivate you to eat well and will keep you motivated until your taste buds adjust and you discover the truly delicious nature of a diet of plant-based, whole, unprocessed foods. You surely won't change for the esoteric love of the planet or because I tell you parsnips are sweetly delicious. You are more likely to change your food if you think it can alter your future, help you avoid disease, or lose weight.

I do not care why you change, just that you do.

It's easy to get started on change. Let's look at the kinds of ingredients you might use every day as examples of ways to upgrade to healthier versions. We'll build from there.

For instance, if peanut butter is a staple in your home, read the label. If there are more ingredients (particularly ones you can't pronounce) than peanuts and maybe salt, then you are not eating peanut butter. Peanut butter doesn't need added oil, sugar, or artificial anything. And yes, before you even ask, natural peanut butter, made from peanuts and only peanuts, may cost you a bit more money, but it will satisfy your desire for peanut butter more easily (since it actually tastes like peanuts) and you'll eat less as a result. So it will last longer. It's real food. Remember that choosy mothers would not, in fact, ever choose Jif. Even their natural line has palm oil, sugar, salt, and molasses. Their traditional line of Jif contains fully hydrogenated oils, mono- and diglycerides, as well as sugar and salt. Choosy, indeed.

Look at each ingredient in your pantry and think about how you can improve the quality of it. Switch from white minute rice to whole grain brown rice (you can even find quick-cooking brown rice . . . not my choice, but if it gets you started, enjoy . . .). Change your pasta to a whole-grain-based pasta for a more robust taste that will stick to your ribs with less volume. Buy jams and jellies without added sugar. Look at the oils and vinegars you have been purchasing and upgrade them to the best quality you can afford.

The cost of cheap ingredients is high. Your food doesn't taste delicious or satisfying, so you eat more, looking for whatever it is you are missing. Food companies win again. You buy more and eat more, looking for taste. And you often do not get what you pay for. It's the old adage of being too good to be true. Why do you think Italians are so committed to the quality of the olive oil they use? Their food is simple, the food of peasants in most cases. The oil enhances the flavors of simple foods, turning any meal into a feast.

In any supermarket, you will find large bottles of "extra-virgin" olive oil for very low prices. Amazing, right? A steal! Is it? Research released by UC Davis in August 2010 showed that popular brands like Bertolli, Pompeian, Carapelli, and Mazola, to name a few, are not what they claim to be. Cut with cheaper and lesser-grade oils, these major brands have sold tons of cheap fat under the veil of extra-virgin olive oil, which we know provides high levels of healthful fats, antioxidants, and low acidity levels . . . all the components of a healthy oil. Problem is that what you are buying for that low price is just fat, just cheap oil.

And then there's salt. You might think the little girl with the umbrella over her shoulder is cute and nostalgic (and the price is right), but what's in the package will kill you. Table salt is at the root of all the trouble we associate with salt consumption: hypertension, high blood pressure, heart disease.

On the other hand, there's natural sea salt. Just look at how both salts are processed and it will be obvious which is better for human health.

Sea salt is made through evaporation of sea water, which leaves behind a natural salt, with sodium and chloride along with twenty-one essential and thirty accessory trace minerals. These additional minerals help balance the sodium and chloride and add subtle nuances of flavor to the salt. Natural sea salt allows moisture to move freely through cell membranes, helping to regulate water in our tissue, assist the absorption of intercellular fluid, and support the kidneys in their work.

Table salt is made by mining salt from underground salt deposits; it is heavily processed to *eliminate* those same trace minerals, leaving only sodium and chloride, and contains an additive, usually silicon dioxide, to prevent clumping. Sometimes iodine is added as well, with stabilizers like sugar. Often, refiners add aluminosilicate of sodium or yellow prussiate of soda as bleaches to achieve the white color we have come to know in salt. This type of salt can create a deficiency in essential minerals and an ion equilibrium imbalance in our cells, causing cell regeneration breakdown.

It's important to remember that salt is the oldest seasoning known to man. It is the single element required for the proper breakdown of plant carbohydrates into digestible human food. Only when salt is added to fruits and veggies can saliva and other gastric secretions break down the fibers so carbohydrates are useable by our bodies.

And last, but certainly not least, natural sea salt closely resembles the chemical makeup of human blood and body fluids . . . so much so that in World War II, navy doctors used seawater for blood transfusions when blood was in short supply, and many lives were saved.

From stabilizing irregular heartbeat to balancing blood pressure to natural antihistamine properties to preventing muscle cramps and aiding in the treatment of diabetes, natural sea salt does more than make our food taste great.

The little girl with the umbrella can't say as much.

Rooting out the processed products in your pantry and replacing them with healthy alternatives will begin the process of rethinking your food. Use of natural sea salt, exquisite olive oils, and other condiments will force you to rethink what you prepare and eat as you discover or rediscover the real flavors in food. It's the little changes that bring us to the big ones.

Looking at what we eat is a process, a journey to natural health and wellness, and everyone has their path. Change is hard, but change we must if we are to survive this modern life we live.

Here's what's in my pantry. I like to keep all my grains on one shelf so I can see them at a glance and all my beans on another. I keep them all sealed in one-quart canning jars so they are uniform and stack easily. My condiments are in their own section as are the dried herbs and other seasonings so I know what I have. Everything in my pantry is within reach and in my sightline. I am never running all over the kitchen with my arms filled with ingredients. It may look cute on a cooking show, but it ain't so much fun when you're trying to get dinner ready.

My fridge is organized, too, with ingredients arranged so I can easily see what I have and what needs replenishing. Make your pantry and fridge work for you. If they are a mess, disorganized with stuff all over the place, you will lose track of what you have, spend money needlessly, and waste food. I'm telling you this because I love you. Get organized.

CLEAN AND DECLUTTER THE KITCHEN

I happen to like symbolism and ritual. I think it conjures powerful images, so one of the things I always advise people to do when they are committing to change is clean. Yup, you heard me, clean. My experience has shown me that when people literally clean the kitchen, it's like creating a clean slate, a blank canvas. It makes you feel renewed. It helps you commit.

When I say clean the kitchen, I mean to clean the kitchen. Empty the cupboards and dust the shelves. Wash everything; scrub the counters and the floors. Get rid of anything you don't use that adds clutter and distracts you. Restock your cupboards with only those things you will use and that serve your new commitment to healthy eating.

Clean the countertops and create a workspace that is functional. Don't clutter them up with stuff like mail or unused gadgets. Create an organized space with only the utensils you use most often at your fingertips. Anything extraneous to cooking needs to have a new home . . . out of the way.

Add Life to the Kitchen

Next, I like to bring some life into the kitchen, with fresh flowers or potted plants . . . or potted herbs on the windowsill. This little act shows you that every single time you walk into the room that life is created and nourished in this room. I also like a bowl of fresh fruit on the counter to encourage healthy snacking.

DECLUTTER YOUR LIFE

With the kitchen cleaned, it's time to declutter your life so you can make the time to cook. So often I am asked how we are expected to find the time to cook in our busy days with all our obligations. Early on in my career, I started asking people to bring me their calendars, filled with their daily "to-dos," and I would help them reorganize their days to find the hour they need to prepare food that nourishes life. In all my years of asking for calendars, no one has brought me one schedule to look over and reorganize. Hmm . . .

Start slowly. Find your way back to the kitchen with small steps. I will guarantee that if you empty your cupboards of all the food that isn't serving your life and start cooking every meal from scratch without a plan to make it work, you will be back to your old ways in a couple of exhausting weeks, convinced that this is just too hard and not worth the work.

The first steps are small ones, but they will help you to feel better, and when you feel better, you will be inspired to do more and more until you are all in, as the saying goes.

The following list of ingredients comprises the basics of both dried and fresh items that are the must-haves you'll need in your pantry to successfully create meals of variety and balanced nutrition.

THE PANTRY

These are what I consider to be the basic staples of a well-stocked healthy pantry. These ingredients are easy to find and versatile, and with them on hand, you will never be at a loss to create a meal. Don't be daunted by the size of the list. You can stock your pantry gradually, but if your cupboard is bare, you won't exactly be able to pull together the meals of your dreams.

To make it even easier, I have placed an asterisk (*) by the most essential ingredients you need to have on hand. The balance of the list can be added as you build your repertoire and confidence.

Almonds: Fruit kernels of the almond tree. They keep best when purchased in their thin brown skins, which protect their freshness and flavor. Also available in their skinned, blanched form, slivered, minced, and ground into a flour for convenience of use. High in antioxidants and good-quality fats for health. I recommend using organic almonds when you can.

Almond milk: Almond milk is a milky drink made from ground almonds. Unlike animal milk, almond milk contains no cholesterol or lactose. It is low in calories, high in fiber and protein, and can be used in any recipe in place of milk. It's completely vegan, with a slightly nutty, sweet flavor. Read the labels carefully and be sure to buy unsweetened almond milk. Otherwise, you're just getting another sugary drink.

Amaranth: A very tiny, brownish-yellow seed, high in protein and lysine, similar to quinoa in flavor. Cooked as a whole-cereal grain, it has an earthy, nutty flavor and cooks quite quickly.

Arrowroot: A high-quality starch made from a tropical tuber of the same name, used for thickening much the same way cornstarch is used. Arrowroot has virtually no taste and becomes clear when cooked, making it ideal as a thickener for puddings, gravies, and sauces. Less expensive than kuzu, it can be used interchangeably in recipes.

Avocado oil: A monounsaturated oil made from pressing whole avocados. Perfect for sautéing, frying, baking, and other cooking. The mild, buttery flavor is perfect for just about any dish, and its stability under heat makes it an essential cooking oil. Its full-bodied texture and light taste give baked goods a moist crumb.

Baking powder: A leavening agent made up of baking soda, cream of tartar, and either cornstarch or arrowroot. Double-acting powder releases carbon dioxide on contact with liquid, creating the air pockets responsible for the light texture in baked goods. Always try to purchase non-aluminum baking powder so that sodium aluminum sulfate is not released into your foods, possibly compromising your health.

Baking powder is more perishable than you might think, not lasting much beyond the expiration date on the can. Store in a cool, dry place and purchase in small amounts for the best shelf life.

Baking soda: Sodium bicarbonate is a white powder used in making effervescent salts and beverages. With a slightly alkaline taste, it is often used in conjunction with baking powder in vegan baking to support leavening in cakes and quick breads.

Balsamic vinegar: Italian vinegar made from white Trebbiano grapes. The vinegar becomes a deep, rich amber color during aging in wooden barrels. The best balsamic vinegars are syrupy, thick, a bit sweet, and a little more expensive than other vinegars, but well worth it. Natural balsamic vinegar is rich in live bacteria and enzymes that aid in digestion.

Barley: Said to be the oldest cultivated grain, barley is native to Mesopotamia, where it was mainly used to make bread and ferment beer. In Europe, barley has been replaced by wheat and rye but is still the staple grain of many countries in the Far and Middle East, Asia, and South America. In modern cultures, barley serves to make everything from livestock feed to malted whiskey to tea to miso. However, by itself, barley is a great, low-fat grain, chockfull of nutrients, and is reputed to aid the body in breaking down fat.

Bay leaf: Also known as laurel leaf, this herb has a delicate aromatic flavor and is used in soups and stews, especially with beans and grains, since they contain compounds that help in the digestion of the fiber of these foods.

Black turtle beans: A sturdy, very satisfying common bean. Earthy and mildly sweet, these beans go well with stronger, spicier seasonings, like those commonly used in Brazilian, Caribbean, and Mexican dishes, and make great, creamy soups and spicy dips.

Brown rice vinegar: A vinegar traditionally made by the agricultural communities of Japan, it is composed of brown rice, cultured rice (*koji*), seed vinegar from the previous year, and well water. The vinegar is then fermented for nine to ten months. Brown rice vinegar has a sharp taste and is used for everything from salad dressings to preserving vegetables. It is also commonly used in sushi rice for flavor and for its preservative properties.

Cannellini beans: Creamy white oval beans most commonly used in the Italian dish pasta e fagioli. Their texture makes them ideal for purees, dips, and creamy soups. Studies show they can help lower cholesterol.

Capers: Little pickled flower buds, most commonly used in Mediterranean cooking. Salty and briny in taste, they really add flavor to sauces and salads. If they taste too strong for you, simply rinse lightly before use.

Chickpeas (garbanzo beans): Beige round beans with a wonderful nutty taste and creamy texture when cooked. Traditionally used when making hummus, a creamy spread combining chickpeas with olive oil, lemon juice, and a bit of garlic. Also wonderful in bean dishes combined with sweet vegetables as well as in soups and stews.

Chiles: Available fresh and dried, they range from mildly spicy to blazing hot. Remember that the real "heat" comes from the capsaicin in the seeds and spines, so removing them reduces the "fire." I recommend you wear rubber gloves when removing seeds so the oil, containing capsaicin, doesn't get on your hands—and then into your eyes when you rub them. It takes several hours, even with washing, to remove this oil. Anchos, chipotles, serranos, habaneros, poblanos, and jalapeños are the most common varieties used in cooking today.

Chile flakes: Dried, flaked chile peppers. Used in cooking, these flakes are quite hot, since the drying has spread the capsaicin throughout the pepper.

Chili powder: A powdered blend of ground chiles, ranging from mild to hot, often combined with oregano, cumin, garlic, and salt. Add it slowly to dishes, adjusting the spicy taste as you go along, as the hot taste increases as you cook it.

Chocolate: Dark chocolate has come into fashion as a healthful ingredient. Rich in antioxidants, iron, and magnesium, chocolate releases "feel good" hormones in the brain, creating a relaxed warm condition in the body. Calorically dense, chocolate is not an everyday staple, but dark chocolate can be a valuable addition to any healthy diet.

Corn: Native to South America, corn has been used for over ten thousand years. It has become the staple grain for the entire North American continent. Today, corn is cultivated worldwide and is one of the most popular grains used in cooking. I recommend organic fresh or frozen corn to avoid genetically modified varieties.

Corn requires hot summer sun and rain to flourish and grows quickly. Often eaten by itself, the popular corn on the cob has practically limitless other culinary uses—flour, meal, grits, tortillas, corn syrup, corn oil, bourbon, and popcorn (from one variety of the grain).

Corn grits: A cracked form of dried corn. Corn grits make a great polenta, creamy breakfast cereal, or texturizer for soups.

Cornmeal: Dried field corn ground into a coarse flour. Used to make creamier polentas, this flour is most commonly used in cornbreads, tortillas, and corn chips.

Couscous: A staple of North Africa, this rolled durum wheat product has been stripped of its bran and germ, made into a thick paste, steamed, and then dried in the form of small granules of pasta. It cooks quite quickly, and its starchy texture makes it a great ingredient for loaves, patties, and soups.

Daikon: A long, white radish root with a refreshingly clean, peppery taste. Commonly used in salads and side dishes, soups, and stews. Frequently served in Asian restaurants with fish or oily dishes, since it is reputed to aid in the digestion of fat and protein as well as to help the body to assimilate oil and cleanse organ tissue. Also available in dried, shredded form to be used in various stews and hearty vegetable dishes.

Garlic: A member of the allium family that also includes onions, leeks, chives, and green onions. Originating in southern Europe and used to flavor foods, garlic has a strong nature that lends itself to being used cooked or raw. Each head of garlic breaks into sixteen to eighteen bulbs and is used to flavor sauces, dressings, soups, stir-fry dishes, tapenades, or rubs. Do not keep garlic in the refrigerator, as it compromises the flavor.

Ginger: A golden-colored, spicy root vegetable with a variety of uses in cooking. It imparts a mild, peppery taste to cooking and is commonly used in stir-fries, sautés, sauces, and dressings. Shaped like the fingers of a hand, ginger has the reputation of stimulating circulation with its hot taste. It is a very popular remedy in Oriental medicine for helping with everything from joint pain to stomach aches and acid indigestion. Do not store it in the refrigerator, as this causes it to rot more easily.

Great Northern beans: Medium-size white beans, they hold their shape very well in cooking, making them ideal ingredients in bean salads as well as in heartier bean dishes that complement their subtle flavor.

Herbs: Simply defined, herbs are the leaves and stems of certain plants used in cooking because of their unique, aromatic flavors. Herbs not only add flavor but have been used for thousands of years for health and wellness. Available fresh or dried, herbs add rich, full-bodied taste to soups, stews, and salad dressings, among other things. When using fresh herbs, remember to use three to four times the amount of dried, as drying concentrates their natural flavor. Try to buy your herbs in their organic form, since you can be assured that these herbs are not irradiated, as most commercial brands are.

Hiziki (hijiki): Sold in its dry form, hiziki resembles black angel hair pasta. It is one of the strongest-tasting of all sea plants, so soaking it for several minutes before cooking can gentle its briny flavor. It is one of the richest sources of useable calcium in the plant kingdom with a whopping 1,350 milligrams of calcium per one-half cup uncooked hiziki, with no saturated fat. So it is worth getting used to. . . .

Kidney beans: Available in a variety of shapes and colors, kidney beans are most commonly recognized in their deep-red All-American shape. Full-flavored and hearty, kidney beans hold up incredibly well in chilies, stews, soups, salads, and casseroles. Their deep color indicates that they are rich sources of magnesium and potassium as well as other minerals.

Kombu (kelp): A sea vegetable packaged in wide, dark, dehydrated strips that will double in size upon soaking and cooking. Kombu is a great source of glutamic acid, a natural flavor enhancer, so adding a small piece to soups and stews deepens flavor. Kombu's glutamic acid also improves the digestibility of grains and beans when added to these foods in small amounts.

Lentils: An ancient legume that comes in many varieties, from common brown-green lentils to red lentils to yellow lentils to lentils *le puys* (a tiny sweet French variety that is great in salads). Very high in protein and minerals and with a full-bodied, peppery taste, lentils are good in everything from stews and soups to salads and side dishes. Studies show that eating lentils once a week can help reduce the risk of heart disease.

Millet: Native to Asia, millet is a tiny grain that once equaled barley as the chief staple of Europe. It was very popular in Japan before the cultivation of rice and is still the staple grain of China, India, and Ethiopia. An effective alkalizing agent, millet is the only whole grain that does not produce stomach acids, so it aids spleen and pancreas function as well as stomach upset. It is also the highest in protein of all whole grains.

Millet is very versatile, making delicious grain dishes, creamy soups, stews and porridges, stuffings and loaves. With its sweet, nutty taste and beautiful yellow color, millet complements most foods well, but goes best with sweet vegetables like squash and corn.

Mirin: A Japanese rice wine with a sweet taste and very low alcohol content. Made by fermenting sweet brown rice with water and koji (a cultured rice), mirin adds depth and dimension to sauces, glazes, and various other dishes and can be used as we would use sherry in cooking.

*Miso: A fermented soybean paste used traditionally to flavor soups but prized in the Orient for its ability to strengthen the digestive system. Traditionally aged miso is a great source of high-quality protein. Available in a wide variety of flavors and strengths, the most nutritious miso is made from barley and soybeans, and is aged for at least two years—this is the miso used most extensively in daily cooking. Other varieties of miso are used to supplement and to create different tastes in different dishes.

Miso is rich in digestive enzymes, but these enzymes are quite delicate and should not be boiled. Just lightly simmering miso activates and releases its strengthening qualities into food.

*Mustard: Mustard in a jar is made by blending dried mustard seeds with vinegar and various spices. The best-quality mustards are Dijon or those that have been stone ground; these are made from coarse seeds and have a rougher texture.

*Noodles: Pasta, macaroni, or noodles are made by combining flour, salt, and water into limitless shapes and sizes. Try to choose pastas made from organic flours, preferably whole-grain. These are made from the endosperm of the wheat and contain protein and carbohydrates as well as essential fiber, minerals, and B vitamins. However, even refined semolina pastas have a place in a whole-foods diet, lending light taste and texture when desired.

Nori (sea laver): Usually sold in paper-thin sheets, nori is a great source of protein and minerals like calcium and iron. Most well-known as a principal ingredient in sushi, nori has a mild, sweet flavor, just slightly reminiscent of the ocean. Great for garnishing grain and noodle dishes or floating in soup.

Nut butters: Thick pastes made from grinding nuts. While rich in fiber and protein, nut butters are also great sources of good-quality fat. Nut butters have intense, rich flavors and are great in sauces, dressings, and baked goods.

Nuts: Nuts are true powerhouses of energy. Bear in mind that, in most cases, nuts have the strength to grow entire trees, so imagine what impact they have on us, giving us great strength and vitality. They are wonderful in small amounts for taste and richness (they are calorically dense) and for a lift of energy. Choose from almonds, pecans, walnuts, hazelnuts, cashews, pistachios, or whatever you like.

Oats: Native to Central Europe and used since Neolithic times, oats are rich in B vitamins and contain one of the highest amounts of protein of any grain in addition to iron and calcium. Reputed to have a high fat content (which they do), oats contain soluble gums, which bind cholesterol in the intestines, preventing its absorption by the body, making it a heart-healthy grain.

Most commonly used in modern cultures as oatmeal, a process by which the oat groats are rolled or steel cut, oats are the most delicious when used in their whole state. I use oatmeal flakes mostly to cream soups and thicken sauces as well as in breads, cookies, and croquettes.

Olives: Olives are native to semitropical climates and are used in Mediterranean cooking to add an appealing punch to grain, vegetable, and bean salads. There are almost limitless varieties available, so you can satisfy your taste by choosing anything from the intensely flavored, oil-cured ripe olives, to purple Greek Kalamata olives, to green Spanish olives. Rich in monounsaturated fats and minerals, pantothenic acid and niacin, olives are a nutritious treat.

Olive oil: Obtained from pressing olives, olive oil is a monounsaturated fat used in cooking, salad dressings, and baking. With production in the Mediterranean, the Middle East, America, and other countries, there is a variety of quality and flavor profiles to enjoy.

Extra-virgin olive oil is the healthiest of olive oils, loaded with antioxidants. Extra-virgin means the oil was pressed with no chemicals added and has an acidity of less than 0.8 percent. It has the most superior quality. Virgin oil is also pressed with no chemicals added, but is higher in acidity. Lesser grades of olive oil are made from various blends of refined and virgin oils and sometimes have other oils added as well. I use only extra-virgin oil.

Onions: The edible bulbs of the lily family, most onions are strongly flavored and are the basis of many recipes from soups to stews to stir-fry dishes. Used cooked or raw, onions are a staple of cooking. Do not refrigerate onions, as it compromises their flavor.

Peanuts: Although considered a nut, peanuts are in fact legumes and are a good source of protein. Unlike other legumes, peanuts are very high in fat. Since peanuts are one of the most chemically treated of all crops, try to choose organic peanuts for use. Peanuts are also prone to a carcinogenic mold called *aflatoxin,* especially if they are stored under humid conditions, so choose peanuts from the arid climate of the Southwest, like Valencia peanuts, to minimize this risk.

Pignoli (pine nuts): Incredibly luscious nuts that are quite expensive, due to the labor-intensive process involved in their harvesting from pinecones. High in oil and rich in taste, pine nuts add great depth to pasta and grain pilafs. Roasting them enhances their rich taste, making them delightful in any dish.

Pinto beans: The most famous Southwestern bean, pintos were actually named by the Spanish, who used the word meaning "painted" for them, because of the red-brown markings on their beige surface. Their nutty taste holds up well in stews, chilies, and baked bean dishes.

Quinoa: A tiny seedlike grain native to the Andes mountains. Pronounced "*keen*-wah," this small grain packs a powerhouse of protein and numerous amino acids not normally found in large amounts in most whole grains, particularly lysine, which aids digestion. Quinoa grains are quite delicate, so nature has coated them with an oily substance called *saponin*. If the grain isn't rinsed well, it can have a bitter taste. Quinoa has a lovely, nutty taste and cooks quickly, qualities that make it a great whole-grain addition to your menus.

Red wine vinegar: An acidic liquid-processed red wine, it possesses a wide range of qualities, because of how long it might be aged. It's always best to choose an organic version of this vinegar, as the acidity is slightly lower and the grapes from which the wine was made were organic, so the quality is superior.

Rice: The staple grain of many cultures, rice is low in fat and rich in vitamins, amino acids, protein, and minerals, like calcium and iron. Rice as we know it was reportedly cultivated in India, spreading from there to Asia and the Middle East.

In its whole form, rice is a near-perfect food. High in moisture, rice acts as a gentle diuretic, balancing the moisture content of the body and encouraging the elimination of any excess. Polished or white rice, while delicious on occasion, is pretty much devoid of nutrition and should be enjoyed occasionally, with brown rice as the staple grain.

The most common strains of rice include short grain, medium grain, and long grain. Short grain, the hardest and most compact variety, is best suited to cooler, temperate climates, while medium- and long-grain rice are used in warmer climates and during the summer months. Other gourmet varieties of rice have become popular in today's cooking. These include arborio, basmati, texmati, wehani, black japonica, and red rice. Sweet brown rice, a glutinous variety of brown rice, is commonly used not only as a grain dish but also in *mochi*, a cake formed by pounding and drying cooked sweet rice.

There are limitless uses for rice in daily cooking: it can be pressure-cooked, steamed, boiled, fried, baked, roasted, sautéed, and used in breads, sushi, casseroles, sautés, pilafs, or stuffings.

Rice syrup (brown rice syrup, rice malt): Rice syrup is a thick, amber syrup made by combining sprouted barley (or other fermentation starter, like enzymes) with cooked brown rice and storing it in a warm place. Fermentation begins and the starches in the rice convert to maltose and some other complex sugars, making this syrup a wonderfully healthy sweetener. Complex sugars release slowly into the bloodstream, providing fuel for the body rather than wreaking havoc on the blood sugar.

Rice syrup's wonderful, delicate sweetness makes it ideal for baked goods and other desserts.

*Salt: All salt is not equal. The best quality of salt to use is white, unrefined sea salt with no additives. Unrefined salts are rich in the trace minerals that are destroyed in processed salt.

*Seeds: In a word, seeds are powerhouses. (Remember that they are the source of entire plants, even trees in some cases.) That's a lot of energy in a little seed. They are good sources of protein and calcium, but because of their high oil content, seeds perish relatively quickly and keep best refrigerated. The most popular seeds in natural foods cooking include pumpkin seeds (pepitas), poppy seeds, sunflower seeds, and sesame seeds.

Seitan (wheat gluten): Most commonly called "wheat meat," seitan is made from wheat gluten. Made by kneading the bran and starch out of flour, raw seitan is rather bland, so most commercial brands are simmered in savory broth before sale. A wonderful source of protein, it is low in calories and fat and is very popular in Oriental "mock meat" dishes as well as in hearty stews and casseroles.

Sesame tahini: A thick, creamy paste made from ground hulled sesame seeds that is used for flavoring everything from sauces to salad dressings to dips, spreads, and baked goods. Available in natural foods stores and Middle Eastern markets, this spread has a delicate nutty flavor that adds luxurious taste to any recipe.

*Shiitake mushrooms: Gaining popularity over the last several years for their power to lower cholesterol and cleanse blood, shiitake mushrooms can be found in just about any natural foods store and gourmet shop. They have an intensely earthy taste, so a few go a long way. It is necessary to soak them until tender, about fifteen to twenty minutes before cooking, and I usually trim off the stem to avoid bitter flavor. They are wonderful in soups, stews, gravies, and sauces and as bouillon flavoring.

Shoyu (soy sauce): A confusing term because it is the generic term for Japanese soy sauce as well as the term for a specific type of traditionally made soy sauce, the distinguishing characteristic of which is the use of cracked wheat as the fermenting starter, along with soybeans. The best shoyu is aged for at least two years. A lighter seasoning than tamari.

Spices: Spices are highly aromatic seasonings that come from the seed, root, bark, and buds of plants, while herbs are obtained from the leaves and stems. Spices generally give food a very strong taste and energy, and can be quite stimulating to our vitality. Use of spices can be very helpful in getting energy moving when stagnant or "stuck." Spices become stale when kept for more than six months, so it is advisable to buy them in small quantities that you will use in that time period. Store spices and herbs in well-sealed containers in a cool, dark place to retain potency.

Tempeh: A traditional Indonesian soy product created by fermenting split, cooked soybeans with a starter. As the tempeh ferments, a white mycelium of enzymes develops on the surface, making the soybeans more digestible as well as providing a healthy range of B vitamins, except B12. Found in the refrigerator or freezer section of natural foods stores, tempeh is great in everything from sandwiches to salads to stews to casseroles.

Tofu (soybean curd): Fast becoming a popular low-fat food in our fat-crazed world, tofu is a wonderful source of protein and phytoestrogens and is both inexpensive and versatile. Rich in calcium and cholesterol-free, tofu is made by extracting curd from coagulated soy milk and then pressing it into bricks. For use in everything from soups and stews to salads, casseroles, and quiches or as the creamy base to sauces and dressings.

Vanilla (pure vanilla extract): A smoky, smooth flavoring made by extracting the essence from vanilla beans and preserving it in alcohol and water, although nowadays you can obtain vanilla preserved without alcohol. Pure vanilla extract is a bit expensive, but a small bit goes a long way, so splurge and get the best. By the way, inexpensive, artificial vanilla is made from vanillin, a by-product of paper making—appetizing, no?

Wakame (alaria): A very delicate member of the kelp family, wakame is most traditionally used in miso soups and tender salads. It requires only a brief soaking and short cooking time and has a very gentle flavor, so it is a great way to add sea vegetables to your diet.

Whole-wheat flour: A flour ground from whole-wheat berries that is high in gluten. Good, stone-ground flour retains much of its germ and bran, and thus much more of its nutrients than its unbleached white counterpart, making it a healthier choice for bread baking.

Whole-wheat pastry flour: A flour ground from a softer strain of wheat that is low in gluten. It is more finely milled than regular whole-wheat flour, making it an excellent choice for pastry, cookie, cake, and muffin baking.

The Extras

This list encompasses the kinds of ingredients that you can add to your basic pantry once you are cooking up a storm and looking for more and more ways to make it exciting and delicious.

Agar-agar: Also called "kanten" in Oriental shops, agar is a gelatinlike food made from various types of red algae. Agar flakes contain concentrated bonding properties and are used to make various types of jelled desserts and terrines.

Apple cider vinegar: Made from apple cider or apple must, this vinegar is brownish in color and is best when sold unpasteurized and unfiltered. Its acidic flavor belies the fact that it's quite alkalizing to the intestines and is used not only in cooking, but in remedies to improve digestion.

Arame: A large-leaf sea vegetable, arame is finely shredded and boiled before drying and packaging for selling. Since it is precooked, it requires far less cooking time than other sea vegetables and can even be marinated for salads with no cooking at all. One of the milder-tasting sea plants, it is a great source of protein and minerals like calcium and potassium.

Buckwheat (kasha): Also known as Saracen corn, buckwheat was reportedly brought to Europe by the Crusaders, although it originated in the Himalayan mountains. In botanical terms, buckwheat is not really a grain; it is actually a member of the rhubarb family, with fruit or groats that resemble tiny, dark-colored nuts.

Grown under adverse conditions in cold weather, buckwheat contains more protein than most other grains as well as iron and B vitamins. A natural source of rutic acid, which aids in arterial and circulatory problems, buckwheat is used by many homeopaths for high blood pressure and other circulatory difficulties.

Cooked by itself, buckwheat makes a great porridge, grain dish, or even a salad. A very traditional recipe involves sautéing onions and noodles and then tossing them together with cooked kasha. Ground into flour, buckwheat is the chief ingredient used to make traditional Japanese soba noodles.

Bulgur (cracked wheat): Made from whole-wheat berries that are cracked into pieces, enabling it to cook quite quickly. A great breakfast cereal, bulgur is most commonly associated with tabouleh, a marinated grain salad combining tomatoes, onions, and cucumbers with an aromatic olive oil dressing.

Burdock: A wild, hearty plant from the thistle family. According to traditional medicine, this long, dark brown root is renowned as one of nature's finest blood purifiers and skin clarifiers. A strong, dense root vegetable, burdock is a rich source of folic acid and is most commonly used in stews, stir-fry dishes, and long-simmered sautés.

Chestnuts: Their rich texture and taste belie the fact that chestnuts are in fact quite low in fat, making them an ideal ingredient in many recipes. At their peak in the fall, fresh chestnuts are a wonderful addition to soups, stews, and vegetable dishes, and their natural sweet taste makes them a great dessert ingredient. Dried chestnuts are available year-round and, with pre-soaking, achieve as creamy and sweet a taste and texture as their fresh counterparts.

Coconut sugar: A relatively new sweetener to hit the market. It's a natural sugar made from the sap of flower buds of the coconut. Also known as palm sugar, coconut sugar comes in crystal or granular form and is delicately sweet, sort of like brown sugar. Low on the glycemic index, it has high mineral content and is low in carbs and fructose. A sucrose-based sweetener, pure coconut sugar has ten calories in a teaspoon, almost identical to any other sugar.

Dulse: From the north Atlantic, dulse has a rich red color, is high in potassium, and comes packaged in large, wrinkled leaves. Its salty rich taste makes it a great snack right out of the package. Because it is so delicate, it actually requires little or no cooking, just a quick rinse to remove any debris on the leaves. It adds depth of flavor to hearty soups, stews, salads, and bean stews.

Kuzu (kudzu): Kuzu is a high-quality starch made from the root of the kuzu plant. A root native to the mountains of Japan (and now in the southern United States), kuzu grows like a vine with tough roots. Used primarily as a thickener, this strong root is reputed to strengthen the digestive tract due to its alkaline nature.

Maple syrup: A traditional sweetener made by boiling sugar maple sap until it becomes thick. The end product is quite expensive because it takes about thirty-five gallons of sap to produce one gallon of maple syrup. The syrup is available in various grades of quality from AA to B: AA and A are quite nice for sauces and dressings, but I use grade B in baking. I have found that the higher grades can result in hard baked goods.

I do not often use maple syrup, since it is a simple sugar, releasing quickly in the bloodstream, thus wreaking havoc with blood sugar. But it also comes in granular form that I sometimes use in baking.

Rice milk: A creamy liquid made by cooking ten parts water to one part rice for one hour, the resulting rice is pressed through a cheesecloth, creating "milk." It is also packaged commercially. Look for rice milk made from whole brown rice, not polished or white rice.

Semolina flour: Made from a yellowish-white whole wheat called durum, it is used in the making of pasta and in cakes to achieve a light, golden end product.

Soba: A noodle made from buckwheat flour. Some varieties contain other ingredients, like wheat flour or yam flour, but the best-quality soba are those made primarily of buckwheat flour.

Somen (Japanese angel hair): A very fine, white or whole-grain flour noodle that cooks very quickly, somen are traditionally served in a delicate broth with lightly cooked fresh vegetables.

Umeboshi plums (ume plums): Japanese pickled plums (actually, green apricots) with a fruity, salty taste. Pickled in a salt brine and shiso leaves for at least one year (the longer, the better), ume plums are traditionally served as a condiment with various dishes, including grains. Ume plums are reputed to aid in the cure of a wide array of ailments—from stomachaches to migraines—because they alkalize the blood. These little red plums (made red from the shiso, which adds vitamin C and iron) make good preservatives. The best-quality plums are the most expensive ones, but they are used in small amounts, so one jar will last a long time.

Umeboshi plum vinegar: A salty liquid left over from pickling umeboshi plums. Used as a vinegar, it is great in salad dressings and pickle-making.

Zest: Also called the peel, the zest is the thin, colored layer of skin on citrus fruit that imparts a fragrant essence of the fruit into cooking.

IN THE FRIDGE

A well-stocked refrigerator means that you never have to worry whether or not you are stocked to make a meal. Your life will change because you always have what you need to cook.

Please think seasonally (see page 119) and alter your list accordingly. Let your taste be your guide, but be adventurous. Try new things. You'll be amazed at how much you will fall in love with fresh food. This list serves to show the nutrition density of Mother Nature's bounty.

Arugula: This delicate green, in season in spring and fall, is slightly spicy and a rich source of protein, vitamin B6, niacin, thiamine, pantothenic acid, zinc, vitamin C, calcium, folate, magnesium, and potassium. It will keep for about a week in the fridge.

Basil: This summer herb can be found year-round, but is at its best in warm weather. In Italian folk medicine, basil was used as a blood purifier because of its rich combination of flavenoids that rid the blood of toxins. On top of that, basil contains compounds that make it antibacterial and anti-inflammatory. Used in pesto, sauces, salads, and stir-fry dishes, basil should be stored with its stems in a glass of water in the fridge with a plastic bag loosely draped over it.

Belgian endive: A member of the chicory family, this delicate vegetable can be eaten cooked or raw. Slightly bitter, endive is a rich source of folate, vitamins C and K, and fiber.

Bok choy: A mildly flavored vegetable that packs a nutritional punch. A rich source of vitamins C and A, bok choy is also a good source of phytonutrients like thiocyanites, which can protect against cancer and lower cholesterol. It is mostly used cooked, but baby bok choy can be shredded raw in a salad.

Broccoli: This cruciferous vegetable should be a staple in every diet. A rich source of protein, calcium, iron, magnesium, and phosphorus, vitamins A,

C, K, B1, B2, B3, B6, and folate, broccoli is one of the most nutrient-dense vegetables known to man. Also a rich source of sulphoraphane, a proven anticancer compound. Best nutritionally when steamed, but can be eaten raw or in a stir-fry as well.

Cabbage (green): This ancient cruciferous vegetable has a mild flavor and is one of the most commonly used and inexpensive vegetables on the market. Famous for its ability to lower cholesterol, cabbage also contains compounds that can help prevent cancer. Cabbage can be applied topically to bruises to relieve pain, and it is said to be the greatest anti-inflammatory of all vegetables.

Carrots: Said to be good for eyesight because of the high content of beta-carotene, carrots bring a lot more than that to the table. A good source of vitamins A, K, C, B6, fiber, and potassium, carrots' sweet taste and crunchy texture make them a winner with kids. Only you need know they are a great source of antioxidants.

Cauliflower: Another member of the cruciferous family, cauliflower's mild flavor belies the fact that it is a rich source of vitamin C, folate, and other essential nutrients. Said to help the body rid itself of toxins, cauliflower's high concentration of antioxidants make it a great cancer fighter.

Celery: You may think celery exists just to dip into hummus, but this rich source of vitamin C has more than crunch going for it. Because it contains 3-n butyl phthalide, a chemical that allows blood vessels to dilate, munching celery is a great way to prevent heart disease.

Chinese cabbage: Mildly flavored, easy to digest, and a rich source of folic acid, it's low in calories and an excellent source of folic acid. Usually found in stir-fry dishes, Chinese cabbage can be shredded and eaten raw in salads to add nutrients and an interesting crunchy texture.

Collards: One of the dark leafy greens essential to health, collard greens, like kale, can help lower cholesterol and protect us against cancer, and they are a rich source of vitamins K, C, folic acid, calcium, and zinc. They hold on to their nutrients best when lightly cooked, like steaming, blanching, or in a stir-fry, but collards can be finely shredded and eaten raw in salads as well.

Cucumbers: There's a reason we love these crunchy, moist veggies in the summer. Their water content keeps our bodies cool and balanced in hot weather, while providing us with plenty of vitamins C and A and fiber. It's said that the silica in cucumbers results in a glowing complexion.

Daikon: This low-in-calorie, peppery tasting root veggie looks like a large white carrot and is a great source of vitamin C and fiber. But its claim to fame is a unique blend of enzymes that aid digestion and help the body assimilate fat, protein, and starches more efficiently. Can be used raw in salads, but the flavor is strong for people. It's best cooked in stews, soups, or stir-fry dishes.

Dandelion: No, not the ones that grow in your lawn, but the delicately bitter leaves we see at the market each spring. A great detox aid, dandelion is a rich source of calcium, vitamins A and K, and lutein to protect our eyesight. Delicious in salads, dandelion can be lightly sautéed with garlic and chili peppers for a great side dish.

Green onions: Green onion is part of the allium family and provides vitamins A, C, and K, as well as folate, copper, manganese, calcium, iron, and fiber. Use in stir-fry dishes, as garnish in soups, in salads, and in any recipe in place of onions.

Kale: Very similar to collard greens in nutritional value, but unlike collards, kale is wonderful when juiced with carrots, cucumbers, and parsley. It's a bit sweeter and lends itself to being eaten raw or lightly cooked.

Lemons (or limes): Either lemons or limes bring a bit of sparkle to any dish, seeming to intensify the flavors. Lime is a wee bit sweeter, but both are rich sources of vitamins A and C, folates, and lutein. All citrus can be used in cooking, from oranges and grapefruit to tangerines, lemons, and limes. Just be advised that you can cook the zest in a dish, but take care not to cook the juice for more than a minute or it will take on a bitter aftertaste. And if you plan on using citrus zest in your cooking, go with organic fruit so you are not grating pesticides in with your sparkling flavor.

Lettuce: Most of us think of lettuce as not so nutrient-dense and a good, bland backdrop for dressing. Romaine lettuce is a good source of calcium, vitamin B6, iron, and other essential nutrients. Even iceberg lettuce has more going for it than crunch. It's a great source of vitamins A, C, K, and B6, as well as iron and potassium. Buy lettuce whole; wash and hand shred it to preserve the most nutrients. They may be easy to use, but shredded salads in a bag have lost a lot of their nutritive value.

Parsley: Much more than a simple garnish, this humble herb is a powerhouse of nutrition. As the world's most popular herb, it is a rich source of vitamins K, C, and A. Its volatile oils contain compounds believed to fight cancer, while its flavenoids, including luteolin, help prevent oxygen damage to cells. Its folic acid content is said to contribute to heart health and the alleviation of arthritis symptoms. Use to enliven cooked dishes, as garnish in soups, as the base for pesto, or in other sauces and dressings.

Parsnips: Not an essential ingredient in your fridge, parsnips add wonderful sweetness and richness to dishes. A great source of fiber, vitamins C and K, folate, manganese, and potassium, parsnips, according to Chinese medicine, can help balance the spleen, pancreas, and stomach and aid in digestion. Great in stews, casseroles, soups, and stir-fry dishes.

Red radishes: Used mostly in salads, radishes have a similar effect in the body as daikon. They help us assimilate protein, fat, and fiber, as well as being a great source of vitamin C. Like other cruciferous veggies, radishes help prevent cancer and in folk medicine are used to treat liver disorders. Use in salads and stews, or pickle in a salt brine.

Seasonal fruits: All fruits are best consumed in season. They provide us with antioxidants, fiber, essential minerals, and vitamins. They are a great sweet snack and an excellent alternative to junk food. However, they are also a rich source of sugar, so best to consume no more than one serving a day of seasonal whole fruit—not the juice, the fruit.

Summer squash: Delicate, soft, creamy flesh belies the fact that summer squashes (including zucchini, patty pans, and yellow squash) are great sources of manganese, vitamins A and C, copper, zinc, and iron. Used in soups, stews, stir-fry dishes, raw in salads, and in quick breads.

Watercress: A member of the mustard family, this peppery green is delicate but provides us with a rich source of vitamins A and C and calcium. Used in salads, lightly blanched, stirred raw into cooked stews for freshness, and in place of lettuce in sandwiches. In Chinese medicine, it is believed that watercress can cleanse the liver.

Winter squash: Includes butternut, buttercup, Hokkaido, kabocha, delicate, acorn, pumpkin. An important source of carotenoids, including lutein and zeaxanthin, as well as vitamins A, C, B1, B3, B5, and B6, potassium, fiber, folate, and copper, these sweet, starchy veggies lend themselves to roasting in the oven, stewing, and in soups, casseroles, and desserts.

Grow Your Own

At the end of the day, with farm markets, CSAs, local markets, preserving, canning, and freezing, there is nothing like growing your own food. Whether you live in a mansion with acres surrounding your estate, a suburban ranch house with a yard, a city row home with a small plot of ground, or an apartment with nothing more than windowsills, grow something. It connects you to your food like nothing else. It creates a reverence for life, for Mother Nature, for all that we have. It will hook you on the flavor of fresh food and ruin you for junk food or compromised ingredients. I know what you're thinking; this is the book that is supposed to make this all so doable, easy, and accessible.

It is. But spare just a wee bit of time and space and grow something. It will change your relationship with food.

11

The Basic Tools

For a stress-free life in the kitchen, you need good tools. You don't need a lot of them, no fancy gadgets or utensils, but you need enough tools to streamline and enjoy your time in the kitchen.

KNIVES

The tool that will serve you best, that is indispensable in the culinary world, is a knife. And not some little wussy, cheap-ass paring knife that you bought from some home-shopping network on a deal . . . or at some cut-rate superstore on a closeout. I'm talking a serious kitchen knife, the kind that can do the job handily.

You don't have to take out a second mortgage on the house to get a knife that will do the job you need to do. Good chef's knives can cost as little as thirty dollars or as much as three hundred dollars or more.

Look for a stainless or carbon steel blade, with a handle that balances well with the weight of the blade. Carbon steel will stain, but will hold its edge longer than stainless and is usually heavier. Depending on how you work and how much you cook, you can decide if you want a heavy knife or a light one.

I am a fan of ceramic knives and can't imagine using anything else. They are light, sleek, and so sharp, they seem to do the work for you. They are expensive, though, but in my view, one of the greatest investments you can make in your kitchen. Women seem to like them a lot because the blades are a little smaller and, of course, for their lightness. Men seem to like bigger, heavier knives to do the job. It doesn't matter in the least. Just buy the knife you like, the one that feels right in your hand. I know that sounds odd, but trust me, when you hold the knife that is for you, you will know it.

I know a lot of people recommend knife sets, with several to choose from. Most home cooks will find that they use the same knife over and over, so invest your money in one good knife. You can always build your collection.

And store your cooking knife in a box or a block; don't just toss it in a drawer with the other stuff in your kitchen. This is your knife . . . your sidekick in cooking.

There is only one exception to the one-knife rule . . . a bread knife. Get one. Don't use your veggie knife on bread. It will dull it quickly, and you will always be sharpening it on the steel instead of slicing and dicing veggies with it.

Next to your knife, the second most important tool in your repertoire is a diamond steel to put an edge on your knife on a daily basis. It's essential to the health of your knife. Each day, before you begin to cook, hone your blade on the steel to keep the edge sharp and your knife ready to go. And once a month or so, take your blade to a kitchen store that sharpens and let them put a good edge on it.

I know this sounds like a lot of effort to care for your knife, but trust me, it's your most important tool and the one you want to baby the most.

CUTTING BOARDS

Next to a knife, you will need a board for prep. And not one of those six-inch free cheese boards you got with a gift basket. Get a cutting board. A wooden cutting board. Before you panic thinking you will have a germ factory on your counter if you use wood, let me tell you that there was a study that reported that natural wood boards held less bacteria and germs than plastic. It seems that wooden boards wick away moisture and the germs with it.

Size matters: While I am a big-board type of girl, you have to take your own kitchen counter space into account when choosing a board. Go as big as you can so you have room to work.

And go for a nice, thick board so you don't have to worry about warping.

An exception is bamboo boards, the newest darlings in the cutting-board world. They are light, durable, antimicrobial, and antibacterial (naturally), and they don't warp. They are a bit hard for my taste, but they are very popular with home cooks, so check them out.

Keep it clean. Your cutting board needs to be clean, but I am not a fan of using soap, because my experience has shown that the board takes on a "soapy" taste in time. I also don't oil my boards because the oil can go rancid over time and the boards will have an odor.

I do clean it. Once a week, I wet my board really well and sprinkle it very generously with salt. I rub half a lemon over the salty wet board and rinse it well. It removes odor and germs and freshens the board for use.

POTS AND PANS

I am a total sucker for gorgeous pots and pans. Most husbands break into a sweat when their wives stop in a jewelry shop. My husband gets chills when I walk into a kitchen shop. Pots and pans have an allure that I can't describe. I am of the view that without pots and pans that are functional and beautiful, you will grow frustrated and depressed with cooking and head back to the drive-through window.

Your pots and pans don't need to be luxuriously expensive, either. They need to be sturdy so they hold up for years of use. Some people like to invest in the latest gourmet brand, but as long as the pots and pans are of good quality, the labels mean nothing.

You will need several pots and pans to function well with cooking. I use a combination of stainless steel, cast iron, porcelain-covered cast iron, and clay cookware. Stainless steel is the most basic and most necessary of all the types of pots and pans on the market. They distribute heat evenly and cook food efficiently. I personally like heavy stainless pots and pans; I have found that they hold up well over time, so I won't be making repeat purchases because I did not invest in the best quality I could afford.

Cast iron is my favorite type of pan to use in cooking. I love the heft of them. I love the even heat. I love the fact that they make me feel warm and cozy when I am cooking on cold winter nights. I love how easily they clean. Cast iron coated with porcelain is up there on my list as well. Casseroles and pots that go stove or oven to table make these indispensable in any kitchen. And they are gorgeous and colorful, so you please your aesthetic sensibilities along with your tummy.

Clay cookware has a light feel, but these are not lightweights when it comes to work. Delicate in that they will chip or break if you drop them, clay pots cook vegetables and beans in a very gentle manner, resulting in succulent stews that do not reduce the veggies to baby food, soups that seem richer and "creamier" without extra work or added ingredients. They move from stove to table, foods don't stick, and the pots and pans have an ageless quality to them (if only people aged so well).

As for nonstick pans, skip them. I had softened my position on them when I discovered that the coating no longer scraped off, ending up in your food. But then someone sent me an article about canaries and parakeets dying in homes where people cooked with nonstick pans. Apparently the chemicals in the coating were emitting fumes that were killing the birds. Dr. Joseph Mercola, the enormously popular health advocate, offers some pretty concrete evidence about the effects of the various chemicals in commercial nonstick cookware, so I am back to my hard-core view. Skip them.

The only exceptions are the new "green" nonstick pans being marketed by both Kitchen Aid and Cuisinart. I have used them and they are okay. They have all the science to tell us that they are safe and they're certainly nonstick. But to be honest, there is something distinctly unsatisfying about cooking with nonstick pans. You can't sear or brown well. That gorgeous, ever so slightly overcooked, syrupy leftover goop in the pan is no longer part of the equation of cooking. And to me, that's a bummer. So use the "green" nonstick if you like, but I say learn to cook well and you won't need them.

OTHER GADGETS

Everyone is trying to sell us gadgets to make our lives in the kitchen easier. In my view, most of them just create more work because we have to figure out how to use them and clean them, and they don't do the job as well as I would prefer.

That said, if gadgets are your thing, then have at them. For me, there are only a few that I think are essential to making life in the kitchen fun, efficient, and satisfying.

Wooden spoons make cooking a dream. They are gentle in the hand, gorgeous, and they don't conduct heat, so you are unlikely to burn yourself while stirring. Size and style don't matter as long as they are comfortable in your hand and are big (or small) enough to do the job.

Whisks, brushes, colanders, sieves, garlic presses, cherry pitters, peelers, measuring cups and spoons, spatulas, zesters, and graters can all come in handy but are not as necessary as a knife and a cutting board, so accumulate your gadgets as you cook and see your needs from experience.

Making Your Life Easy

I am not one to advocate for packaged foods of any kind; I want you in the kitchen, cooking from scratch. But I live in the real world and I know that for most of us living a busy, modern life, eating well is a process. I know we live in a world that doesn't encourage us to cook. We are encouraged to buy, heat, and eat. We live in a grab-and-go culture. We have to break that stranglehold. So make it easy on yourself, not too easy, but a little easy.

Cooking dinner is not splitting the atom, so relax and take advantage of some of the conveniences we have to make pulling a meal together a little smoother until you become more comfortable at the stove.

Organic canned beans make any salad a protein powerhouse, so keep a variety of your favorites on hand for those times when you do not have the time to cook them from scratch (which takes about an hour). You can sprinkle them on your salad right out of the can; add them to soups with fresh veggies that will cook in minutes; puree them with seasonings of your choice to make dips and spreads. With their high fiber content for digestion and protein for strength, beans are a must-have addition to your diet. Just remember to rinse them well before using, as the stale water they are stored in can result in you being . . . well . . . musical after eating them.

To be perfectly frank, salad-in-a-bag aggravates me no end. When did we get too busy to rinse lettuce under water and shred it into a bowl? But . . . but . . . if you live that busy a life, then go for it and buy the salad in a bag. However, choose an organic version, please. The commercial salads in a bag lose about two-thirds of their nutritive value in the nitrogen flush process (that leads to such a long shelf life for these delicate shredded leaves), and the veggies are not washed in chlorinated water in the organic varieties. Yes, Virginia, like in a swimming pool. Yuck, right? Organic salads in a bag will not last as long, so you will be forced to eat more veggies so you don't waste money and food. A win-win in my book.

One thing that seems to make people the most insane about cooking is the prep work, the slicing and dicing to get the veggies ready for cooking. While for me that is part of the joy of creating the meal and I am quite efficient at my chopping, for some of us, well, that part of the job is slow and causes the process of getting a meal on the table to be tedious. For you, there are frozen, chopped veggies . . . ready to go, from bag to wok, so to speak. Keep a bag or bags of assorted sliced or chopped vegetables in the freezer for those times when dinner needs to be ready fast. Skip the fresh already-chopped veggies, as they have lost most of their nutritive value and taste flat. The frozen versions retain more of their nutrients and have more intense flavors.

But don't get too dependent on these babies. One of the joys of cooking is the skill that develops the more you cook. So take one or two nights a week and chop your veggies fresh for that meal. The more you chop, the more efficient and proficient you become, and you will fall in love with cooking. Trust me on this one.

Other convenience foods, natural or not, from potpies to frozen dinners to breakfast burritos to canned and shelf-stable soups have to be carefully considered before you buy them and add them to your diet. In a pinch they may work, but unless you have made recipes with your own hands, there are likely ingredients in these foods that you might not choose. At the very least, they will provide more calories, salt, sugar (of some kind), and fat than you need . . . or want. Don't be fooled.

12

Kitchen Techniques and Tips

I am always amazed at how challenged people are at the thought of cooking. It's not a judgment; maybe it's because I have been cooking all my life. However, more than twenty years of teaching has taught me that people need to relearn this most instinctual of life skills because our society has taken us so far from it.

Going back to the kitchen is not a big deal; nothing to stress over. The thought of taking your health back in your own hands in your kitchen with the foods you choose to prepare each day should, in fact, excite you. This is the ultimate adventure with a most delicious outcome.

That said, I would never mislead you. Cooking is work. Sometimes, it's even hot and sweaty. Sometimes it's frustrating and things don't turn out quite like you had planned. But most of the time, unlike the Lean Cuisine commercial that tells us slicing and dicing at the end of the day is anything but relaxing, you will find cooking to be fulfilling, satisfying, enjoyable . . . and relaxing. You may even become passionate about it.

There are things you can do to make cooking more enjoyable, too. You can cook with friends or family members. The social aspect of the evening will make the chores associated with cooking fly by. You can play music to enlist another of your senses in the process. I can't tell you how well these will work for you. My students tell me that these are tried-and-true methods of relaxation during cooking. I cook with my husband or by myself. Either way, I am a quiet cook, letting the "music" of the kitchen seduce me. I do not like music or television or distractions when I am cooking. I want to listen to my food doing its thing. This style allows me to be very present when I am cooking. But that's me.

There are basics of cooking, just like any skill. Not mastering those skills will leave you chronically flustered and at odds with creating meals. You will hate the very idea of going into the kitchen and preparing food.

VEG PREP

This part of the cooking process can be the most time-consuming and the most challenging for those people not all that familiar with the kitchen and its skills. And while I will describe the basic skills needed here, there is really only one way to get really, really good at cooking . . . you must cook!

So grab your brand-new knife and practice these basic cutting styles so you can be efficient and comfortable at your cutting board.

Dicing

I am not a peeler. It's the rare occasion that I take the outer skin off a veggie, not even for nonorganic items. You can't peel the pesticides off and why lose those nutrients? The exceptions are acorn squash or anything that is obviously waxed. Otherwise, I like keeping the fiber from the skin, the surface nutrients, like vitamin C, intact. I also don't feel the need to add another step to the job of cooking. There is absolutely nothing wrong with the skin, even if the veggies are not organic, unless, again, it's waxed.

To dice, wash the vegetable and wet your cutting board with a sponge or a wet cloth. Wetting the board prevents nutrients from the cut veggies from absorbing into the wood.

For round vegetables, cut them in half lengthwise and lay each half on its flat side on the board. Slice the vegetable lengthwise into slices (the thickness depends on how large or small the dice you want). Stack the slices and cut into spears. Gather the spears and cut crosswise to create a dice. This method works for any round veggie, from turnips to cabbage to onions to beets.

For long vegetables, like cucumber, carrot, and parsnip, trim the tips as needed. Slice the veggie in half lengthwise and lay each half on its flat side on the board. Cut each half into long spears. Gather the spears and cut crosswise to create a dice.

Remember that the size of your dice depends on how thick or thin you cut the spears. The average dice is about ¼-inch. Mincing is just very small dicing.

Julienne/Matchstick

This delicate cut is so easy, you will surprise yourself. I don't teach this method in the traditional French style, as there are a lot of steps and it can get frustrating. Instead I use a method known as the "domino cut."

Trim the tips off the carrot or other vegetable you are planning to julienne. Lay the vegetable on the cutting board, on an angle, holding the thicker end. Thinly slice the veggie into diagonal pieces. If your knife is sharp, the slices will fall onto themselves, resembling fallen dominoes. You may need to rearrange the slices slightly to achieve this effect as you practice. Once the vegetable is sliced, hold the overlapped pieces in place with your hand, spreading your fingers to hold as many of the pieces in place as possible. Cut lengthwise across the pieces to create long, slender matchstick pieces.

For round vegetables, simply cut in half lengthwise and lay each half on its flat side on the board. Thinly slice lengthwise; stack the slices and slice into thin spears.

Shredding

Used for slaws and salads, shredding is easy. Not as precise as julienne and dicing, shredding gives you more leeway as you practice.

To shred veggies like cabbage, you have two choices. Pull off a few outer leaves, roll them into cylinders, and thinly slice crosswise to create long threads. You may also cut the vegetable in half and lay the flat side on the board and slice crosswise into threads. This is more challenging because the cabbage can be large and unwieldy to hold.

For leafy greens, simply trim off the tips of the stems (do not cut the stem out and throw away. The stems are loaded with valuable minerals). Roll the leaves into cylinders and slice them crosswise into threads. If the stems are very thick, simply fold each leaf in half, exposing the stem. Slice the stem out of the green and cook separately. Continue with the method to shred the leaves after removing the stem.

Chunk or Roll Cut

When making stews, casseroles, and hearty soups, you sometimes prefer that the vegetables are cut into larger pieces so that they grow sweet and soft in the recipe. Large chunks take longer to cook, but the better to make a stew with, my dears.

To cut round vegetables into chunks, cut the vegetable in half lengthwise and lay the flat side on the board. Cut into thick wedges; gather the wedges and cut crosswise to create the size chunk you want.

For long vegetables, trim the ends and lay the vegetable on the board, holding on to the thicker end. With your knife at an angle, cut crosswise, taking a chunk off the end. Roll the vegetable ninety degrees and cut again. Keep rolling and cutting until you have cut the entire vegetable, adjusting the degree of rolling so that the pieces are similar in size when you are through.

Although you want to become efficient in the kitchen, while you practice, the goal is not speed but accuracy. Your goal is to create cuts that are the same size and same thickness so that the dish you prepare cooks evenly and is aesthetically pleasing to the eye. People eat with their eyes before they taste anything. Speed will come as you gain experience slicing and dicing.

Other Stuff You Should Know About Vegetable Prep

Now that you have the basic skills to practice your cutting, there are a few more tips before we get to the stove and begin cooking.

When you buy produce, don't wash it before putting it in the fridge. It will shorten the life of whatever you buy. And don't wrap things in paper towels or plastic bags. That method dries out the produce and wastes paper. (In my view, there is no need to even buy paper towels, save for once a year when you wash your windows . . . Just use rags and wash them. We need to stop wasting paper and killing trees, but I digress . . .)

Before you pop your produce in the fridge, remove any rubber bands or binders on the bunches so air can circulate. Leave the bags loosely open. You will get about four days out of delicate vegetables like fresh basil, arugula, spinach, and parsley and at least a week of freshness from kale, collard greens, bok choy, and broccoli. Heartier vegetables like cauliflower, cabbage, and most roots will last for at least two weeks.

You also don't need to be crazy with the fridge either. Foods like onions, tomatoes, winter squash, apples, pears, oranges, peaches, grapefruit, bananas, lemons, limes, and avocados should not be in the fridge. It compromises their flavors, so I like to have big bowls of these fresh foods around the kitchen. They look gorgeous and bring life to the room. They will inspire you to cook.

I also keep fresh pots of herbs growing on my windowsills year-round so that I can add fresh life to any dish with a pinch of my fingers. I usually grow the basics that I use almost daily: flat-leaf parsley, basil, and rosemary. Oh, and the perfume of the fresh herbs in your kitchen. If it doesn't inspire you to cook, then you might be a lost cause.

One last thing. When you are cooking, you don't always use the whole carrot, parsnip, squash, onion, or cabbage. Simply wrap the unused piece in the same produce bag it came from (or plastic wrap) and return it to the fridge. Once cut, everything has to be refrigerated, including onions or they will rot quickly. And when you split a winter squash, be sure to remove the seeds from both halves, even if you are not using the whole squash. Storing cut squash with the seeds inside will cause it to sour quickly. Remove the seeds, wrap the unused piece in a produce bag, and you will get at least ten days' life out of each squash.

AT THE STOVE

There is a certain magic to the kitchen, an alchemy like no other when it comes to orchestrating ingredients into the perfect meal. The sensuality of coaxing every nuance of flavor from food overwhelms my senses. Simmering pots, steam rising, aromas filling the air. Delicately cooked vegetables, satisfying soups, pasta and grains heady with the fragrance of fresh herbs, crisp fresh salads vital with life all come together under the hand of the cook to create the meals that nourish us to health and well-being.

Comfort in the kitchen allows you to move from task to task, smoothly and efficiently, intoxicated as the colors and perfumes of the dishes come together. There is little in life more lusty than cooking.

Most of us have come to think of cooking as something we watch on television or some dreaded chore to be endured at the end of a long day. In truth, cooking is life. An art form rapidly being lost in this modern connected world, cooking is the foundation upon which you build your life. No matter what you choose to prepare, your competence in cooking determines whether or not your meals are delicious or pedestrian; sublime or just a way to feed yourself because you must.

Cooking is simple, elegant, and satisfying. You only need to master some basic techniques to create a great meal—no matter what chefs or molecular gastronomists tell you.

Braising is a slow cooking process where the ingredients are seared or browned in fat or oil and then simmered in a small amount of liquid until tender. Braising is usually done in deep skillets or in a Dutch oven–style pan so that the juices accumulated in the braising combine to create a richly flavored sauce in the cooking process.

Grilling is a style of cooking where high heat is applied directly to the food . . . below the food, like a barbecue or in a grill pan over high heat on the stove top. Grilling seals in the flavor of the food and at the same time creates a rich, smoky taste that everyone loves. Of course, use a gas grill; no need to cook your food in a chemical haze of lighter fluid and coal.

Broiling is also a high direct heat that seals in the flavor and imparts a glorious browning that is without compare. The heat is above the food in close contact and cooks very quickly, so you need to be diligent when broiling. It is used a lot as a finishing style of cooking, to brown a food once it's been baked or roasted.

Roasting is a slow cooking style done in the oven. The enclosed, dry, intense heat of the oven surrounds the food and drives the sugars of the vegetables to the surface, making them so-o-o-o sweet, they could stand in for dessert. I dress the veggies I am roasting in olive or avocado oil, salt, and pepper. That's it. (Okay, sometimes I use cinnamon on squash or sweet potatoes . . .) I cover the casserole dish tightly and roast for forty-five minutes to an hour. Then I remove the cover and return the dish to the oven to brown the edges of the veggies. Yum.

Baking is a technique reserved for oven-cooking breads and pastries. Many chefs would have you believe that to bake well you need to join a secret society and take a blood oath of secrecy. Hardly. Just follow recipes until you have mastered the techniques, the textures, the ingredients, and then you can venture off on your own.

Poaching is a simple method by which you simply cook food in simmering liquid, imparting a sweet tenderness and resulting in a dish that is the perfect comforting texture.

Stewing is a moist-heat cooking process a bit like braising except that braising is done in fat or oil, while stewing is done in a broth-style liquid. The food is cooked in a small amount of liquid and served in the gravy that results from the combination of the juices of the vegetables and cooking broth.

Sautéing is a method of cooking that uses a small amount of fat in a shallow pan over relatively high heat. The oil is heated and the ingredients added in succession. The ingredients are usually cut into small pieces or thinly sliced to facilitate quick, even cooking. The ingredients are stirred together, constantly moving, allowing steam to escape so that the veggies don't stew and maintain their crispness. A sauté is seasoned toward the end of the cooking process.

Shallow- or pan-frying is different from sautéing, although it is often confused with it, as is stir-frying. Shallow-frying uses more oil, and larger pieces of food are cooked until browned and then turned once for even cooking.

Stir-frying is the term used for two styles of cooking, one similar to a sauté and the other starting with a hot wok to which the oil is added and then the veggies and seasonings in rapid succession and cooked, stirring constantly, to crisp perfection.

Frying or deep-frying is cooking food over high heat completely submerged in hot oil. The result is crisp, light, and richly flavored food. If the food is oily-tasting, then your oil wasn't hot enough. If the oil is hot, the food will sink and immediately rise to the top and brown. It will be in and out of the oil in a minute or two. A hint: bring your oil to the proper temperature (350–375°F) over low heat to ensure that the oil is hot enough and doesn't smoke.

Boiling and blanching are methods of cooking in water. Boiling foods involves the food being submerged in water for several minutes to achieve the tenderness desired. Blanching involves a quick dip into boiling water just to remove some of the "raw"-ness or bite of a delicate vegetable. A pinch of salt is added to the water before cooking in either of these styles so that the vegetables hold on to more of their nutrients and do not bleed them into the water.

Steaming is a method of cooking where the food is cooked above boiling water so it actually cooks in the steam that rises off the water. The result is very crisp, brightly colored vegetables that hold a lot of their nutrients. The resulting vegetables are light, fresh, and drier than food cooked submerged in water.

With these basic cooking and prep techniques, there's nothing you can't achieve in the kitchen.

PART FIVE

Recipes Just Like Mama Used to Make, Only Healthier

I t used to be that adapting recipes took the creativity of da Vinci to come up with substitutions to make a dish healthier. And even then, the results were often disappointing and flat.

But the world you are cooking in is different. The demand for healthy foods has opened a floodgate of creative thinking, and the market abounds with healthier versions of the foods you love. But remember to read labels carefully. Often what seems to be a healthy option is just smoke and mirrors designed to trick you into buying more processed junk food under the guise of healthy eating.

You know the drill. If food won't rot or sprout, throw it out.

13

Changing Ingredients Because There's No Substitution for Health

In order to make a recipe over, you need to understand the ingredients that are in the original and the ingredients you want to substitute. Don't panic. You don't need a degree in biochemistry to pull this off. Just use the simple tips here and you will do fine.

EGGS

This is a big one for people, particularly in baking, but also in cooking. Scrambled eggs without the eggs? Yup. Recipes exist that are so delicious, you won't miss the cholesterol.

In general, understanding the "job" of eggs in a recipe will help you decide which substitute to use. Eggs perform different functions in recipes, so it's important to know what you need for the final recipe result.

In cakes, eggs are used to create a light and fluffy texture, so it's a leavening agent. In cookies, they add moisture and act as a binder holding all the ingredients together. For quiche or mayonnaise, eggs are central to the recipe so a lot of consideration is needed.

There are also commercial egg replacers like Ener-G, a very popular choice among vegans for baking and binding. It is flavorless and easy to work with, although you will need to compensate for its dryness with a bit more moisture in your batters and dough. It's not my personal choice, but it is vegan and there's no bad news about it, so if you want to give it a go, have at it.

Bananas and applesauce are used very often in baking to replace eggs because they lend sweetness as well as moisture. They work great, but my favorite is grated zucchini. It adds moisture, binds just a wee bit better, and adds no flavor at all. None of these replacements help the cakes or pastries rise. You will need baking powder and soda to do that.

Baking powder and soda are essential to vegan baked goods rising, creating that light, fluffy texture we all love in desserts. The rule of thumb is 1 teaspoon baking powder and ½ teaspoon baking soda for each egg in a recipe.

Tofu works as a great egg substitute in dishes like quiche, frittata, egg salad, or scrambled eggs. Soufflé is a bit of a challenge, but with tofu, baking powder, and sparkling water, you can pull off a reasonable facsimile, if you desire. And in baking, tofu lends moisture, binds a little, and imparts no flavor, so it's great in certain recipes. But keep in mind that tofu can make your batter heavy and thick, resulting in a heavy end product, so use it wisely.

The king of all egg replacers for baking, in my humble view, is chia. These tiny seeds, sprouted in a small amount of the liquid of your recipe, will help your cakes, cupcakes, and other pastries rise; they will help bind, like eggs (especially helpful when baking with gluten-free flours); and they produce a soft, moist, delicate texture in pastries that is out of this world. I just soak a tablespoon of chia seeds (per recipe) in a small amount of liquid for fifteen minutes before I begin to assemble my ingredients. I whisk them and add them into the batter.

You will see how to use all these substitutes in the recipes that follow, and once you see the "formula," you will be able to branch out and adapt all your own favorite recipes.

MILK

This one is easy, with all the milk replacements on the market today. It's a matter of finding the one that you like best or the flavor that serves your recipe the best.

Soy milk is the most commonly known non-dairy milk. It has become a hugely marketed and, in many cases, compromised product, but there are still some great brands out there for use. Go for the unsweetened, made from whole certified organic soybeans, and you will do just fine. If the ingredient panel on your soy milk (or any other product) reads like a Russian novel, skip it. Soy milk is loaded with protein, low in fat, and mild in flavor. In my opinion, it can make baked goods a bit heavy, but I like it in sauces and soups.

Rice milk is another alternative to dairy milk, but if the brand you are considering is made from white rice, take a pass. White rice is a simple carb, and the resulting "milk" is no better for you than sugar water. Rice milk made from brown rice will provide nutrients and fiber. Delicate, almost translucent, rice milk can be watery in soups and casseroles, but is well-suited to baking when you are trying to cut the fat a bit.

Oat milk is a creamy, rich alternative to milk. It's much more popular in Europe than in the United States, but you can find it in natural food stores. It lends a silky, gorgeous texture to soups and a moist crumb to cakes and pastries. Its mild flavor is perfect in just about any dish where you use cream.

Almond milk rules in my world. There are other nut milks, but almond milk has stolen my heart. It's mild and creamy, but not heavy. It has fiber, protein, and good-quality fats and is low in calories. I love it for cakes, pastries, cupcakes, cookies, soups, stews, casseroles, biscuits, and in any recipe where I would have used milk in the past.

BUTTER

Butter is a well-loved ingredient. It's easy to work with, versatile, creates stunning texture, and is, well, delicious. It's stable under heat and browns beautifully. It creates a moist tender crumb in baking.

It will kill you.

So what do we do? Suffer a grim existence of fat-free, cardboard-like treats that could double as the soles to shoes? Nope. I have your back . . . even on something as glorious as butter.

Interestingly, there are a number of substitutes for butter for any cooking or baking. Some, as you can imagine, are of better quality than others. It's important to read labels (yes, again . . .) to be sure the product you choose has no saturated, trans, or hydrogenated fats; the sodium is reasonable; and the ingredient panel doesn't read like *War and Peace*, in its original Russian.

My favorite butter substitutes are **extra-virgin olive oil** and **avocado oil**. I use them both for various tasks and have achieved gorgeous, silky buttery results with no saturated fats. Sure, there are calories and we'll get to the low-fat subs in a minute, but for now, let's revel in the indulgence of oils, shall we?

There are a lot of olive oils available, from extra virgin to light. In my view, there is one olive oil worth using: **extra virgin**. Don't even bother with the rest of them. Extra virgin is the first press of the olives and is the richest in antioxidants, nutrients, and flavor. I use it for everything, from sautéing to baking, particularly in piecrusts.

There is some controversy about whether or not you can cook with olive oil healthfully. According to the experts at www.oliveoilsource.com, the most important thing about cooking with oil is to not exceed its smoke point—the temperature at which oil or fat begins to break down, creating an unpleasant flavor. In some cases, the oil becomes unhealthy.

As well, there is not a consensus about what the smoke point of olive oil actually is. The important point to remember, and one reason that I prefer high-quality extra-virgin olive oil (with low free fatty acids): it has a high smoke point. Extra-virgin olive oil smokes roughly between 365°F and 400°F, depending on the quality. It may be more expensive than the lower-quality, mass-produced oil, but, frankly, even those oils are safe to cook with.

The International Olive Oil Council says: "When heated, olive oil is the most stable fat, which means it stands up well to high frying temperatures. Its high smoke point (410°F) is well above the ideal temperature for frying foods (356°F). The digestibility of olive oil is not affected when heated, even when it is reused for frying."

Now there's nothing I can do to take the calories out of olive oil (120 per tablespoon), but I can promise you fabulous results in your cooking and salad dressings if you invest in some good-quality extra-virgin olive oil.

Rich, buttery, and delicious, **avocado oil** is a relative newcomer to the oil scene and a welcome newcomer at that. A monounsaturated fat, with a smoke point of 491°F, avocado oil is nutrient-dense and has a very mild flavor. It's rich and satisfying as a fat to use in cooking and baking. I also love that its mild taste doesn't compete or conflict with any other strong flavors in a recipe. For instance, I am not a fan of the flavors of olive oil and soy sauce together. So I use avocado oil when I am stir-frying as a mild counterpart to the strong flavor of soy sauce.

I also love it as the seasoning when I am roasting sweet vegetables like winter squash and sweet potatoes, since I often use cinnamon in these kinds of dishes and, again, the avocado oil gives me richness but doesn't compete with the strong taste of the cinnamon.

In baking, avocado oil has no peer in my view. It results in a delicate, moist crumb and adds nothing in terms of taste. It's light and doesn't weigh my cakes and pastries down; it won't leave you with an oily film on your lips after eating it. It tastes like everything you bake is richly flavored with butter. Only you need know the truth.

Solid Butter Substitutes

There are a lot of solid fats that can be used in the place of butter. I remember, as a kid, my mother thought she was making a move toward healthier cooking when she switched from butter to Crisco and margarine. She was wrong. Both of these products, unless otherwise stated, contain fully hydrogenated oils and fats. So you can skip those, in my view.

There are brands like Smart Balance and Earth Balance that offer us alternatives to butter, margarine, and shortenings with non-hydrogenated solid oil blends for cooking and baking. Earth Balance is the natural-food brainchild of the people who make Smart Balance and, in my view, is a better product for use. While not a fan of eating a lot of solid oil, I don't want to have to read labels, and Smart Balance has two shortcomings: some of their items contain fish oil, and none of them guarantee that the ingredients are not genetically modified.

Earth Balance, on the other hand, is a line of vegan products, some organic, some not, but all guarantee that no genetically modified ingredients are used. I like Earth Balance products and use them now and again in my cooking. They taste remarkably like butter and are much healthier for you than hydrogenated and saturated fats. Are they perfect? Nope, but they can work in an occasional recipe to achieve the results you seek and not compromise your health.

COCONUT OIL

I wish I had a nickel for every time someone asked me whether I thought they should cook with extra-virgin coconut oil. I will say, for the record, that the jury is out for me on this one. Personally, I do not like the flavor, but that's not a reason for me to advise against the use of coconut oil.

The use of coconut oil for health is a subject of great controversy, and I can just tell you what I know from my own research and experience with it.

Proponents say that virgin coconut oil is antiviral, antibacterial, and antimicrobial. They also cite the health and longevity of the tropical populations who consume it regularly as a ringing endorsement. In truth, there are a lot of reasons that these same populations enjoy good health and long lives, more than eating coconut oil.

They also tell us that we need some saturated fat in our diets. True. They also explain that coconut oil is a medium-chain fatty acid, which can increase metabolism and is more easily digested. They say that coconut oil is processed directly in the liver and converted into energy, so it doesn't store in the body as fat.

However, the American Medical Association says that Americans do not need another source of saturated fat in their diets and that the studies claiming benefits have not been extensive enough or were inadequately controlled to be completely valid in their claims. Many were done by the industry making the oil. What do we think they will say?

Dr. Mary Enig, PhD, a biochemist and strong advocate of virgin coconut oil, says that the body uses coconut oil to produce monolaurin, a disease-fighting compound. She also cites the need for saturated fat in our diets to balance HDL/LDL cholesterol. But according to the Mayo Clinic, coconut oil contains more saturated fat than do butter and lard, so it's hard for me to see how the benefits outweigh the risks here.

Add to that the fact that everything you cook tastes like suntan lotion and that we have other options for healthy oils and, for me, coconut oil is off the table.

There are a lot of oils and fats on the market. It can make you crazy. From canola to sunflower and safflower to nut oils, peanut oil, soy oil, grapeseed oil, flax oil, hemp oil, and others; for me, I have narrowed my options to include extra-virgin olive oil, avocado oil, and a wee bit of Earth Balance. I know what I am getting with each of them and I know my results.

Feel free to experiment, but don't get trapped in all the confusion around fat. There are three kinds of fat: saturated, monounsaturated, and polyunsaturated. Saturated fats (carbon atoms are saturated with hydrogen atoms), like those found in high concentrations in animal food, are very stable under heat and challenging to digest, so they build up in the body and result in obesity. Polyunsaturated fats (long carbon chains with many double bonds unsaturated with hydrogen atoms), like sesame seed, safflower, canola, sunflower, and corn oil, are very easy to digest but are not so stable under heat, so we need to use these oils carefully in cooking. Monounsaturated fats (long chains of carbon with only one unsaturated double bond), like extra-virgin olive oil and avocado oil (along with peanut and other nut oils), are stable under heat, and that one little break in the molecular chain makes them easier on digestion. "Monos" are a win/win for your health.

My advice? Keep it simple with the oils you choose and work with what you know is healthy and will give you glorious flavor and texture.

SUGAR

We all know that sugar has been implicated in all manner of ills, including diabetes and obesity. It messes with our blood chemistry, resulting in a roller coaster of energy throughout our days. There are indications that it exacerbates the symptoms of conditions from ADD-ADHD to autism. Yet, many will agree that sugar is glorious—and it's natural. So what's the problem?

We eat too much of it.

The truth is that refined sugar is addictive. It is quickly digested, landing in your bloodstream, altering your blood sugar on impact, so to speak. You get that sensational sugar rush, followed by the inevitable crash. You need more sugar, and the cycle of disaster has begun. And marketers cash in big on this one.

With 194 calories in three tablespoons (¼ cup), the calories alone make sugar bad news, but it's the unbridled consumption of sugar that makes the story so scary. The average American eats about 156 pounds of sugar each year, more than 700 calories every day—and that's just from sugar. High-fructose corn syrup is consumed at a rate of about sixty-three pounds per person on average. See where this is going?

Not only calorically devastating to any healthy life, sugar also robs the blood of minerals, the bones of calcium, and suppresses immune function, making you tired, lethargic, and more likely to get and stay sick.

But here is where it gets tough. Sugar and high-fructose corn syrup are hard to eat in moderation. And not because they are both so yummily sweet. They are in just about everything we eat, from soda and sweets to salad dressing, bread to tomato sauce, salsa to canned vegetables. Now I am not absolving us from all responsibility here. It's not a case of "the big marketers made me do it." But we are fighting an uphill battle, and it takes will and ingenuity to beat these guys at a game designed to have only one winner . . . them.

In 1970, the average American was consuming a modest half pound of high-fructose corn syrup in a year. The food industry made a conscious choice to substitute this cheaper sweetener for sugar. It's twice as sweet (and addicting, in my view) and has a long shelf life. Plus, the one thing we can produce in this country is corn. According to Greg Critser, author of *Fat Land: How Americans Became the Fattest People in the World*, the federal government set this into motion with policies that led to a glut of corn in the '70s, which led to the invention and production of high-fructose corn syrup. So now manufacturers could increase the size and amount of sweet foods and drinks along with their profits while they robbed you of your health.

The Corn Refiners Association is changing the name of high-fructose corn syrup to "corn sugar" in an attempt to rid themselves of the stench that comes with the manufacture and use of this product. They are trying to convince the public that the body reacts to corn syrup in the same way it does to sugar. "Corn sugar or cane sugar; your body can't tell the difference" is their sell-tag. But that's not exactly the truth.

Certainly, calorically, these two sweeteners are similar. But that's where it ends. Most medical experts agree that fructose is processed by the liver, unlike sucrose and glucose. It adds an additional burden on this much over-worked gland and changes the way metabolic-regulating hormones function, resulting in the release of more fat into the bloodstream (which raises triglycerides, among other things).

What to do?

There are other choices to make for sweet living. *Brown rice syrup* and *barley malt* top my list, as they are complex carbohydrate sugars, meaning that they digest slowly and don't lead to sugar highs and lows or insulin resistance. *Honey, maple syrup*, and *fruit juice* are all better for you than sugar (organic or not, raw or not), but they are largely simple sugars, so they digest quickly and make you crave more sugar.

Of these, brown rice syrup is my personal favorite and the one you will see used most often in my recipes. Its butterscotch flavor is delicate, it's about half as sweet as sugar, and it works just great in most of the desserts I make. It has about 170 calories in that same quarter cup, so you need to be careful to control your intake. Just because it's healthy doesn't mean it has no calories. I got myself into trouble with too many desserts and I was making them from all the right ingredients.

Let's look at some other options.

Coconut sugar is a great option when only a granular sweetener will do.

Agave rose to fame quickly as a result of its popularity in the raw cuisine movement and its claim that it's a low-glycemic sweetener. While it's natural, just cooked down syrup from the agave cactus, the processing results in a sweetener that's about 80 percent fructose . . . higher than high-fructose corn syrup (which comes in at about 55 percent fructose). Yikes, right? It is very sweet and has a runny liquid texture. Used in small amounts, it's not likely to damage your health. It's natural, not invented, so that's an advantage, but that level of fructose will result in an overworked liver and weight gain pretty quickly. So think about it before you use it.

Stevia is an intensely sweet herb whose leaves are ground and powdered for use. Indigenous to South America, stevia is a great choice when looking for a natural, no-calorie sweetener. It's safe for diabetics and works well in baking. One teaspoon is equal to three cups of sugar in terms of sweet flavor. I don't know about you, but that is just too sweet for me. Should you decide that stevia is your choice, you can cook with it, bake with it, stir it into your tea. You will need to play with your recipes to see about the amount to use. My experience has been that about a tablespoon of stevia is worth about a cup of sugar. It has an odd sweet aftertaste that takes some getting used to, but it's a great choice when you are watching your weight or controlling diabetes.

Erythritol is a polyol or sugar alcohol that is a natural sweetener made by fermenting naturally occurring plant sugars. While there are several polyol-type sweeteners on the market, this one has the best flavor, in my opinion. Unlike some of the other polyols, erythritol is absorbed into the bloodstream in the small intestine, but it is quickly excreted in the urine, so it does not affect blood chemistry at all, nor does it create any stomach distress unless eaten in substantive amounts.

With about 80 percent of the sweetness level of sugar, erythritol behaves in cooking and baking much as sugar does, but because it is not absorbed, it has no caloric effect on you. There are some little quirks I have learned in cooking with it to ensure that there is no grainy texture in the final dessert, but that is a small thing compared to how well it does the job of sweetening with no compromise to your health or waistline. I have done a lot of research on this because it seemed to be too good to be true. I have not found any bad news, so I am hopeful that I have found a no-calorie sweetener that is safe for diabetics and has a pleasant flavor as well.

As I previously stated, I am a fan of **brown rice syrup**. It's glucose based, with a high percentage of complex carbs in its makeup. Yes, there are calories, but the desserts you make with rice syrup are sweetly satisfying and won't spike your blood sugar, so you are less likely to binge. How sweet is that?

You will need to play with it in recipes because it is a liquid sweetener and it will affect the texture of your batter and dough, but after trying out some of the recipes in this book, you will have no trouble adapting any recipe to be sweetly healthy.

SALT

In a word, table salt will kill you and has no place in your life. Use a white, unrefined sea salt for daily use and you will create better-tasting food with no impact on your cardiovascular health.

There are other salt options, like pink **Himalayan salt**, which is fabulous and healthy, but **white unrefined sea salt** is the most compatible with your blood chemistry and what I recommend for daily use in cooking—never at the table, just in cooking to create flavor.

You can also use *miso* and *soy sauce* in cooking when you are looking for an Asian flair in a recipe. These fermented products provide the salt you need to bring out the flavor in a dish, but also aid in digestion by way of being fermented.

MEAT

There is no real substitute for meat. It sucks. But it's time to get it out of your life. There are so many yummy options, you won't miss meat or all the health-compromising stuff that goes with it. I don't care what Michael Pollan says (as much as I love him) about needing to keep the farmers in business. They can grow other things, like veggies and fruit.

Use beans, tofu, tempeh, and seitan to give your body the protein it needs to grow big and strong.

These basic substitutions should be enough for you to begin to experiment. So pull out the shoebox of Grandma's recipes, and let's adapt them.

RECIPE ADAPTATION

Making healthy versions of your favorite foods can be easy but sometimes a little tricky. Many recipes are just fabulous once they have been tweaked, and some of them, well, not so much—or they require too many processed foods. Some recipes are impossible to re-create, and some products simply don't have direct substitutions. So pick your battles and start easy. You will be experimenting, so be prepared for some disappointments as well as soaring successes.

To adapt any recipe, you must first know how to make the original recipe.

It's hard to know what you are going for if you have never gone for it before. It's important that you master something so you understand it, and then you can play with the ingredients to alter the original recipe.

Do some research to discover what the various ingredients do in the recipe. Once you know this, you can figure out how and what can be altered to yield a delicious result. Some things can't be changed or removed successfully, and some things can be changed and yield a different result, but one that is no less delicious. So you have choices.

When adapting a complex recipe, change one or two things at a time and see how it works out. If you change too many things at once and you are unhappy with the results, then you won't know what worked and what didn't.

Look at other recipes and how the ingredients work. There are combinations that are matches made in heaven, and then there are those that will have you scratching your head and wondering what you were thinking. For instance, chocolate goes brilliantly well with coffee and/or cinnamon, but not so well with lemon or lime. Orange flavor, yes, but not other citrus. Looking at other successful recipes will help you adapt and invent with ease.

Look at adaptations of recipes that already exist. When I searched for how to adapt a recipe to be vegetarian, 141,000 results popped onto my laptop screen. And vegetarian websites that give great advice? Thirteen million results. Vegan cooking? More than 615,000. The point is that there are lots of websites offering advice on how to adapt a not-so-healthy recipe to be good for you. You don't have to reinvent the wheel here. With the abundant advice you will find online and the tips from this book, you will be converting recipes faster than your loved ones can feast on them.

And finally, don't be attached to the original recipe. It's unlikely that your adaptation will turn out exactly like the original. The point is not to re-create the original recipe, but to adapt it to be familiar enough. If you are thinking you'll get results just like Mama used to make, then why adapt? A lot of those recipes are how and why we got into trouble in the first place. Adapting makes the transition to eating a diet of whole unprocessed foods fun, comfortable, accessible, and in many cases more delicious (in a different way) than the original version.

So have some fun and allow yourself to be surprised and delighted at the outcome.

PART SIX

The Recipes

I t's time to cook. This section of the book is divided into two parts. The first is dedicated to making over some of America's favorite main courses to be healthy, and the second places the focus on simple, healthy recipes that will help you expand your repertoire as your tastes change and your skills sharpen. In the previous section of the book I've provided lots of information about substitutions and adapting recipes in general, so if you skipped right to this part of the book, do yourself a favor and read Part 5, "Recipes Just Like Mama Used to Make, Only Healthier."

In the makeover section, I have made over lots of America's favorite foods, from burgers to pizza, and paired them up with other recipes in the book to create balanced, nutritious meals. I know it's a big thing to make one-dish meals. Rachael Ray has built an empire on making dinner in one skillet. I think it's really hard to get variety—in ingredients, tastes, and textures—and I think it's boring at best. It's more challenging to create meals with the visual appeal you want in order to convert your family without a hassle. But that's me.

Throughout the recipes, I've included items like canned organic beans, tofu, tempeh, and other naturally convenient foods. While all the ingredients may not be familiar to you, you can get each and every one of them in a supermarket. Even tofu and tempeh, both soy foods, and seitan, packed with nutrients, versatile in recipes, and fast and easy—oh, and yummy—have found their way into mainstream consciousness and onto supermarket shelves.

These recipes are designed to set your feet on the path of healthy eating without breaking a sweat. With a combination of freshly cooked foods and some healthy prepared or convenience foods, these dishes will help you gain confidence, win over your family, and move you forward to slowing down, enjoying time in the kitchen, and cooking from scratch.

About Nutritional Analysis

This book is intended to inspire you to reconnect with real food and turn away from the processed junk food that is threatening the collective health of our modern world.

You may wonder why I have not included nutritional analyses for these recipes. By virtue of being plant-based dishes, you have little to worry about in terms of excesses. And my own view is that the standard nutritional information only tells us the bad news, painting a negative picture of an otherwise healthy recipe. They do not, for example, tell you how much vitamin C or carotenoids or polyphenols exist in a dish; only the calories, fat, and carbs. Of course, there are some ingredients, such as oils, that are dense in calories, but for the most part these are used sparingly. And you will use your own common sense to determine what is best for you and your needs. I want these recipes to free you to create delicious healthy meals, not create more neuroses around food.

A plant-based diet is naturally low in fat, less calorically dense, and incredibly nutrient-rich. Eating this way will allow your body to settle into its perfect weight, and you will enjoy robust health.

14

Main Course Makeovers

In this chapter, we'll look at some of America's favorite foods. With a few tweaks and by substituting healthier ingredients for the ones that don't serve us, they turn into powerhouses of nutrition that won't steal your vitality.

Using some of the tips and techniques from Chapter 13, you will see how easily you can adapt a recipe to be healthier without losing the familiar feel and flavor you love.

I hope you use these recipes as a springboard to adapting your own family favorites to be healthier versions of the foods they love.

MAC AND CHEESE

There are lots of vegan recipes for mac and cheese, but a lot of them have ingredients that I don't really like. They're complicated, and the results make the dish seem unfamiliar. In this version, the techniques are the same, but the ingredients are healthier and just as delicious.

Makes 4–5 servings

3 tablespoons vegan buttery spread (Earth Balance)

2 tablespoons whole-wheat pastry flour

1 (8-ounce) package shredded vegan mozzarella (Daiya)

2 cups unsweetened almond milk

Sea salt

1 tablespoon garlic powder

1 tablespoon paprika

1 tablespoon turmeric

Cracked black pepper

1 pound elbow macaroni

Topping

2 tablespoons vegan buttery spread (Earth Balance)

½ cup whole-wheat bread crumbs

½ cup almond meal

Preheat oven to 350°F and bring a pot of water to a boil with a generous pinch of salt.

Place vegan spread in an oven-proof Dutch oven over medium heat. As the spread melts, stir in flour, vegan cheese, and almond milk. Whisk into a smooth paste. Season to taste with sea salt and whisk in garlic powder, paprika, turmeric, and black pepper to taste. Whisk very well.

While the sauce cooks and when the water boils, cook macaroni until about 80 percent done. Stir pasta into sauce, mixing gently to coat evenly. Pour into casserole dish.

In a small saucepan, melt vegan spread and mix in bread crumbs and almond meal. Top the macaroni mixture with the bread crumb mixture and bake for 30–35 minutes, until the cheese is bubbling and the topping is browned.

Serve this family-friendly dish with Crisp Watercress Salad for a grown-up dinner, with French Fries for the kids (made from the recipe in this book, of course), and Berry Crumble for a sweet ending for everyone.

PORTOBELLO BURGERS WITH GUACAMOLE

These decadent burgers have none of the saturated fat of meat but all the "meaty" goodness of a burger and will have even the most committed carnivores coming back for more. And the guacamole adds omega-3, so these fun burgers become powerhouses of nutrition.

Makes 4 servings

Extra-virgin olive oil

4 medium Portobello mushrooms, stems
removed

1 red onion, thinly sliced into half-
moons, from top to bottom

3 cloves fresh garlic, minced

Sea salt

Cracked black pepper

Balsamic vinegar

Guacamole

2 avocados, halved, pits removed,
mashed

2 plum tomatoes, diced

Juice of ½ fresh lemon

Generous pinch chili powder

4 whole-grain burger buns, lightly
toasted

4 romaine lettuce leaves

2 large tomatoes, cut into thick slices

Brush mushrooms with oil and sprinkle lightly with salt and pepper. Heat a large skillet over medium heat. Lay mushrooms in the hot skillet and cook until tender, about 4 minutes per side. Transfer to a plate, cavity side up, and cover lightly with foil to keep warm.

In the same skillet, place a small amount of oil, onions, and garlic over medium heat. When the onions sizzle, add a pinch of salt and pepper and sauté until soft, about 5 minutes.

While the onions cook, make the guacamole. Combine the mashed avocado with tomatoes, lemon juice, and chili powder with salt to taste.

Spread the guacamole on the bottom half of each burger bun. Lay a slice of lettuce on the guacamole, add a tomato slice and then the Portobello. Lay the top half of the bun on top. Serve immediately.

Serve these burgers with Crunchy Tuscan Kale Salad to add some crispy texture and plenty of antioxidants.

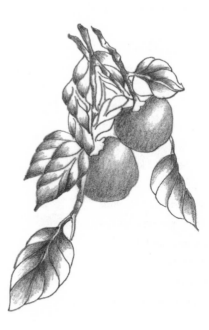

SPICY BLACK BEAN BURGERS

There's something wonderfully meaty and satisfying about a burger made from beans. And the spice in these babies is just the ticket to getting meat off the table without much of a fuss. The lack of saturated fat and the density of nutrients make these burgers the perfect entrée.

Makes 4 burgers

1 (15-ounce) can of black turtle beans, drained and rinsed well

½ red onion, finely diced

3 cloves fresh garlic, crushed

1 teaspoon hot sauce

½ red bell pepper, roasted, peeled, and diced

½ teaspoon cayenne pepper

½ cup silken tofu, pureed

Sea salt

Cracked black pepper

1 cup whole-wheat bread crumbs

Avocado oil for frying

Romaine lettuce leaves for serving

2 tomatoes, diced

3 sprigs fresh flat-leaf parsley, coarsely chopped

1 tablespoon extra-virgin olive oil

Mash the beans with a fork in a large bowl and mix in onions, garlic, hot sauce, red pepper, cayenne, tofu, and salt and pepper to taste. Fold in bread crumbs in small amounts to hold the burgers together (you may not need the whole cup). As soon as the burger mixture holds together, stop adding bread crumbs or the burgers will be too dry. Form the bean mixture into thick patties.

Heat about ½ inch oil in a deep skillet and fry the patties until firm, about 4 minutes on each side. You can also grill them over medium heat on a gas grill.

To serve, arrange lettuce leaves on plates with the burger in the middle of the leaf. Mix together the tomatoes, parsley, and olive oil. Mound the tomato mixture in the center of each burger and serve.

◆ **Note**

You can also serve these in the traditional manner on a bun with the usual condiments.

◆ **Serving Suggestion**

I love to serve these burgers with Sweet Potato Chips and the Mother of All Tomato Salads for the perfect balance of textures, colors, and nutrients.

PINTO BEAN AND MUSHROOM BURGERS WITH SALSA

I love serving these burgers at parties. They're richly flavored and have a great texture. They have a nice density without being heavy. I love them. They are really burger-y with no saturated fat.

Makes 4 full-size burgers or 8 miniature burgers

2 tablespoons extra-virgin olive oil

1 red onion, diced

3 cloves fresh garlic, crushed

4–5 whole green onions, coarsely chopped

Sea salt

Cracked black pepper

½ teaspoon ground cumin

½ teaspoon paprika

½ teaspoon chili powder

1 cup coarsely chopped fresh mushrooms

1 (15-ounce) can pinto beans, drained and rinsed well

3–4 sprigs fresh basil, leaves removed, finely minced

Avocado oil

4 whole-wheat pita breads, split open

Dijon mustard

Romaine lettuce leaves

2 tomatoes, cut into slices

Handful of broccoli sprouts (optional)

Place oil, red onion, and garlic in a deep skillet over medium heat. When the onions begin to sizzle, add the green onions and a pinch of salt and pepper and sauté for 2–3 minutes. Add cumin, paprika, chili powder, chopped mushrooms, and another pinch of salt and sauté until the mushrooms are tender, about 5 minutes. Transfer to a mixing bowl and set aside.

Mash the beans with a fork or potato masher until well smashed. Stir into the mushroom mixture and add basil and salt and pepper to taste. Mix very well.

Form the mixture into patties that are traditional burger-size. Heat about ¼ inch oil in a deep skillet and fry the burgers for 4 minutes on each side, turning once to ensure even browning.

To serve, split pita breads and spread one side with mustard. Lay lettuce leaves and a tomato slice in each pita. Slide the burger into the pita, top with sprouts, and serve.

These elegant burgers make a great lunch or brunch main course when served with refreshing Cucumber Salad . . . and a Sweet Almond Chocolate Milkshake for fun (made from the recipes in this book, of course).

PASTA POMODORO

You wouldn't think that pasta with tomato sauce could be unhealthy, but have you read what's in some of those jars of sauce you buy? Sugar, additives, and other stuff Mother Nature would frown upon . . . once you make this easy recipe, you'll never buy it again.

Makes 5–6 servings

Extra-virgin olive oil

1 small red onion, diced

2 cloves fresh garlic, crushed

Sea salt

½ cup dry white wine (optional)

Cracked black pepper

2 cups crushed tomatoes

1 cup tomato puree

2 tablespoons tomato paste

Spring or filtered water

1 carrot, left whole

3–4 sprigs fresh basil, leaves removed,
    coarsely chopped

1 pound spaghetti

Bring a pot of water to a boil with a generous pinch of salt.

While the water boils, make the sauce. Place a small amount of oil, along with onion and garlic, in a saucepan over medium heat. When the onions begin to sizzle, add a pinch of salt and sauté for 1–2 minutes. Add wine, if using, and a pinch of black pepper. Stir in crushed tomatoes, tomato puree, and tomato paste. Add 1 cup water and season to taste with salt and pepper. Submerge the carrot in the sauce. Cover and cook over low heat until the pasta is cooked.

When the water boils, cook the spaghetti al dente, 8–9 minutes, and drain. When the pasta is ready, remove the carrot from the sauce (it helps reduce the acidity of the quickly cooked tomato sauce) and discard. Transfer the pasta directly into the sauce and stir well to coat the pasta. Transfer to a serving platter and garnish with fresh basil. Serve hot.

I am not a fan of serving just a big bowl of pasta for dinner. I feel the meal needs more balance. In my house, I serve it with Italian Lentil Soup and Bitter Green Salad with Sweet Orange Dressing to strike a perfect balance.

CHICKPEA CUTLETS

Who would think chickpeas could create meaty patties? The carnivores in your life won't miss the meat, and the veg heads will love you because they are not weirdly meaty but have a great texture. High in fiber, protein, vitamins, and minerals, these make a great main course.

Makes 4 patties

1 cup cooked or canned organic
   chickpeas

2 tablespoons avocado oil, plus more for
   pan-frying

½ cup high-gluten flour

½–¾ cup whole-wheat bread crumbs

Spring or filtered water

2 cloves fresh garlic, crushed

½ red onion, finely minced

1–2 tablespoons soy sauce

½ teaspoon smoked paprika

¼ teaspoon rubbed, dried sage

Cornmeal, for breading

Place chickpeas and 2 tablespoons oil in a mixing bowl and mash to form a creamy texture and break the beans. Stir in flour and bread crumbs. Slowly add water, mixing, until a stiff texture forms. Knead for 2 minutes to activate gluten. Fold in garlic, onion, soy sauce to taste, paprika, and sage.

Form the mixture into 4 patties and dredge them in cornmeal.

Heat a generous amount of oil in a flat-bottomed skillet. When the oil is hot, pan-fry the patties, turning them once to ensure even browning and a crisp crust at the edges, 6–7 minutes per side. Turn them when the edges are browned and the patties are firm. Drain on paper and serve.

◆ **Note**

High-gluten flour can be purchased in natural food stores or online at Bob's Red Mill.

◆ **Variations**

You can also bake these if you do not want to fry, but they are not as satisfying. You simply brush the patties with oil and bake at 375°F for 20 minutes; flip and bake 8–10 minutes on the other side.

You may also use sweet paprika, but the smoked imparts a flavor you will love.

◆ **Serving Suggestion**

I serve these cutlets with Braised Asparagus and Baby Carrots and Crispy Potatoes for an elegant but simple supper.

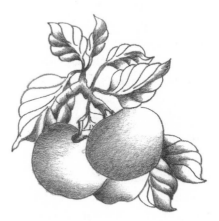

WISE GUY CHILI

My Uncle Ralph, a true wise guy, used to make the best chili. And served with my aunt Laura's home-baked bread, it was the "hit" of the "family." My vegan version is just as spicy as Uncle Ralph's but won't shorten your lifespan, since it has no saturated fat to clog your arteries.

Makes 3–4 servings

Extra-virgin olive oil

3 cloves fresh garlic, minced

1 red onion, diced

Sea salt

3–4 teaspoons chili powder (or to your taste)

Scant pinch smoked paprika

1 stalk celery, diced

1 small can chopped green chiles

1 (32-ounce) can diced tomatoes

2 tablespoons tomato paste

2 squares dark chocolate (non-dairy), coarsely chopped

½ cup quinoa, rinsed well

1 cup dried pinto or borlotti beans, rinsed well

1 bay leaf

Spring or filtered water

Cracked black pepper

2–3 sprigs fresh flat-leaf parsley, coarsely chopped

Place a small amount of oil along with garlic and onion in a soup pot over medium heat. When the onion begins to sizzle, season with a pinch of salt, chili powder to taste (it gets hotter as it cooks), and paprika and sauté for 2–3 minutes. Stir in celery and a pinch of salt and sauté for 1 minute. Add chiles, tomatoes, tomato paste, and chocolate and stir well. Add quinoa, beans, bay leaf, and 3 cups of water. Cover and bring to a boil. Reduce heat to low and cook for 1 hour or until the beans are soft. Season to taste with salt and pepper and simmer for 3–4 minutes more. Remove bay leaf and serve garnished with fresh parsley.

This chili is perfect served with Raw Beet and Pear Salad. The cool nature of the salad helps us manage the heat of the chili and adds some light, crisp texture to the meal.

VEG HEAD POTPIE

Loaded with antioxidants and none of the ingredients we don't want, like saturated fats, hormones, or steroids found in meat, this truly is comfort food. If your family isn't wild about veggies, then this is the recipe for you. Who can resist veggies topped with a flaky crust in their own individual cup?

Makes 3–4 servings

Crust

1¼ cups whole-wheat pastry flour

Pinch sea salt

⅓ cup avocado oil or vegan buttery
    spread (Earth Balance)
Cold spring or filtered water

Filling
2 cups spring or filtered water
4–6 small new or fingerling potatoes,
    unpeeled and diced
½ head cauliflower, broken into small
    florets
4 medium carrots, diced
1 zucchini, diced
½ cup frozen corn
2 slices packaged baked tofu
⅓ cup whole-wheat pastry flour
Sea salt
Cracked black pepper
Generous pinch rubbed, dried sage
Generous pinch cumin

Preheat oven to 425°F and lightly oil four 10- to 11-ounce ramekins, including the top rim.

To make the crust, combine flour with salt and cut in oil with a fork to create the texture of wet sand. Slowly add water to create a crust dough that just holds together. Knead a couple of times; gather into a ball and wrap in plastic. Set aside while preparing vegetables.

Bring water to a boil and cook potatoes for 5–6 minutes. Remove with a slotted spoon and transfer to a mixing bowl. In the same water, cook cauliflower for 4–5 minutes. Remove with a slotted spoon and transfer to the bowl

with potatoes. In the same water, cook carrots for 3–4 minutes. Drain, reserving the broth, and transfer the carrots to the bowl with the potatoes and cauliflower. Gently stir in zucchini, corn, and baked tofu. Set aside.

Place broth on low heat. Combine flour with salt and pepper to taste, sage, and cumin. Whisk flour mixture into broth and cook, whisking constantly until it thickens, about 3–4 minutes. Pour thickened broth over vegetables and mix gently to combine. Spoon vegetables evenly into ramekins.

Divide the crust into 4 equal pieces and roll them out to be slightly bigger than the ramekins. Lay a crust over the top of each filled ramekin and pleat the outer edges of the crust. Make 4 small slits in the crust to allow steam to escape.

Place ramekins on a baking sheet and bake until the crust is golden brown and the filling is bubbling, about 25 minutes. Serve hot.

◆ **Note**
You can purchase ready-made whole-wheat piecrusts and cut them into the sizes needed for these individual potpies or use the crust as they are to create full-size pies.

◆ **Serving Suggestion**
This is such a warming dish. I love to serve it with Corn Chowder and

Italian-Style Greens to bring some vitality to all this calming comfort.

SO-O-O-O EASY PIZZA

Everyone thinks the fastest way to get pizza is to call Domino's, but once you have made this recipe and see how easily it comes together, you'll toss the take-out menus in the recycle bin . . . where they belong. No more compromised ingredients for you.

Makes 6–8 servings

Dough
1 tablespoon active dry yeast
½ cup lukewarm water
1 teaspoon sea salt
2 tablespoons extra-virgin olive oil
1 cup whole-wheat pastry flour
¼ cup semolina flour

Topping
1 recipe Pasta Pomodoro sauce
  (see page 216)
2 cups shredded vegan mozzarella
  (Daiya or Follow Your Heart)
10–12 fresh cherry tomatoes, halved
2–3 sprigs fresh basil, leaves removed,
  left whole

Preheat oven to 425°F. Mix yeast with warm water until it dissolves. Set aside for 2–3 minutes. Stir in salt and oil. Mix in flours to form a soft dough. Roll out dough and transfer to a lightly oiled pizza tin or to a lightly floured pizza stone. Bake for 5 minutes. Remove from oven and spread sauce over the surface of the pizza, leaving about half an inch around the rim exposed. Add vegan cheese and return to the oven to bake for 15–20 minutes, until the crust is browned and firm.

Remove the pizza from the oven and sprinkle with fresh cherry tomatoes and basil leaves. Serve hot.

◆ **Note**
You may vary the toppings to your taste: onions, peppers, mushrooms, etc.

◆ **Serving Suggestions**
I like to make sure we are always getting some lovely veggies, so I serve this with Decadent Greens and Beans with the Best Chocolate Chunk Cookies as a real treat.

TEMPEH REUBEN

The key to a good reuben is the thousand island dressing, in my view, anyway. A traditional reuben is loaded with meat and cheese, but it's really the oozy dressing we love so much . . . in this vegan version,

you'll whip up a creamy dressing in no time with none of the stuff in the bottled versions that you might not want.
Makes 2 sandwiches

Dressing
1 cup vegan mayonnaise (Vegenaise)
⅓ cup natural ketchup (no sugar or artificial additives)
½ teaspoon garlic powder
½ teaspoon onion powder
Generous pinch sea salt
3 tablespoons natural sweet pickle relish

Reuben
Avocado oil
8-ounce tempeh block, sliced in half and then in half thicknesses, making 4 pieces
4 slices whole-grain rye bread
2 slices vegan Swiss cheese
2–3 tablespoons natural sauerkraut

Make the dressing, adjusting seasonings to your taste. Set aside.

Place oil in a skillet to cover the bottom of the pan. Lay tempeh slices in the oil over medium heat and cook until browned, about 4 minutes. Turn and brown on the other side, about 4 minutes. Transfer to a plate. In the same skillet, lay the bread slices with the cheese on 2 of them. Allow the cheese to melt as the bread toasts.

Remove the bread from the skillet and spread with dressing. Place 2 pieces of tempeh on top of the cheese.

Spoon sauerkraut on top of the tempeh. Lay bread with melted cheese on top to close the sandwich. Slice diagonally and serve hot.

◆ **Serving Suggestions**
I like to serve this as a perfect lunch or brunch with Instant Veggie Soup and Simple Steamed Greens to strike the right balance of richness and simplicity.

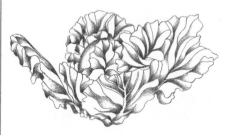

PHILLY "CHEESESTEAK"

"Wit or Witout" is the phrase most associated with Philly cheesesteaks, and refers to with or without onions. My version is "witout" meat and "witout" Cheese Whiz (God forbid)—no saturated fat or compromised ingredients but "wit" all the flavor and texture you love.

Makes 4 sandwiches

Extra-virgin olive oil
1 red onion, thinly sliced into half-
    moons, from top to bottom
Sea salt
3 roasted red peppers, thinly sliced
1-pound package seitan, shredded
4 whole-grain hoagie rolls, split
    lengthwise
1 (8-ounce) package shredded vegan
    cheese (Daiya)
Almond or soy milk

Place a small amount of oil in a skillet over medium heat. Sauté onion with a pinch of salt until wilted, about 2 minutes. Stir in roasted red peppers, season with salt to taste, and sauté for 2 minutes more. Transfer to a bowl and wipe out skillet.

Place a small amount of oil in the same skillet. Sauté seitan, with a light seasoning of salt until browned, about 4 minutes. Transfer to a plate and wipe out skillet one more time.

Lay rolls, cut side down, in the oily skillet and cook over medium-low heat until the bread browns lightly. Remove from skillet.

While the rolls brown, make the sauce. Place cheese, enough milk to cover, and salt to taste in small saucepan and cook, whisking, until cheese is melted and the sauce is thick and creamy.

To assemble, lay rolls open, mound seitan, pepper, and onion on each and spoon cheese sauce over top.

◆ **Serving Suggestions**
I know, I know: cheesesteaks go with cheese fries, but to make for a healthier meal, I serve this sandwich with Crunchy Tuscan Kale Salad.

GRILLED CHEESE SANDWICH

When I was a kid, the only meal my mother could be sure I would eat was a grilled cheese sandwich. In this version, whole-grain bread and vegan cheese do the job deliciously.

Makes 2 sandwiches

4 slices whole-grain bread
Vegan buttery spread (Earth Balance)
4 slices vegan cheese (mozzarella)
4 slices ripe tomatoes

Preheat a lightly oiled skillet or griddle pan over low heat.

Lay two slices of bread on a dry work surface and lightly spread both sides of the slices with buttery spread. Arrange two slices of cheese on the bread and top with two slices of tomato. Lightly cover the remaining bread with buttery spread on both sides and press onto the cheese and tomatoes. Lay the two sandwiches in the skillet and press down firmly with a spatula. Allow to grill until lightly browned, 2–3 minutes. Turn sandwiches and press with spatula again and cook until lightly browned, 2–3 minutes. Remove from pan, slice in half diagonally, and serve immediately.

◆ **Serving Suggestions**

The perfect sandwich needs the perfect soup to go with it, so serve this with the Quickest Tomato Soup and Hot Fudge Sundaes to bring back all the nostalgia of childhood with grown-up dishes.

BEEFCAKE STEW

My dad was a butcher, so when I was growing up, our dinner table was all about meat. Not cool for me, but I did love the veggies—the potatoes, the tomatoes (we're Italian; there were tomatoes in everything!)—in the beef stew. There's no beef (so no saturated fat, growth hormones, or steroids) in this version, but it will make you look and feel like a pinup.

Makes 3–4 servings

1 pound seitan, cut into 1-inch cubes
⅓ cup arrowroot
Sea salt
Cracked black pepper
3 tablespoons extra-virgin olive oil
3 red onions, quartered
4 carrots, chunk cut
2 parsnips, chunk cut
1 large (16-ounce) can diced tomatoes
2 bay leaves
Spring or filtered water
4 medium Yukon gold potatoes, cubed
1 cup frozen peas

Cube seitan. Combine arrowroot with a generous pinch of salt and pepper. Dredge seitan in arrowroot mixture and set aside.

Heat oil in a heavy pot and pan-fry seitan pieces until the coating is crispy, about 5 minutes. Add onions, carrots, parsnips, tomatoes, and bay leaves. Season lightly with salt and pepper and add water to almost cover ingredients. Bring to a boil, cover, reduce heat to low, and cook for 20 minutes. Add potatoes, adjust seasonings to your taste, and cook until potatoes are tender, about 20 minutes more. Add more water, if needed, to keep a stewlike consistency. Remove bay leaves, stir in peas, and cook 5 minutes more. Stir gently to combine and serve hot.

This is a hearty stew, so I lighten the meal by serving it with Sautéed Zucchini Crostini and Marinated Eggplant Bruschetta to add a few more veggies to the meal.

EGGLESS SALAD

If you have your doubts about tofu, then this is the recipe for you. With the texture of egg salad and all the flavor you expect, well, you could become a convert in no time. Your heart will thank you!

Makes 3–4 servings

1 pound extra-firm tofu, hand-crumbled
2 roasted red bell peppers, diced
2 stalks celery, diced
1 small carrot, shredded
4 whole green onions, diced
½ cup vegan mayonnaise (Vegenaise)
2–3 sprigs fresh flat-leaf parsley, finely
   chopped
1 teaspoon garlic powder
¼ teaspoon turmeric
1 tablespoon Dijon mustard
1 teaspoon sea salt
½ teaspoon cracked black pepper

Combine tofu with peppers, celery, carrot, and green onions.

Make the dressing by mixing mayo, parsley, garlic powder, turmeric, mustard, salt, and pepper. Adjust seasonings to taste. Stir into tofu mixture to combine. Chill completely before serving on bread or crackers.

◆ **Serving Suggestions**

This is the perfect lunch at home or as a brown bag. I like to serve this with Broccoli Pâté and baby carrot sticks on the side.

LIGHT-AS-AIR PANCAKES

My husband's simple recipe has pleased every guest, every child, every Doubting Thomas in our lives. Made from whole-grain flours so there's some fiber, no eggs or sugar, these pancakes are as healthy as they are delicious.

Makes 12 pancakes

1 cup whole-wheat pastry flour
1 teaspoon baking powder
Pinch sea salt
¾–1 cup unsweetened almond milk
1 teaspoon red wine vinegar
1 tablespoon extra-virgin olive or
   avocado oil

Whisk dry ingredients very briskly, for about a minute. Whisk wet ingredients, blending well.

Mix wet ingredients into dry, whisking briskly for 1 minute, adding more almond milk, if necessary, to create a spoonable batter.

Lightly oil (with olive oil) a griddle or skillet and warm over medium heat.

Spoon batter onto hot griddle by ¼ cups and cook until golden. Flip each pancake and cook until golden.

To serve, heat ⅓ cup brown rice syrup with 3 tablespoons fruit preserves or with 1 tablespoon pure maple syrup to create a maple flavor. Spoon over pancakes and serve hot.

◆ **Variation**
Use ¾ cup whole-wheat pastry flour with ¼ cup spelt flour, cornmeal, or buckwheat flour to create different versions of the basic pancake.

◆ **Serving Suggestions**
These pancakes go well with Apple and Berry–Scented Quinoa and some fresh cut seasonal fruit to create the perfect brunch.

BO-BO-BOLOGNESE SAUCE

People love meat sauce. Meat sauce doesn't love people's hearts. What are we to do? Make this easy-to-make, richly flavored sauce, and everyone's tickers and tummies will rejoice.

Makes 3–4 servings over pasta

2 tablespoons extra-virgin olive oil
2 cloves fresh garlic, minced
1 red onion, diced
Sea salt
Cracked black pepper
Generous pinch dried oregano
1 cup coarsely chopped seitan
1 (28-ounce) can crushed tomatoes
2 tablespoons tomato paste
1 bay leaf
2–3 sprigs fresh flat-leaf parsley, coarsely chopped

10 ounces whole-wheat spaghetti

Place oil, garlic, and onions in a saucepan over medium heat. When the onions begin to sizzle, add a pinch of salt and pepper and sauté for 2–3 minutes. Add oregano, seitan, tomatoes, and tomato paste. Stir well to combine. Add bay leaf, cover, reduce heat, and cook for about 15 minutes. Season to taste with salt and simmer for 5 minutes more. Remove the bay leaf.

While the sauce cooks, bring a pot of water to a boil with a generous pinch of sea salt. Cook the spaghetti al dente, 8–9 minutes. Drain and transfer right to the sauce. Mix well to combine. Stir in parsley and serve immediately.

◆ **Variation**

If your family doesn't like whole-wheat pasta, use semolina pasta.

◆ **Serving Suggestions**

Since this pasta dinner is packed with protein . . . and hearty, I like to serve it with Pronto Pomodoro and Pane as a side salad and some Sicilian Fruit Cookies to keep the Italian theme going.

FRITTATA

I know what you're thinking. How can she make a frittata without eggs? No saturated fat, all the antioxidants and essential nutrients of vegetables, and the versatile protein of tofu, that's how.

Makes 4–5 servings

¼ cup extra-virgin olive oil

2 cloves fresh garlic, thinly sliced

1 small red onion, thinly sliced into half-moons, from top to bottom

1 small zucchini, diced

2 ripe tomatoes, diced, with their seeds

1 teaspoon sea salt

½ teaspoon cracked black pepper

1 pound firm tofu

4 tablespoons sweet white miso

¼ cup unsweetened almond milk

2 cups baby spinach or baby arugula

Preheat oven to 325°F.

Use a large skillet that can go directly from stove top to oven, like cast iron. Place olive oil, garlic, and onion in the skillet over medium heat. When the onions begin to sizzle, add a pinch of salt and sauté for 2–3 minutes. Stir in zucchini and tomatoes; season with salt and pepper and stir well. Reduce heat to low and cook, stirring, for 5–7 minutes.

While the veggies cook, puree tofu with miso and almond milk in a food processor until smooth and creamy. The mixture will be thick.

Stir baby greens into veggies and fold tofu mixture into the veggies. Using a spatula, spread the mixture evenly over the pan and transfer to the oven. Bake for 40–45 minutes, until the top of the frittata is golden brown and the edges are firm. It's okay if the center is a little soft. It will firm as it cools. Slice into wedges and serve.

◆ **Serving Suggestions**

Most often served for breakfast or brunch, the frittata can be a main course for any meal. I like to serve it with Apple-Braised Greens for brunch and Lemon-Scented Brussels Sprouts with Roasted Walnuts for a simple dinner.

GENERAL TSO'S "CHICKEN"

Got a hankering for Chinese takeout? What if you could cook your favorites from column A and B with natural ingredients and not have to worry about all the chemicals, fat, salt, and sugar you know you are getting with most of it? Well, now you can. . . . I will grant you that one ingredient, yuba, is a bit exotic, but it's so worth searching for at an Asian market or in some health food stores.

Makes 4–5 servings

2 cups spring or filtered water

2 teaspoons soy sauce

2 cups yuba (dried tofu skin)

1 cup arrowroot flour

Avocado oil

3 cloves fresh garlic, thinly sliced

5–6 whole green onions, cut into 2-inch pieces

2 roasted red peppers, sliced into ribbons

2 cups snow peas, tips trimmed

Sauce

3 tablespoons soy sauce

3 tablespoons brown rice syrup

1 tablespoon red chili paste

2 tablespoons white wine or sake

2 teaspoons arrowroot flour

1–2 tablespoons brown rice vinegar

Mix water and soy sauce and warm over low heat for 1–2 minutes, until just warm. Remove from heat and soak yuba in it until soft, about 15 minutes.

Prepare the veggies while the yuba soaks.

To make the sauce, combine soy sauce, syrup, chili paste, and wine in a saucepan over low heat. When the mixture is warm, stir in arrowroot and cook, stirring until it thickens, about 3 minutes. Reduce heat to very low and allow sauce to simmer while finishing recipe.

When the yuba is soft, heat 1 inch oil in a deep skillet. While the oil heats, towel-dry the yuba so you don't get water in your oil and burn yourself. Dredge the soaked yuba in arrowroot to cover it completely. Fry until golden brown and crispy, turning once, about 4–5 minutes. Drain well on paper or a kitchen towel.

While you are frying the yuba, heat a small amount of oil in a skillet and sauté the garlic, green onions, roasted peppers, and snow peas until the snow peas are bright green and crisp-tender, about 3 minutes.

When the yuba is fried, mix it in with the veggies. Whisk rice vinegar into the sauce and gently stir sauce into yuba and veggies to coat.

◆ **Serving Suggestions**

This makes for a yummy main course over or with Forbidden Rice with

Snow Peas and Simple Steamed Greens that balance out the oil in the dish.

LASAGNETTES

Love lasagna but hate the work, the calories, the saturated fat, and the mess? Then these are for you. I adapted this recipe from my good friend Nick Stellino, whose take on Italian food is fresh and innovative.

Makes 4 servings

4–6 dry lasagna noodles
2 cups Pasta Pomodoro sauce (see page 216)
Extra-virgin olive oil
4–5 cloves fresh garlic, thinly sliced
1 medium red onion, diced
Sea salt
Generous pinch crushed red pepper flakes
1 medium carrot, diced
1–2 medium zucchini, diced
2–3 sprigs fresh basil, leaves removed, coarsely chopped
1 sprig fresh rosemary, leaves removed, coarsely chopped
½ cup white wine
Cracked black pepper
Vegan Parmesan cheese (optional)

Preheat oven to 450°F and lightly oil four 3 x 5 gratin dishes. You may also use four 4-inch ramekins.

Bring a pot of water to a boil with a generous pinch of sea salt. Cook the lasagna noodles al dente, about 8 minutes. Drain and arrange flat on a wet cutting board. When cool enough to handle, cut the pasta to fit the dishes: 4-inch squares for the ramekins or 3 x 5-inch rectangles for the gratin dishes. You will need 3 pieces of pasta per dish. Place pasta in a bowl of cold water.

Place a small amount of oil, garlic, and onion in a skillet over medium heat. When the onions begin to sizzle, add a pinch of salt and red pepper flakes and sauté for 1–2 minutes. Stir in carrot and a pinch of salt and sauté for 2 minutes. Stir in zucchini and a pinch of salt and sauté for 2 minutes. Add herbs, wine, and salt and pepper to taste. Reduce heat to low and simmer for 5–7 minutes, stirring occasionally, to reduce the wine to a syrup. Stir in half the Pomodoro Sauce and simmer for 3–5 minutes.

Assemble the lasagnettes. Spoon a small amount of Pomodoro Sauce on the bottom of each dish. Top with a sheet of pasta. Spoon 2–3 tablespoons of veggies and sauce on top. Layer pasta and veggies twice more, ending with veggies and sauce on top. Sprinkle with Parmesan, if using.

Bake for 10–15 minutes, until the edges are browned. Cool 3–5 minutes before serving.

◆ **Note**

For those of you not "all in" with being vegan, choose a grass-fed, organic Parmesan cheese for your topping.

◆ **Serving Suggestions**

Start the meal with Spring Vegetable Barley Soup and accompany the lasagnettes with Grilled Eggplant and Cannellini Beans.

CHICKPEA MCNUGGETS

Now I know you have all gone the route of the Golden Arches, but now that you know what's really in those little fried nuggets of nonsense, what's a mother to do when the kids are calling for their nugget fix? This version is all natural and crispy, and the kids in my world love it.

Makes 12 servings

½ cup unsweetened almond milk
½ teaspoon fresh lemon juice
2 cups cooked or canned organic
  chickpeas
½ cup whole-wheat bread crumbs
1–2 tablespoons Dijon mustard
2 tablespoons brown rice syrup
1 teaspoon soy sauce (use low sodium
  if cooking for kids under four
  years old)
Generous pinch garlic powder
Generous pinch rubbed, dried sage
½ cup high-gluten flour
Spring or filtered water
2 cups organic unsweetened cornflakes
½ teaspoon poultry seasoning, not
  powder

Preheat oven to 350°F and line a baking sheet with parchment paper.

Whisk almond milk and lemon juice together until bubbly. Set aside.

In a mixing bowl, mash the chickpeas with a fork, breaking the beans so they are not whole but not enough to puree them. Mix in bread crumbs, mustard, syrup, soy sauce, spices, and gluten flour. Stir in ¼ cup spring or filtered water and mix well. The gluten should form almost immediately, binding the mixture. Turn out onto a dry work surface and knead for 2–3 minutes, until gluten strands form. Gather mixture into a ball and set aside.

Place cornflakes in a bowl and crush into a coarse meal, a little more coarse than bread crumbs. Set aside.

Re-whisk almond milk and lemon juice and transfer to a shallow bowl. Pull off nugget-size pieces of the chickpea mixture. Dip in almond milk mixture to coat and then in cornflake crumbs to coat completely. Arrange nuggets on lined baking sheet. Repeat with balance of ingredients.

Bake for 10 minutes; turn the nuggets and return to the oven for 15 minutes more or until crispy. Serve hot with ketchup or mustard.

◆ **Note**

High-gluten flour can be purchased in natural food stores or online at Bob's Red Mill.

◆ **Serving Suggestions**

To make these as authentic as possible for your family, serve these babies with French Fries and a Sweet Almond Chocolate Milkshake (made from the recipes in this book, of course).

SLOPPY JOE THE VEGAN SANDWICH

There is something about a messy, meaty sandwich that has stolen America's heart . . . and health. In this version, the filling is lean, meat- and saturated-fat-free, but loaded with the taste and texture we have come to adore . . . and the nutrients we need.

Makes 4 sandwiches

2 tablespoons avocado oil
½ small red onion, finely chopped
2 cloves fresh garlic, minced
Sea salt
1 (8-ounce) package tempeh, crumbled
1 roasted red pepper, diced
¼ cup tomato sauce (no sugar added)
1 tablespoon soy sauce
2 tablespoons brown rice syrup
Scant pinch chili powder

Scant pinch cayenne pepper
¼ teaspoon celery seed
¼ teaspoon ground cumin
½ teaspoon ground coriander
½ teaspoon dried oregano
½ teaspoon sweet paprika
Sea salt
Cracked black pepper
4 whole-grain hamburger buns

Heat oil in a deep skillet over medium heat. Sauté the onion and garlic with a pinch of salt for 2–3 minutes. Stir in crumbled tempeh and cook, stirring until the tempeh begins to brown. Add peppers and sauté for 1 minute. Stir in tomato sauce, soy sauce, syrup, spices, and salt and pepper to taste. Simmer, uncovered, stirring occasionally for 10–15 minutes.

While the tempeh mixture cooks, heat a lightly oiled griddle and lay the hamburger buns, cut side down, on the hot griddle to lightly toast them.

To serve, spoon hot tempeh mixture onto buns and serve with lots of napkins.

◆ **Serving Suggestions**

I usually have these for a casual dinner with Carrot Coconut Soup to start and alongside Crispy Baked Kale Chips to get all the nutrients we need from greens.

MAIN COURSE CHOW MEIN

Everyone loves a good platter of chow mein, but no one loves the excessive calories, additives, salt, and sugar that weigh you down after the indulgence. My version is lighter, fresher, and just as tasty . . . and you can cook it in your slow cooker all day!

Makes 3–4 servings

1 pound seitan, chopped into chunks

2–3 stalks celery, diced

1 small leek, split lengthwise, rinsed free
   of dirt, diced

½ inch fresh ginger, minced

2 cloves fresh garlic, minced

2–3 small carrots, diced

6–8 whole green onions, cut into 1-inch
   pieces

1 cup spring or filtered water

¼ cup soy sauce

½ cup mung bean sprouts

1 (8-ounce) can water chestnuts, drained
   and rinsed

¼ cup arrowroot flour

2 teaspoons light sesame oil

2 cups snow peas, rinsed well, left whole

Combine all ingredients except arrowroot, oil, and snow peas in a slow cooker. Cover and allow to cook over low heat for 6–8 hours.

When you are ready to serve, dissolve arrowroot in a small amount of cold water and stir it, along with sesame oil and snow peas, into seitan and vegetables. Stir until arrowroot thickens and clears and snow peas turn bright green.

◆ **Serving Suggestions**

Kick off this feast with a light Instant Veggie Soup. I like chow mein with cooked brown rice instead of noodles to add whole grain to the meal.

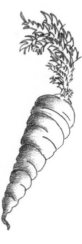

BAKED ZITI

Who doesn't love baked ziti? Cheesy, gooey, and rich, this complete indulgence is loaded with fat, right? Not my version—and not one ounce of flavor was lost in the translation. Plus it's fast and easy.

Makes 6–8 servings

1 pound whole-wheat ziti, cooked until 80 percent done, drained; do not rinse
1 recipe Pomodoro Pasta sauce or 1 (32-ounce) jar unsweetened tomato sauce
2 cups shredded vegan mozzarella (Daiya or Follow Your Heart)
Dried basil
Dried oregano

Preheat oven to 350°F and lightly oil a 9 x 13-inch casserole dish.

Mix cooked ziti with pasta sauce, 1 cup of the cheese, and spices to taste. Cover tightly and bake for 25 minutes. Remove cover, sprinkle the top of the pasta with the remaining cheese, and bake for 10–15 minutes more, until the top is browned and bubbling. Serve hot.

◆ **Serving Suggestions**
Start with Cauliflower Soup with Roasted Red Peppers and set out the Crisp Watercress Salad to aid in digesting this hearty dish.

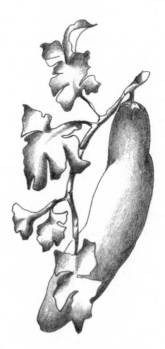

15

Recipes for the Rest of Your Life

You can mix and match the following dishes to create an endless array of tasty feasts. With meals that consist of soups, whole grains, beans and bean products, and lots and lots of veggies cooked a variety of ways (as well as raw), you have the freedom to create meals that best suit your tastes and lifestyle.

BREAKFAST DELIGHTS

I know that everyone is looking for a quick breakfast—except maybe for a leisurely weekend brunch—but if standard dry cereals or fast food are usually your first meal, I urge you to take this one small step and spend a few extra minutes in the morning to get the day started right. (In Chapter 3, I do recommend some dry cereal alternatives that will fit with a healthier lifestyle, but nothing beats a breakfast cooked from scratch.) See also the Frittata and Light-as-Air Pancakes in Chapter 14, "Main Course Makeovers."

SOFT RICE PORRIDGE

Breakfast sets the tone for your day, and this soft morning porridge is just perfect for keeping your energy stable, giving you the stamina of an endurance athlete . . . and you can cook it all night in a slow cooker, so there's no added stress in your chaotic morning. Steam some greens and you are good to go!

Makes 3–4 servings

1 cup short-grain brown rice
5 cups spring or filtered water
Pinch sea salt

Combine ingredients in a slow cooker and cook all night (7–9 hours) on low heat. In the morning, remove the lid and if the porridge is thinner than you like, just cook it for a few more minutes, stirring.

◆ **Variation**

There are so many variations on this recipe for breakfast porridge. You can cook whole-oat groats with a cinnamon stick; millet with corn and cauliflower; brown rice with cubes of butternut squash; rice mixed with millet, or oats or barley and corn; quinoa and corn. All of these combos will take the same amount of water and time to produce a creamy and satisfying porridge.

MORNING VEG STEW

If you think veggies in the morning are weird, think again. You've had a Western omelet, right? Start your day with antioxidant-rich vegetables (without the eggs) and watch as they work their magic on your health. This dish can be prepared ahead of time.

Makes 3–4 servings

1 red onion, large dice
1 medium carrot, large dice
¼ head green cabbage, large dice
Sea salt
1 bay leaf

Layer veggies in the pot in the order listed. Add a pinch of salt, the bay leaf, and ¼ inch water. Cover and bring to a boil over medium heat. Reduce heat to low and cook until carrots are tender, about 15 minutes. Season to taste with salt and simmer for 5 minutes more. If any liquid remains, remove cover and allow to simmer until the liquid dissipates. Remove bay leaf and stir gently to combine.

◆ **Serving Suggestions**

This makes an ideal accompaniment to Soft Rice Porridge.

◆ **Note**

Vary the vegetables to suit your taste and to avoid boredom. Leftovers can be used as the base for soup.

APPLE AND BERRY-SCENTED QUINOA

I was enlisted to create a healthy breakfast cereal that kids would actually eat and that moms could easily afford and make on a busy morning. It's high in complete protein, contains fresh fruit, and the added protein of walnuts. Tested on lots of kids, this recipe has won raves every time!
Makes 3–4 servings

1 cup quinoa, rinsed well
2 cups unfiltered apple juice
Pinch sea salt
Pinch ground cinnamon
1 pint fresh blueberries
1 pint fresh raspberries
½ cup coarsely chopped walnuts (or other nuts)

Place quinoa and apple juice in a saucepan over medium heat. When the quinoa boils, add salt and cinnamon, cover, reduce heat, and bring to a boil. Cook over low heat for 15–20 minutes, until the quinoa has absorbed all the juice.

While the quinoa is hot, stir in the berries and nuts. Serve hot.

◆ **Variations**
You can use any fruit, but harder fruits like apples and pears, or dried fruit, like raisins or cranberries, should be cooked in with the quinoa and not stirred in at the end. Fruits like peaches, plums, and apricots can be stirred in at the end, just like the berries.

THE BEST SCRAMBLED TOFU

What is it about scrambled eggs that makes everyone so happy? The saturated fat? The cholesterol? This vegan version is a hit with all the flavor and none of the stuff we don't want. My challenge was to create a texture that was as tender and moist as eggs. You can build on this to develop your own masterpiece.
Makes 4–5 servings

1 pound firm tofu (extra-firm is too dry)
1 teaspoon avocado oil
¼ yellow onion, diced
2–3 fresh whole green onions, minced
1 cup fresh baby spinach or arugula
1 roasted red bell pepper, diced
⅛ teaspoon turmeric
¼ teaspoon soy sauce
Sea salt
Cracked black pepper

Cut tofu in half so that it is half its original thickness. Press each half between your hands over the sink to expel some water. Using your fingers, crumble tofu into a bowl. Set aside.

Place oil and onion in a skillet over

medium heat. When the onions begin to sizzle, sauté for 2–3 minutes. Add green onions, greens, and pepper, stirring to combine. Stir in turmeric and soy sauce, stirring until an even golden color forms. Season to taste with salt and pepper and cook, stirring, for 3–4 minutes more. Serve immediately.

ELIXIRS OF LIFE

Soup is the perfect first course to any meal, warming our digestive tract so that we assimilate food more efficiently. It helps us eat less. Soup delivers nutrients to the cells efficiently. It's easy to make. You can make it in large batches, freeze portions, and have soup almost on demand. It's deeply nourishing and satisfying. It comforts us like nothing else.

Think I'm crazy? Make a pot of soup. You'll see what I mean.

INSTANT VEGGIE SOUP

This quick soup is a great first course for any meal. Its fresh taste and light consistency whets your appetite for the meal to come without weighting you down, and it's jam-packed with nutrition. Varying the veggies make the possibilities just about endless.

Makes 4–5 servings

Extra-virgin olive oil
½ yellow onion, thinly sliced into half-moons
Sea salt
1 medium carrot, thinly julienned
½ cup shredded cabbage
½ cup frozen organic corn kernels
4–5 cups spring water
2 whole green onions, thinly sliced, for garnish

Place a small amount of oil and onion in a soup pot over medium heat. When the onion begins to sizzle, add a pinch of salt and sauté for 1 minute. Add carrot and a pinch of salt and sauté for 1 minute. Add cabbage, corn, and a pinch of salt and sauté until the cabbage just wilts. Add water, cover, and bring to a boil. Reduce heat to low and cook for 7 minutes. Add salt to taste and simmer for 5 minutes more. Serve garnished with green onions.

ITALIAN LENTIL SOUP

This is the soup of my childhood. I had no idea that my mother was nourishing us with protein, fiber, and antioxidants to keep us healthy! I just knew it was delicious.

Makes 4–5 servings

Extra-virgin olive oil
2 cloves fresh garlic, minced
1 small red onion, diced
Sea salt
Crushed red pepper flakes
2 stalks celery, diced
2 medium carrots, diced
1 (14-ounce) can diced tomatoes
1 cup green or brown lentils, rinsed well
4 cups spring or filtered water
1 bay leaf
Cracked black pepper
2–3 sprigs fresh flat-leaf parsley, coarsely
  chopped, for garnish

Place a small amount of oil, garlic, and onion in a soup pot over medium heat. When the onion begins to sizzle, add a pinch of salt and a generous pinch of crushed red pepper flakes. Sauté for 2–3 minutes. Stir in celery and a pinch of salt and sauté for 1 minute. Stir in carrots and a pinch of salt and sauté for 1 minute. Add tomatoes and lentils and stir well. Add water and bay leaf and bring to a boil, covered. Reduce heat to low and simmer for 45–50 minutes or until lentils are soft and the soup is "creamy." Remove bay leaf and add salt and pepper to taste. Simmer 5 minutes more. Serve garnished with fresh parsley.

THE QUICKEST TOMATO SOUP

This tomato soup usually simmers for hours and gets rich and creamy as the bread "melts." In this quick version, the soup has a chunky texture that is incredibly satisfying; cooks in just minutes; and is loaded with vitamins, minerals, protein, and fiber.

Makes 3–4 servings

Extra-virgin olive oil
1 small red onion, diced
Sea salt
2 (28-ounce) cans diced tomatoes
½ loaf whole-wheat bread, cut into
  cubes
Cracked black pepper
2–3 sprigs fresh basil, leaves coarsely
  chopped

Place a small amount of oil and onion in a soup pot over medium heat. When the onion begins to sizzle, add a pinch of salt and sauté for 2 minutes. Stir in tomatoes and bread; season to taste with salt and pepper and cook for 15 minutes. Add water in small amounts to create a thinner soup texture. Simmer 5 minutes more if you add water. Stir in basil and serve hot.

TOMATO SOUP

Who doesn't love tomato soup? It's Campbell's bestselling soup by far, even surpassing Chicken Noodle. And why not? There's something sexy and sunny about tomato soup. In my version, which is easy and quick to make, you get to keep all the antioxidants in luscious tomatoes, since they did not come out of a can!

Makes 4–5 servings

Extra-virgin olive oil
1 red or yellow onion, diced
Sea salt
Cracked black pepper
1 (32-ounce) can diced tomatoes
   (or 3½ cups diced fresh tomatoes,
   in season)
3 cups spring or filtered water
1 carrot, left whole
1 bay leaf
2–3 sprigs fresh basil, leaves removed
   and coarsely chopped, for garnish

Place a small amount of oil and onion in a soup pot over medium heat. When the onion sizzles, add a pinch of salt and pepper and sauté for 2–3 minutes. Stir in tomatoes and water; season to taste with salt and pepper. Add carrot and bay leaf and bring to a boil. Cover and reduce heat to low. Cook for 15–20 minutes. Remove carrot and bay leaf and discard.

Transfer soup to a food processor and puree until smooth. Return to the soup pot and keep soup on low heat until ready to serve. You may also use an immersion blender to puree the soup. Stir fresh basil into soup just before serving.

◆ **Note**

You can spice up the soup with chili powder or cayenne.

CAULIFLOWER BISQUE WITH ROASTED RED PEPPERS

Creamy, smooth soups are the perfect first course when a meal is more like a feast, with lots of flavors and textures to come. This soup is eye candy as well as being richly flavored and loaded with the cancer-fighting compounds we know come from cruciferous vegetables.

Makes 4–5 servings

3 tablespoons avocado oil
1 yellow onion, diced
Sea salt

⅛ teaspoon saffron threads, soaked in
  2 tablespoons water
2 small potatoes, unpeeled, diced
1 head cauliflower, broken into small
  florets
1 cup unsweetened almond milk
3 cups spring or filtered water
Cracked black pepper
2 roasted red bell peppers, diced
2–3 sprigs fresh flat-leaf parsley, coarsely
  chopped

Place oil and onion in a soup pot over medium heat. When the onion begins to sizzle, add a pinch of salt and sauté for 2–3 minutes. Add saffron (and soaking water) and potatoes and a pinch of salt and sauté for 2 minutes. Add cauliflower and stir well. Add milk and water; cover and bring to a boil. Reduce heat to low and cook until cauliflower is quite soft, about 20 minutes. Season to taste with salt and pepper and simmer for 5 minutes more.

Transfer soup to a food processor and puree until smooth. Return to the soup pot and keep soup on low heat until ready to serve. You may also use an immersion blender to puree the soup.

To serve, ladle soup into bowls. Mix roasted peppers and parsley together and use to garnish soup.

RED LENTIL SOUP WITH CORN

This is one of my all-time favorite summer soups (but I make it year-round). It's light and cooks quickly, but has enough body, protein, and substance to sustain us through all our activities.

Makes 4–5 servings

Avocado oil
2 cloves fresh garlic, minced
1 red onion, diced
Sea salt
½ teaspoon curry powder
1 stalk celery, diced
1 medium carrot, diced
2 ripe tomatoes, diced, with their seeds,
  or 1 (14-ounce) can diced tomatoes
Cracked black pepper
1 cup red lentils, rinsed well
4 cups spring or filtered water
½ cup fresh or frozen organic corn
1 bay leaf
2–3 whole green onions, sliced thinly on
  the diagonal, for garnish

Place a small amount of oil, garlic, and onion in a soup pot over medium heat. When the onion begins to sizzle, add a pinch of salt and the curry powder. Sauté for 2–3 minutes, until the onions are golden from the curry. Stir in celery and a pinch of salt and sauté for 1 minute. Stir in carrot and a pinch of salt and sauté for 1 minute.

Add tomatoes and a pinch of pepper. Stir in lentils, water, corn, and bay leaf. Cover and bring to a boil. Reduce heat to low and cook until lentils are quite soft, about 25 minutes. Season to taste with salt and pepper, remove bay leaf, and simmer for 5 minutes more. Serve garnished with green onions.

CORN CHOWDER

Corn chowder can be made at any time of year using frozen organic corn, but truthfully, it's only really yummy in the summer when organic corn is fresh and sweet. Loaded with fiber, B vitamins, and folate, this sweet whole grain creates vitality and strength.

Makes 4–5 servings

Extra-virgin olive oil

1 yellow onion, diced

Sea salt

3–4 new or fingerling potatoes, unpeeled, diced

2 stalks celery, diced

3 ears fresh corn, kernels removed, cobs reserved

2 cups unsweetened almond milk

2 cups spring or filtered water

2 cubes vegetable bouillon

Cracked black pepper

3–4 fresh chives, minced, for garnish

Place oil and onion in a skillet over medium heat. When the onion begins to sizzle, add a pinch of salt and sauté for 2–3 minutes. Stir in potatoes and a pinch of salt and sauté for 1 minute. Stir in celery and a pinch of salt and sauté for 1 minute. Add corn and a pinch of salt and sauté for 1 minute.

While cooking the veggies, bring almond milk and water to a boil with bouillon cubes and reserved corn cobs (to sweeten the broth). When the bouillon cubes dissolve, remove the cobs and discard. Stir in sautéed veggies and return to the boil. Cover and reduce heat to low. Simmer for 15 minutes. Season to taste with salt and pepper and simmer for 5 minutes more. Serve garnished with fresh chives.

◆ **Note**

Vegetable bouillon cubes can be purchased at any supermarket. You may also use vegetable stock in this recipe and eliminate the step that dissolves the bouillon.

SPRING VEGETABLE BARLEY SOUP

This light and airy soup is as fresh as the season. The barley helps to refresh and serves as a tonic to the liver, so we move easily from cold to warm weather without discomfort. And since it cooks quickly, you can make healthy soup on the busiest of days!

Makes 4–5 servings

1 tablespoon extra-virgin olive oil
1 small leek, split lengthwise, rinsed free
   of dirt, diced
Sea salt
2 medium carrots, diced
2 cups sliced fresh shiitake
   mushrooms
2 new potatoes, unpeeled, diced
1 small zucchini, diced
½ cup pearled barley, rinsed well
4 cups spring or filtered water
2 tablespoons sweet white miso
Several leaves fresh dandelion, coarsely
   chopped
Grated zest of 1 fresh lemon

Place oil and leek in a soup pot over medium heat. When the leek begins to sizzle, add a pinch of salt and sauté for 2 minutes. Stir in carrots and a pinch of salt and sauté for 1 minute. Stir in mushrooms and a pinch of salt and sauté for 2 minutes. Stir in potatoes and a pinch of salt and sauté for 1 minute. Stir in zucchini and a pinch of salt and sauté for 1 minute. Add barley and water and bring to a boil. Cover; reduce heat to low and simmer for 15–20 minutes, until the barley is soft. Remove a small amount of broth and dissolve miso in it. Stir back into soup and simmer (do not boil) for 3–4 min-

utes more. Stir in dandelion and lemon zest just before serving.

WHITE BEAN BISQUE WITH SAUTÉED GREENS

I love white beans in any form. If there was a white bean gelato, I would be all over it. Instead, I use them to create all kinds of yummy dishes, like this richly flavored decadent soup that I love to serve as the starter to a pasta dinner. And it's just icing on the cake that white beans contain compounds that can help lower cholesterol.

Makes 4–5 servings

Extra-virgin olive oil
2 cloves fresh garlic, minced
1 yellow onion, diced
Sea salt
2 stalks celery, diced
2 cups diced butternut squash
2 cups cooked or canned organic
   cannellini or Great Northern beans
4 cups spring or filtered water
Cracked black pepper
3 leaves broccoli rabe, cut into small
   pieces
Grated zest of 1 fresh lemon

Place a small amount of oil, garlic, and onion in a soup pot over medium heat. When the onion begins to sizzle, add a pinch of salt and sauté for 2–3 minutes. Stir in celery and a pinch of salt and sauté for 1 minute. Stir in butternut squash and a pinch of salt and sauté for 1 minute. Add beans and water, cover, and bring to a boil. Reduce heat to low and cook for 15–20 minutes, to allow beans to get creamy and the squash to soften. Season to taste with salt and pepper and simmer for 5 minutes more.

Transfer soup to a food processor and puree until smooth. Return to the soup pot and keep soup on low heat until ready to serve. You may also use an immersion blender to puree the soup.

While the soup simmers, place a small amount of oil in a skillet and sauté greens with a pinch of salt until just wilted, about 3 minutes. Stir in lemon zest.

To serve, ladle the soup into individual bowls and garnish with greens.

◆ **Note**

You can use dried beans for this soup. It just means cooking it for 1–1½ hours before pureeing, but it results in a totally yummy soup.

BLACK BEAN AND CORN SOUP

I love bean soups. As a vegan, I find that they are a delicious way to get the protein I need in life. They also freeze well, making life easier. This one is a little spicy, so it's strengthening and good for circulation, as well as a good source of protein, folate, and fiber; low in fat; and beneficial to digestion (because they contain compounds, including butyric acid, which aid in the digestion of protein).

Makes 4–5 servings

Avocado oil

3–4 cloves fresh garlic, minced

1 jalapeño pepper, minced, seeds and spine included

1 red onion, diced

Sea salt

1 stalk celery, diced

1 medium carrot, diced

1 zucchini, diced

2 ripe plum tomatoes, diced, with their seeds

1 cup dried black turtle beans

4 cups spring or filtered water

1 bay leaf

½ cup fresh or frozen organic corn kernels

1 cup vegan sour cream (optional)

2–3 sprigs fresh flat-leaf parsley or cilantro, coarsely chopped, for garnish

Place a small amount of oil, garlic, jalapeño, and onion in a soup pot over medium heat. When the onion begins to sizzle, add a pinch of salt and sauté for 2–3 minutes. Stir in celery and a pinch of salt and sauté for 1 minute. Stir in carrot and a pinch of salt and sauté for 1 minute. Stir in zucchini and a pinch of salt and sauté for 1 minute. Stir in tomatoes and beans. Add water and bay leaf; cover and bring to a boil. Reduce heat to low and cook for about an hour or until the beans are soft. Stir in corn and season soup to taste with salt. Simmer for 5 minutes more. To serve, ladle soup into individual bowls with a dollop of "sour cream" on top and a sprinkle of parsley or cilantro.

◆ **Notes**

You can use canned organic beans (rinsed and drained) and shorten the cooking time of this soup to 30 minutes.

Vegan sour cream can be purchased in most natural food stores. You may also make your own by pureeing 1 cup silken tofu with a pinch of salt and the juice of ¼ fresh lemon.

CINNAMON-SCENTED BUTTERNUT SQUASH SOUP

When the weather outside is frightful, there is nothing more delightful than winter squash. It's sweet, comforting, warming, centering, and loaded with antioxidants to ward off colds and flu. In this soup, I add cinnamon to up the ante on the warmth, increase sweetness, and help to stabilize blood sugar.

Makes 4–5 servings

Avocado oil
1 yellow onion, diced
Sea salt
3 cups diced, unpeeled butternut squash
Generous pinch ground cinnamon
1 cup unsweetened almond milk
3 cups spring or filtered water
Whole nutmeg, to be grated for garnish

Place oil and onion in a soup pot over medium heat. When the onion begins to sizzle, add a pinch of salt and sauté for 2–3 minutes. Stir in squash and cinnamon to taste. Add milk and water, cover, and bring to a boil. Reduce heat to low and cook for 35 minutes or until squash is tender.

Transfer soup to a food processor and puree until smooth. Return to the soup pot and keep soup on low heat until ready to serve. You may also use an immersion blender to puree the soup.

To serve, ladle soup into individual bowls and garnish with a few grates of nutmeg.

LEEK, POTATO, AND PARSNIP SOUP

This creamy, slightly sweet soup is elegant, but not so fancy that you have to reserve it for special occasions. A rich source of B vitamins, vitamin C, copper, folic acid, and pantothenic acid, this soup is sweet on many levels.

Makes 4–5 servings

Extra-virgin olive oil
½ yellow onion, diced
1 leek, split lengthwise, rinsed free of dirt, diced
Sea salt
2 medium parsnips, diced
3 medium Yukon gold or russet potatoes, unpeeled, diced
1 cup unsweetened almond milk
3 cups spring or filtered water
2 tablespoons sweet white miso
2–3 sprigs fresh flat-leaf parsley, coarsely chopped, for garnish

Place oil, onion, and leek in a soup pot over medium heat. When the onion begins to sizzle, add a pinch of salt and sauté for 2–3 minutes. Stir in parsnips and a pinch of salt and sauté for 1 minute. Stir in potatoes and a pinch of salt and sauté for 1 minute. Add milk and water, cover, and bring to a boil. Reduce heat to low and cook for 35 minutes, until the potatoes are soft. Remove a small amount of broth and dissolve miso in it. Stir back into soup and simmer 3 minutes more.

Transfer soup to a food processor and puree until smooth. Return to the soup pot and keep soup on low heat until ready to serve. You may also use an immersion blender to puree the soup.

To serve, ladle soup into individual bowls and garnish with parsley.

CARROT COCONUT SOUP

This quirky soup is so cool. I love this combination. Coconut milk and carrots have a complementary sweetness that works together perfectly in this soup. It's simple, yet rich, loaded with nutrients like beta-carotene as well as the good-quality fats of coconut!

Makes 4–5 servings

Avocado oil
1 yellow onion, diced
Sea salt
6 carrots, diced
2 sweet potatoes, unpeeled, diced

1 tablespoon brown rice syrup

2 cups coconut milk (regular or low-fat)

1 cup unsweetened almond milk

1 cup spring or filtered water

Grated zest of 1 fresh lemon

Heat a small amount of oil and onion in a soup pot over medium heat. When the onion sizzles, add a pinch of salt and sauté for 2–3 minutes. Do not let the onions darken. Stir in carrots, sweet potatoes, and syrup. Add milks and water, cover, and bring to a boil. Reduce heat to low and simmer for 35 minutes, until the carrots are soft.

Transfer soup to a food processor and puree until smooth. Return to the soup pot and keep soup on low heat until ready to serve. You may also use an immersion blender to puree the soup.

To serve, ladle soup into individual bowls and garnish with lemon zest.

RAW CREAMY CORN SOUP

When the summer is at its hottest and corn at its sweetest, this soup is perfection. This cold blender soup is luscious and easy to make. The fiber from the corn and the protein in the almond milk make this soup as powerfully nutritious as it is yummy.

Makes 3–4 servings

6 ears fresh organic corn, husks removed

½ cup raw cashews or almonds

1 cup unsweetened almond milk

1 cup spring or filtered water

2 teaspoons sea salt

4–5 tablespoons extra-virgin olive oil

2 tablespoons brown rice syrup

2–3 sprigs fresh basil, leaves removed, coarsely chopped, for garnish

Remove the kernels from the corn cobs and then, holding the cob by its stem over a bowl, run the back side of your knife along the cob to extract the "cream" left behind when you removed the kernels.

Place the kernels, the "cream," nuts, milk, water, and salt in a food processor or blender and puree until smooth. Add oil by the tablespoon to achieve the texture and flavor you like. Add syrup slowly to achieve the sweetness you like.

Serve chilled or at room temperature, garnished with fresh basil.

ISRAELI CHICKPEA SOUP

I learned to make this soup when I was in Israel teaching cooking. I love how the vegetables work with the double whammy of protein that comes from red lentils and chickpeas, resulting in a nutrient-dense first course.

Makes 4–5 servings

2 tablespoons extra-virgin olive oil

2 tablespoons red wine

2 red onions, diced

Sea salt

4 small sweet potatoes, unpeeled, diced

3 beets, peeled, diced

⅔ cup red lentils, rinsed well

1 (14-ounce) can organic chickpeas, rinsed well

4 cups spring or filtered water

1 teaspoon ground cumin

Juice of ½ fresh lemon

3–4 fresh chives, minced, for garnish

Place oil, wine, and onions in a soup pot over medium heat. When the onions begin to sizzle, add a pinch of salt and sauté for 2–3 minutes. Stir in sweet potatoes and beets. Add lentils and chickpeas. Stir in water and cumin, cover, and bring to a boil. Reduce heat to low and simmer for 30 minutes, until the beets are soft. Season the soup with salt to your taste.

Transfer soup to a food processor and puree until smooth. Return to the soup pot and keep soup on low heat until ready to serve. You may also use an immersion blender to puree the soup. Stir in lemon juice just before serving garnished with chives.

ZUPPA DI CIPOLLE

Traditional onion soup in Tuscany comes loaded with pancetta and is made with beef broth with all the accompanying artery-clogging fat and calories. Mine is made with onions, onions, and more onions and is loaded with flavenoids and polyphenols, chromium and vitamin C so it lands lightly on our hearts and our hips.

Makes 4–5 servings

Extra-virgin olive oil

5 large yellow onions, thinly sliced into half-moons

½ cup red wine

2 tablespoons brown rice syrup

4–5 cups spring or filtered water

Sea salt

Cracked black pepper

5 slices thickly sliced whole-grain bread

2–3 sprigs fresh basil, leaves removed, coarsely chopped

Place about 5 tablespoons oil and onions in a large soup pot over medium heat. When the onions begin to sizzle, add red wine and syrup and sauté until the onions just wilt. Cover and cook over low heat, stirring occasionally for 15 minutes.

Pour in water and season to taste with salt and pepper. Cover and bring to a boil. Reduce heat to low and cook for 30 minutes.

While the soup cooks, heat a small amount of oil in a flat-bottomed skillet over medium heat and quickly toast the bread on both sides.

To serve, lay a slice of bread in 4–5 individual bowls and ladle soup over top. Serve garnished with fresh basil.

ROASTED FENNEL AND TOMATO SOUP

This soup is uncommon in this country, but absolutely celebrated in Italian cuisine. The fresh, clean taste of the fennel is the perfect complement to the sweetness of the tomato. Both are loaded with vitamin C and when you pair that with the lycopene in tomatoes and the anise-flavored compounds in fennel that help with digestion, you have the perfect first course.
Makes 4–5 servings

1 fennel bulb, trimmed, diced
8 ounces cherry tomatoes
1 medium carrot, diced
2 whole cloves garlic
Extra-virgin olive oil
Sea salt
4 cups spring or filtered water
1 bay leaf
1 tablespoon balsamic vinegar
2–3 sprigs fresh flat-leaf parsley, coarsely chopped, for garnish

Preheat oven to 350°F.

Mix fennel, tomatoes, carrot, and garlic with a generous drizzle of oil and salt to taste. Toss to coat the veggies and transfer them to a baking sheet with sides, spreading them out to avoid overlap. Roast, uncovered, for about an hour, until soft and lightly browned.

Transfer roasted veggies to a soup pot and add water and bay leaf. Bring to a boil, covered. Reduce heat to low and simmer for 15 minutes. Season with salt to taste, and simmer 5 minutes more.

Transfer soup to a food processor and puree until smooth. Return to the soup pot and keep soup on low heat until ready to serve. You may also use an immersion blender to puree the soup. Serve garnished with a drizzle of balsamic vinegar and parsley.

ENERGY TO BURN!

Whole grains are the foundation of a healthy life and are powerfully rich in nutrients, like complex carbohydrates for energy, fiber for digestion, and vitamins and minerals essential for life. Want to glide through your day with energy to spare? Then this is the section for you.

CURRIED QUINOA WITH CURRANTS

I love the combination of the nutty flavor of quinoa with the delicate sweetness of currants. The curry provides a little heat and a lot of interest to this grain, which provides us with the same complete protein as an egg without the downside of saturated fat and cholesterol.

Makes 3–4 servings

Avocado oil
½ yellow onion, diced
2 teaspoons curry powder
1 cup quinoa, rinsed very well
2 cups spring or filtered water
Sea salt
½ cup currants
½ ripe mango, finely diced
2 fresh whole green onions, diced

Place about a teaspoon of oil and onion in a saucepan over medium heat. When the onion begins to sizzle, stir in curry powder and sauté for 2–3 minutes. Add quinoa and water and bring to a boil. Add a pinch of salt and currants, reduce heat to low, cover, and cook for 15–20 minutes, until liquid has been absorbed. When the quinoa is cooked, stir in mango and green onions. Serve warm or at room temperature.

QUINOA WITH PISTACHIO PESTO

A student of mine, Deb Hayes, said this recipe helped her family fall in love with this high-protein ancient grain. Adding the fiber, good-quality fat, and other nutrients in pistachios and olive oil makes this a powerfully energizing dish.

Makes 3–4 servings

1 cup quinoa, rinsed well
2 cups spring or filtered water
Sea salt

Pistachio Pesto
1½ cups fresh basil
½ cup fresh flat-leaf parsley

1 cup dry, shelled, unsalted pistachios

3 cloves fresh garlic, chopped

½ cup extra-virgin olive oil

1 teaspoon fresh grated lemon zest

2 tablespoons sweet white miso

1 teaspoon brown rice syrup

Bring quinoa and water to a boil in a saucepan over medium heat. When the quinoa boils, add a pinch of salt, cover, and reduce heat to low. Cook for 15–20 minutes, until all the liquid has been absorbed.

While the quinoa cooks, make the pesto. Combine all ingredients in a food processor and puree until a coarse but creamy texture develops. Adjust seasonings to your taste. Set aside.

When the quinoa has cooked, fluff with a fork and allow to cool for 10 minutes before stirring in 1–2 tablespoons of pesto. You want the quinoa to turn a lovely light green, but at the same time, you do not want so much pesto that the grain becomes gooey.

You will have much more pesto than you need. It will keep, refrigerated in a sealed jar, for a couple of days. It's great on pasta or salad.

QUIRKY QUINOA SALAD

Quinoa will bite you on the butt. It's a whole grain with all the goodness that goes with that, is a complete protein, is gluten-free, and cooks quickly, so you have no excuses not to cook and eat whole grains. And this salad? Ay, ay, ay, it's good.

Makes 3–4 servings

1 cup quinoa, rinsed well

2 cups spring or filtered water

Pinch sea salt

1 cup snow peas, tips removed

½ roasted red pepper, sliced into ribbons

½ cucumber, unpeeled and diced

2–3 sprigs fresh flat-leaf parsley, coarsely chopped

2–3 whole green onions, minced

2 sprigs fresh mint, coarsely chopped

Dressing

3 tablespoons extra-virgin olive oil

1 teaspoon fresh lemon juice

Generous pinch sea salt

Generous pinch ground pepper

Generous pinch garlic powder

Cook the quinoa. Place quinoa and water in a pot and bring to a boil. Add salt, cover, and reduce heat to low. Cook for 15 minutes, until liquid has been absorbed.

While the quinoa cooks, make the dressing. Whisk ingredients together and adjust seasonings to your taste.

This may look like a tiny amount of dressing, but too much of it will make the quinoa mushy.

When the quinoa is ready, stir in veggies. The heat of the quinoa will cook them just a bit, making them tender. Fold in dressing and serve. You may serve this hot, warm, or at room temperature.

QUINOA WITH WILD RICE AND HAZELNUTS

I love the flavors in this dish. It's a bit of work because you cook the grains separately, but once you taste it, you won't mind that one extra pot to clean up. All the protein, complex carbohydrates, antioxidants, and aid to digestion make it worth the effort.
Makes 3–4 servings

⅓ cup wild rice, rinsed well
Spring or filtered water
Sea salt
½ cup quinoa, rinsed well
½ cup hazelnuts, pan-toasted, skins left on, coarsely chopped
¼ cup dried, unsweetened cranberries
3–4 fresh whole green onions, minced
3–4 sprigs fresh flat-leaf parsley, coarsely chopped
2 teaspoons extra-virgin olive oil
1 teaspoon apple cider vinegar
Cracked black pepper

Place wild rice in a small saucepan. Bring 1 cup water to a boil. Pour boiling water over rice to just cover. Keep balance of water hot. Add a pinch of salt and turn heat to medium. When the rice boils, reduce heat to low and cook, adding more boiling water as needed to cook the rice. It will take about 35 minutes. You know the rice is done when the water is absorbed and the grains are cracked and tender. Fluff with a fork and set aside.

While the rice cooks, cook the quinoa. Place quinoa and 1 cup water in a saucepan over medium heat. When the quinoa boils, add a pinch of salt, reduce heat, cover, and cook for 15–20 minutes, until the liquid has been absorbed.

When both grains are cooked, mix them together with the nuts, cranberries, green onions, and parsley.

Whisk together oil and vinegar with salt and pepper to taste. Fold dressing gently into warm grain to incorporate it throughout. Serve warm.

FORBIDDEN RICE WITH SNOW PEAS

Forbidden rice has a dramatic color and nutty flavor that makes this the perfect side dish to any meal. I cook the rice in green tea to increase the antioxidants and give a hint of unique and elegant flavor to the dish. Loaded with iron and said to aid in circulation, black rice is gluten-free, making it a must-have in any pantry.

Makes 3–4 servings

1 green tea bag
1¾ cups spring or filtered water, boiled
1 cup black forbidden rice, rinsed well
Sea salt
2½ cups (8 ounces) fresh snow peas, washed, ends trimmed, cut into 1-inch pieces
3–4 green whole green onions, minced
2 teaspoons brown rice vinegar
1 teaspoon brown rice syrup
Chia seeds, for garnish

Place tea bag in a heat-resistant bowl and pour boiled water over top (cool water for 2 minutes after boiling before pouring over tea bag to avoid a bitter taste). Set aside to steep for 5 minutes.

Place rice and brewed tea in a saucepan over medium heat and bring to a boil. Add a pinch of salt, reduce heat to low, cover, and cook for 30–35 minutes, until the liquid has been absorbed and the rice is tender. Fluff with a fork and cool slightly before stirring in snow peas, green onions, vinegar, and syrup. Serve with chia seeds on the side for garnish.

FARRO WITH CAULIFLOWER

Farro is the best thing since sliced bread, in my view. It cooks quickly and is completely delicious. It's versatile and goes with any meal. Rich in fiber, with more protein than wheat (although it is similar to spelt) and high in complex B vitamins, farro is an ancient grain with a low-gluten content that can be traced by to 5000 BC.

Makes 3–4 servings

Extra-virgin olive oil
2 cloves fresh garlic, minced
½ red onion, diced
Sea salt
¼ head cauliflower, broken into small florets
Grated zest of ½ fresh lemon
1 cup farro, rinsing not needed
2 cups spring or filtered water
2–3 sprigs fresh basil, leaves removed, coarsely chopped.

Place oil, garlic, and onion in a saucepan over medium heat. When the onion begins to sizzle, add a pinch of salt and sauté for 2–3 minutes. Stir in cauliflower and lemon zest. Add farro and water and bring to a boil. Add a generous pinch of salt, cover, and reduce heat to low. Cook until all liquid has been absorbed and farro is tender, about 20–25 minutes. Stir in fresh basil and serve warm or at room temperature.

SAFFRON-SCENTED RISOTTO

This simple dish is a classic with roots in Milan. The rice cooks to creamy, chewy perfection, and the saffron tints it with a color worthy of royalty . . . and adds just a wee bit of spicy taste. So even though this dish is made with nutrient-deficient white rice, we amped the nutrition right back up with the antioxidants in butternut squash and the carotenoids in saffron.

Makes 4–5 servings

2½ cups spring or filtered water
¼ cup dry white wine
⅛ teaspoon saffron threads
Extra-virgin olive oil
2 shallots, diced
2 cloves garlic, minced
Sea salt
1 cup unpeeled, diced butternut squash
1 cup Arborio rice (do not rinse)
Cracked black pepper

2–3 sprigs fresh flat-leaf parsley, coarsely chopped, for garnish

Place water and wine in a saucepan over medium heat and bring to a boil. Reduce heat to low and stir in saffron threads. Keep this mixture over very low heat.

Place about a tablespoon of oil, shallots, and garlic in a deep skillet over medium heat. When the shallots begin to sizzle, add a pinch of salt and sauté for 2–3 minutes. Stir in butternut squash and sauté for 2 minutes. Add rice and cook, stirring for 2 minutes. Reduce heat to medium low and begin adding warm saffron broth ¼ cup at a time, stirring frequently, adding liquid as it absorbs into the rice until all the liquid has been used. When you add the last ladle of liquid, season to taste with salt and pepper and cook, stirring, until the liquid has been absorbed and the rice is creamy. The whole process takes 25–30 minutes. Remove rice from heat and stir in parsley. Serve immediately.

QUINOA AND BLACK BEAN SALAD

Quinoa and beans go together like Romeo and Juliet without the tragedy. The quinoa serves as the background for the combination known as the "Three Sisters"—corn, beans, and squash that made up the foundation of ancient Latin cuisine—and provides us with antioxidants, protein, fiber, and essential vitamins and minerals.

Makes 3–4 servings

1 cup quinoa, rinsed well
½ cup fresh or frozen corn kernels
1 jalapeño, minced (with seeds and
   spines to make it spicier, without to
   make it milder)
2 cups spring or filtered water
Sea salt
½ cup cooked or canned organic black
   turtle beans
1 tablespoon red wine vinegar
3–4 fresh whole green onions, minced

Dressing
3 tablespoons avocado oil
2 tablespoons fresh lime juice
Cracked black pepper

Place quinoa, corn, jalapeño, and water in a saucepan over medium heat. When it comes to a boil, add a pinch of salt and reduce heat to low. Cover and cook for 15–20 minutes, until the quinoa has absorbed all the liquid.

While the quinoa cooks, toss the beans with the vinegar and set aside.

Make the dressing by whisking the ingredients together; season with salt and pepper to taste.

When the quinoa is cooked, fold in beans, green onions, and dressing. Serve salad warm or at room temperature.

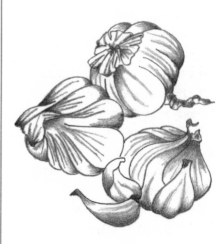

BRAZILIAN BEANS AND RICE

Tropical weather and the combo of rice and beans go together like love and marriage. Steeped in tradition, this ancient duo gives you the endurance that comes from whole grains, while making you big and strong with the protein in the beans . . . and skips the beef and pork normally found in this dish.

Makes 3–4 servings

Extra-virgin olive oil
3 cloves fresh garlic, minced
1 yellow onion, diced
1 tablespoon minced fresh ginger
Sea salt
3 ripe but firm bananas, peeled, cut in
    half crosswise and then lengthwise
8 ounces tempeh, crumbled
½ teaspoon ground cumin
Pinch cayenne pepper
1½ cups cooked or canned organic
    kidney beans
1 (14-ounce) can diced tomatoes
2–3 sprigs fresh flat-leaf parsley, coarsely
    chopped
Several leaves shredded lettuce
2 cups cooked, hot brown rice

Place about 2 tablespoons of oil, garlic, onion, and ginger in a skillet over medium heat. When the onion begins to sizzle, add a pinch of salt and sauté for 2–3 minutes. Push onion mixture to the side of the skillet and lay banana slices in the center of the skillet. Braise them on both sides until lightly browned at the edges, turning once. Remove bananas to a plate.

Stir tempeh, cumin, and cayenne into onion mixture and sauté until tempeh is browned, about 3–4 minutes. Stir in beans and tomatoes, cover, reduce heat to low, and cook, stirring frequently, for about 30 minutes. Season to taste with salt and pepper and simmer 5 minutes more. Remove from heat and stir in parsley.

To serve, arrange shredded lettuce on a platter. Mound hot rice on top and spoon bean mixture over the rice. Arrange bananas on the side of the platter. Serve hot.

BARLEY WITH SWEET RICE AND CORN

This simple rice combo makes for an elegant side dish that will leave you feeling refreshed and vital. The barley helps relax the liver, and the corn and rice provide energy to burn. All provide us with complex carbohydrates, complex B vitamins, folate, and protein for strength.

Makes 3–4 servings

½ cup whole barley, rinsed well, soaked
    for 1 hour

½ cup sweet brown rice, rinsed well, soaked for 1 hour
1 cup fresh or frozen corn kernels
Grated zest of ½ fresh lemon
2 cups spring or filtered water
Sea salt
3–4 fresh whole green onions, minced

Soak barley and sweet rice together. Drain well and place in a pressure cooker with corn and lemon zest. Add water and bring to a boil. Add a pinch of salt per cup of grain and seal the lid of the pressure cooker and bring to high pressure over medium heat. Reduce heat to low and cook for 25 minutes. Turn off heat and allow pressure cooker to stand, undisturbed, for another 25 minutes. Remove the lid; stir in green onions and serve warm or at room temperature.

TANJUN'NA GOMOKU (SIMPLE RICE STEW)

This stewed rice dish will warm you on the chilliest of days. Most definitely a cool-weather dish, it is also used in Chinese medicine and macrobiotics when someone is feeling weak or sickly. So imagine how powerful you'll feel eating it just because it's delicious.

Makes 3–4 servings

3–5 shiitake mushrooms, soaked in 2 cups spring or filtered water
Avocado oil
1 yellow onion, diced
4–5 slices fresh ginger, minced
1 medium carrot, diced
1 small lotus root, diced
1 small burdock, diced
2 tablespoons mirin
1 cup short-grain brown rice
2 squares dried tofu, soaked till soft, cubed
Soy sauce
3–4 fresh whole green onions, minced

Soak shiitake in water until soft. Drain, reserving soaking water, and squeeze excess liquid from shiitakes. Dice the mushrooms.

In a heavy pot, place oil, onion, and ginger over medium heat. When the onion begins to sizzle, sauté for 2 minutes. Stir in carrot, lotus root, and burdock and sauté for 2 minutes. Add mirin, rice, dried tofu, and soaking water. Bring to a boil. Season lightly with soy sauce and cook, covered, over low heat for 45–50 minutes, until the liquid has been absorbed into the rice and it has become creamy. Stir in green onions and serve.

POLENTA WITH CIAMBOTTA CON CARCIOFFI

(Polenta with Artichoke Stew)

More than just an Italian tradition, this stew is loaded with complex B vitamins in the corn, and the stew contains artichokes, one of the most antioxidant-rich veggies we know. Along with the rest of the nutrient-dense veggies, this dish is more than just comfort food.

Makes 4–5 servings

Polenta

1 cup fine corn grits
5 cups spring or filtered water
Pinch sea salt
Extra-virgin olive oil
Unsweetened almond milk

Ciambotta con Carcioffi

½ pound eggplant, unpeeled and cut into 1-inch cubes
1 tablespoon extra-virgin olive oil
1 large onion, thinly sliced
5 large cloves garlic, minced
1 stalk celery, thinly sliced
Large handful of fresh basil, stems removed, chopped
1 (14-ounce) can diced tomatoes
¾ pound new potatoes, or any waxy potato, scrubbed and cut into 1 x 2-inch pieces
½ pound canned artichoke hearts (in water, not oil)
1 large or 2 small sweet red or yellow peppers, seeded and cut into 1 x 2-inch strips
Salt and freshly ground black pepper

To make the polenta, place all ingredients except oil in a saucepan over medium heat. Cook, whisking constantly, until it boils. Reduce heat to low and cook, whisking frequently, until the center of the polenta bubbles or heaves, about 25 minutes. Stir in a drizzle of oil and almond milk and spoon into a bowl. Keep warm so the polenta stays soft.

Toss the eggplant cubes in a colander with 2 teaspoons salt. Let it sit in the sink until it starts to sweat out the bitter juices. Rinse, drain, and pat the eggplant dry, squeezing a little.

In a large pot, heat the oil. Add the onion, garlic, and celery. Add a pinch of salt and sauté over high heat for about 5 minutes, adding a little water as necessary to prevent sticking and burning.

Add the basil and sauté for 2 minutes; then add the tomatoes. When it comes to a simmer, add the eggplant, potatoes, and ½ teaspoon salt. Stir, bring to a boil, then turn down and simmer, covered, for 15 minutes.

Add the artichoke and peppers and simmer 15 minutes more, or until all of the vegetables are tender. Taste for salt and pepper, transfer to a warm serving bowl, and allow to stand 15 minutes before serving.

To serve, spoon polenta into individual bowls with stew mounded on top.

◆ **Note**

You can make this spicy by adding crushed red chili flakes when sautéing the onions and garlic.

SPINACH AND BASIL CONCHIGLIONI

This baked pasta dish is rich in protein, calcium, and iron and unlike other baked pasta dishes is low in fat, contains no saturated fat, and is lower in calories than other cheese-laden pasta dishes.

Makes 4–5 servings

1 pound firm tofu
5 ounces frozen spinach, thawed,
    steamed for 2 minutes,
    squeezed dry
⅓ cup pine nuts
⅓ cup loosely packed fresh basil leaves
1 teaspoon white miso
2 cloves fresh garlic
Generous pinch ground nutmeg
Generous pinch cracked black pepper
Extra-virgin olive oil
1 recipe Pomodoro Presto

1 box Conchiglioni (large shell macaroni)

Crumble tofu coarsely into a bowl. Chop spinach and mix into tofu. Set aside.

Place pine nuts, basil, miso, garlic, nutmeg, and a pinch of black pepper in a food processor. Pulse to form a coarse paste, slowly adding oil to create a thick, creamy texture (up to 2 tablespoons). Add tofu mixture to the pine nut mixture and puree until smooth, scraping the sides down as needed.

Preheat oven to 350°F. Bring a pot of water to a boil with a generous pinch of salt. Cook the shells al dente, about 9 minutes, stirring occasionally to prevent sticking. Drain shells and lay them out on a kitchen towel to cool to room temperature before handling.

Spoon sauce over the bottom of a large casserole dish. Spoon filling abundantly into each shell and arrange them to fit tightly in the dish. Spoon sauce to generously cover stuffed shells; cover tightly and bake for 20–25 minutes. Serve hot.

PENNE POMODORO PRESTO

There is nothing yummier, easier, or more welcome on any dinner table than pasta, and this quick sauce is loaded with flavor; antioxidants; vitamins C, A, and K; and lycopene. Spice it up . . . or not; add more veggies . . . or not; add vegan cheese . . . or not . . . olives and capers . . . or not. I love options.

Makes 4–5 servings

Extra-virgin olive oil
2 cloves fresh garlic, minced
½ red onion, diced
½ teaspoon dried oregano
Sea salt
Cracked black pepper
1 (28-ounce) can of diced tomatoes
   (organic, if possible)
3–4 sprigs fresh basil or parsley, coarsely
   chopped

1 pound whole-wheat or semolina
   penne or ziti pasta

Place a generous amount of oil, garlic, and onion in a deep skillet over medium heat. When the onion begins to sizzle, add oregano, a pinch of salt and pepper. Sauté for 2–3 minutes, but do not let the onions brown. Stir in tomatoes, season lightly with salt and pepper, cover, and simmer for 3–4 minutes. Remove cover and simmer for 4–5 minutes more. Stir in parsley just before combining with pasta.

While the sauce cooks, bring a large pot of water to a boil with a generous teaspoon of salt. When the water boils, cook pasta al dente, about 9–10 minutes. Drain pasta, but do not rinse. Combine with sauce and serve.

SWEET PEA RAVIOLI

I love these elegant ravioli. I use wonton wrappers so I don't always have to make pasta dough from scratch. The fact that peas contain antioxidants and are famous for their anti-inflammatory properties makes them all the more sweet.

Makes 4–5 servings

1 package eggless wonton wrappers

Filling
Extra-virgin olive oil
3 shallots, minced
Sea salt
3 cups petite peas, fresh or frozen
4 ounces soft tofu, not silken
2 teaspoons brown rice syrup
Cracked black pepper

Chili Oil
1½ cups extra-virgin olive oil
1 shallot, minced

3 cloves fresh garlic, minced

Sea salt

1 teaspoon crushed red chili flakes

1 teaspoon chili powder

1 teaspoon sweet paprika

4–5 fresh whole green onions, minced

2–3 sprigs fresh basil, leaves removed, coarsely chopped

1 cup petite peas, steamed until bright green, for garnish

4–5 tips of basil sprigs, for garnish

To make the filling, place a small amount of oil and shallots in a saucepan over medium heat. When the shallots begin to sizzle, add a pinch of salt and sauté for 2–3 minutes. Add peas and tofu and cook over low heat until the peas are bright green. Stir in syrup and salt and pepper to taste. Transfer to a food processor and puree until smooth, slowly adding oil by the teaspoon as needed to create a smooth, thick texture. Set aside to cool before proceeding.

Make the oil while the filling cools. Combine all ingredients except green onion and basil in a saucepan over low heat, whisking occasionally, for 10 minutes to develop the flavors. Take care not to brown or burn the spices. Turn off heat and reheat oil when ready to serve.

To make the ravioli, place a wonton wrapper on a lightly floured, dry work surface. Spoon 1 generous tablespoon of filling onto the center of the wonton. With a wet finger, moisten the outer rim of the wonton. Lay another wrapper on top, aligning it with the bottom layer. Press the edges lightly to seal the ravioli. Repeat with remainder of ingredients.

While making the ravioli, bring a pot of water to a boil with a generous pinch of salt.

When the ravioli are ready to cook, reheat the oil on very low heat. Cook the ravioli in boiling water until they rise to the top of the pot, about 3–4 minutes. Do not overcook. Drain and transfer to a serving platter.

Stir green onions and basil into hot oil and spoon over ravioli. Garnish with peas and basil sprigs and serve immediately.

◆ **Note**

You can make tiny ravioli by using one wonton wrapper. Simply spoon a teaspoon of filling onto one corner of the wonton; moisten the edges; fold the corner over, forming a triangle. Press to seal and proceed with the recipe.

CHINESE-STYLE NOODLES WITH PEANUT SAUCE

These noodles are so great for families. Kids love them; fussy eaters love them; everyone loves them. As a simple lunch or dinner, this is my go-to dish on a night when I need a satisfying meal . . . now! And since it's loaded with protein and complex carbohydrates, I know the simple nature of the dish doesn't compromise on nutrition.

Makes 2–3 servings

8 ounces soba noodles or whole-wheat
    spaghetti

Peanut Sauce
½ cup all-natural crunchy peanut butter
¼ cup soy sauce
1 tablespoon brown rice syrup
4 teaspoons light sesame oil
2 teaspoons brown rice vinegar

Veggies
Avocado oil
2 cloves fresh garlic, minced
3–4 fresh whole green onions, cut into
    1-inch pieces
Soy sauce
½ fresh cucumber, unpeeled and cut into
    long, thin matchstick pieces
1 roasted red pepper, sliced into thin
    ribbons
½ cup coarsely chopped roasted peanuts

Bring a pot of water to a boil with a generous pinch of salt and cook noodles al dente, about 9 minutes. Drain well, rinse, and place in a bowl. Cover and chill thoroughly before proceeding.

To make the sauce, whisk all ingredients together. Adjust seasoning to your taste. Set aside.

Place oil, garlic, and green onions in a deep skillet or wok over medium heat. When the green onions begin to sizzle, season lightly with soy sauce and sauté for 2 minutes. Remove from heat and mix in cucumber and roasted pepper.

To serve, toss cold noodles with peanut sauce and arrange on a platter. Spoon hot veggies over top and garnish with roasted peanuts. Serve immediately.

ORECCHIETTE ALLA PUGLIESE

I learned this recipe from Salvatore Di Cristofaro, one of the finest and most knowledgeable Italian chefs I have had the honor to work with over my career. Loaded with antioxidants, vitamins, and nutrients like folate, this dish will be on your table all the time, and you'll rest easy knowing everyone is well fed.

Makes 4–5 servings

Extra-virgin olive oil

1 long hot pepper, minced

2–3 cloves fresh garlic, crushed

2 small Italian eggplants, diced

1 cup diced canned tomatoes

4 ounces pitted black olives

5–6 sprigs fresh parsley, coarsely chopped

5–6 sprigs fresh basil, coarsely chopped

Sea salt

Cracked black pepper

1 pound whole-wheat or semolina orecchiette, cooked al dente, about 8–9 minutes

Start a large pot of water boiling, with a generous pinch of salt and a drizzle of oil.

Place about ¼ cup oil, pepper, and garlic in a deep skillet over medium heat. Sauté until garlic is lightly golden, about 3 minutes. Stir in eggplant and a pinch of salt and sauté for 2 minutes. (You may need to add a touch of oil, as the eggplant soaks it up.) Stir in tomatoes, olives, parsley, basil (reserving about 1 teaspoon of each for garnish), and salt and pepper to taste. Simmer for about 8 minutes.

While the sauce simmers, cook pasta al dente, about 8–9 minutes. Using a slotted spoon, transfer pasta to the skillet with the sauce and stir gently to combine. Serve hot, garnished with a bit more fresh parsley and basil.

PENNE FRA DIAVOLO

Daring and spicy, this pasta sauce will make for a smokin' hot dinner! The fact that it's loaded with antioxidants and stimulates circulation, which promotes heart health, just adds to its "heat."

Makes 4–5 servings

Extra-virgin olive oil

5 cloves fresh garlic, crushed

3 cups whole peeled tomatoes with liquid, coarsely chopped

1 teaspoon sea salt

1 teaspoon crushed red pepper flakes

1 tablespoon capers, drained but not rinsed

½ cup oil-cured black olives, pitted, left whole

1 pound whole-wheat or pure semolina penne

3–4 sprigs fresh basil, leaves removed, coarsely chopped

Place a generous amount of oil (about 3 tablespoons) and garlic in a deep skillet over medium heat. Sauté garlic for 30 seconds. Do not let it brown. Stir in tomatoes, salt, red pepper flakes, capers, and olives. Cover, reduce heat to low, and simmer 25–30 minutes to fully develop the flavors.

While the sauce simmers, bring a pot of water to a boil with a generous pinch of salt. Cook the penne al dente, 8–9 minutes. Using a slotted spoon, transfer the penne right to the sauce and stir well. Remove from heat and stir in fresh basil. Serve hot.

POWER FOODS!

Beans and bean products provide protein and other nutrients essential to building a strong body. They keep us sated, give us powerful endurance, help build new muscle and other tissue, and don't weigh us down. Beans are humble, but don't let their Clark Kent personalities fool you. They are Supermen of nutrition.

TEMPEH WITH CABBAGE AND ONIONS

This simple main course is perfect for those nights when you need to get dinner on the table . . . now! Satisfying, filling, and nutrient dense, this easy-to-make recipe will become a go-to in your busy life. And the fermented nature of the tempeh helps strengthen digestion.

Makes 4–5 servings

3 tablespoons avocado oil
3 cloves fresh garlic, thinly sliced
1 red onion, thinly sliced into half-moons
8 ounces tempeh, crumbled
Soy sauce
2 teaspoons brown rice syrup

¼ head green cabbage, shredded
½ cup fresh or frozen corn kernels

Place oil, garlic, and onions in a skillet over medium heat. When the onion begins to sizzle, add tempeh, a splash of soy sauce, and the rice syrup. Sauté for 3–4 minutes, until the tempeh is beginning to brown and the onions are soft.

Stir in cabbage and corn and season to taste with soy sauce; cover, reduce heat to low, and cook until the cabbage is quite soft, 10–15 minutes. Stir well to combine, and serve.

TOFU AND SPINACH GALETTE

This recipe looks fancy, but it's so easy. The term galette *is used in some parts of France to refer specifically to crepes made with buckwheat. But my version uses a simple packaged whole-wheat pizza dough. And if you have any tofu haters in your household, this could change their minds. High in protein and low in fat, tofu is an essential ingredient in your kitchen when you want to create easy, healthy meals.*

Makes 4 servings

Crust

1 package whole-wheat pizza dough

Filling

1 pound extra-firm tofu, crumbled
3 tablespoons extra-virgin olive oil
2 tablespoons fresh lemon juice
1½ teaspoons sea salt
½ teaspoon cracked black pepper
1 teaspoon garlic powder
3 cups frozen spinach, thawed

Onion Topping

2 tablespoons extra-virgin olive oil
1 red onion, thinly sliced into half-moons
Sea salt

Preheat oven to 350°F and line a round pizza tin with parchment paper.

Between parchment sheets, roll out the prepared pizza dough to be slightly smaller than the perimeter of the pizza tin. Roll evenly. Set aside.

Combine tofu, oil, lemon juice, salt, pepper, garlic powder, and spinach. Set aside.

Place oil and onion in a skillet over medium heat. When the onion begins to sizzle, add a light seasoning of salt and sauté until wilted, about 4 minutes. Set aside.

Assemble the pie. Spoon tofu mixture evenly over the crust, leaving one inch of dough exposed around the rim. Spoon onions on top of tofu mixture. Fold the rim up over the filling, leaving the filling exposed. Using your fingers, pleat the crust to form a rim around the filling, but leaving the filling mostly exposed.

Bake for 35 minutes, until lightly browned. Slice into wedges and serve hot.

◆ **Note**

Whole-wheat pizza dough can be found at natural food stores, Trader Joe's, and Whole Foods Markets. You may also make your own or use phyllo dough, although I prefer the whole wheat.

COCONUT BLACK BEANS

Coconut is a great source of medium-chain saturated fats and can be used in cooking to create rich flavor and provide us with some of the fat we need to be healthy. Combined with beans, like in this dish, it provides a powerful combination of protein and fat that can keep you satisfied for a long time and help manage sweet cravings.

Makes 4–5 servings

Avocado oil
3–4 cloves fresh garlic, minced
½ red onion, diced
Sea salt
2 jalapeño peppers, minced (seeds and spines included for more spice)
2 teaspoons dried cumin
1 (15-ounce) can coconut milk (you can use regular or low-fat)
1 (15-ounce) can (or 2 cups cooked) organic black turtle beans
1 bay leaf
Cracked black pepper
1 ripe avocado, halved, pitted, peeled, sliced into thin wedges
1 ripe mango, halved, seeded, peeled, sliced into thin wedges
2–3 sprigs fresh cilantro, coarsely chopped

Place oil, garlic, and onion in a skillet over medium heat. When the onion begins to sizzle, add a pinch of salt and sauté for 2–3 minutes. Add jalapeño and cumin and stir well. Add coconut milk and simmer for 3–5 minutes before proceeding. Add beans and bay leaf and bring to a boil. Cover and reduce heat to low. Cook for 10–15 minutes. Remove the bay leaf; season to taste with salt and pepper, and simmer for 7–10 minutes more.

While the beans cook, prepare the avocado and mango. To serve, arrange avocado and mango around the rim of a shallow bowl. Stir cilantro into beans and spoon into the center of the bowl (it will be a little soupy). Serve hot with soft tortillas.

◆ **Note**
To work with cooked beans, you will need to cook them 3 parts water to 1 part beans for 45 minutes to 1 hour before proceeding with the recipe.

FAGIOLI NERI

My Nonna knew nothing about nutrition, but she knew that beans, cooked with herbs, vegetables, and olive oil, kept us strong. Protein-packed and energizing, this dish makes a great main course, light lunch, or . . . after-school, after-work, or after-gym snack.

Makes 4–5 servings

Extra-virgin olive oil
3 cloves fresh garlic, minced

1 red onion, diced

Sea salt

Crushed red pepper flakes

2 cups coarsely chopped mushrooms; cremini, oyster, or Portobello work best

¼ cup dry white wine

1 teaspoon dried oregano

2 cups canned, diced tomatoes

3 cups cooked or canned organic black turtle beans

Cracked black pepper

2 cups baby arugula, rinsed well

Place oil, garlic, and onion in a large saucepan over medium heat. When the onion begins to sizzle, add a pinch of salt and a generous pinch of crushed red pepper flakes. Sauté for 2–3 minutes. Add mushrooms and white wine and sauté until the edges of the mushrooms are lightly browned, about 3 minutes. Stir in oregano and tomatoes. Add beans and bring to a boil. Cover and reduce heat to low. Cook for 10–15 minutes. Season to taste with salt and pepper and simmer 5 minutes more. Remove from heat and stir in baby arugula. Transfer to a serving bowl. Serve hot over pasta or brown rice, or mounded on hot whole-grain bread.

◆ **Note**

To work with cooked beans, you will need to cook them 3 parts water to 1 part beans for 45 minutes to 1 hour before proceeding with the recipe.

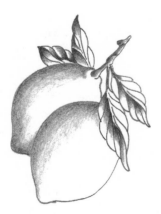

SPICY BLACK BEAN PATTIES WITH CORN SALSA

These are a bit of work, but they are so satisfying and so complete as a meal that you can whip up a crisp, fresh salad to accompany them and you're good to go. Black beans provide us with protein, fiber, phytonutrients, and other essential nutrients, proving that Nonna knew her stuff.

Makes 3–4 servings

1½ cans (15-ounce) or 2 cups organic black turtle beans
¼ cup whole-wheat bread crumbs
2 shallots, diced
4 sprigs fresh flat-leaf parsley, coarsely chopped
1–2 fresh jalapeño peppers, seeded, minced
4–5 cloves fresh garlic, minced
3 roasted red bell peppers, diced
Sea salt
Cracked black pepper

Corn Salsa
1 cup pan-roasted fresh or frozen corn kernels
3 sprigs fresh flat-leaf parsley, minced
¼ red onion, diced
1 roasted green pepper, diced
Juice of 1 fresh lime

Avocado oil, for frying

To make the patties, place beans in a mixing bowl and mash them with a fork to create a thick paste, breaking all the beans. (You can also use a food processor.) Stir in bread crumbs to create a thick texture that can be formed into patties. Stir in shallots, parsley, jalapeño (to taste), garlic, and roasted peppers. Season to taste with salt and pepper. Set aside.

Make the salsa by placing corn in a hot, dry skillet over medium heat and dry-roasting until the corn is lightly browned. Combine corn, parsley, onion, pepper, and lime juice with salt and pepper to taste. Cover and chill while forming and cooking patties so flavors can develop.

To cook the patties, place a generous amount of oil in a flat-bottomed skillet (the oil should cover the bottom of the pan) over medium heat. When the oil is hot, drop large spoonfuls of bean mixture in the oil and flatten them with a spatula. Fry until golden on both sides, turning once, about 2 minutes per side. Drain on paper or kitchen towels and transfer to a parchment-lined baking sheet. Place finished patties in a warm oven to stay warm while cooking the remaining patties.

To serve, arrange patties on a platter with a dollop of salsa on each patty.

Serve hot with cold salsa.

◆ **Note**

To work with cooked beans, you will need to cook them 3 parts water to 1 part beans for 45 minutes to 1 hour before proceeding with the recipe.

DECADENT GREENS AND BEANS

This is the greatest side dish—there are so many possibilities with this recipe! Vary the greens seasonally; try different beans and season to your own taste and style. High in protein, rich in antioxidants, and ready in minutes. It's perfection.
Makes 4–5 servings

Extra-virgin olive oil
1 red onion, thinly sliced into half-moons
Generous pinch crushed red chili flakes
Sea salt
Cracked black pepper
1 can organic cannellini, garbanzo, or
    Great Northern beans, drained and
    rinsed well
1 bunch kale, collards, escarole, bok
    choy, or other dark greens, rinsed well
    and cut into bite-size pieces
Fresh lemon juice

Place a small amount of oil and onion in a deep skillet over medium heat. Add a pinch of salt and pepper and sauté for 2–3 minutes. Stir in beans and ¼ cup water; season lightly with salt and cook over low heat until the beans are warmed through. Stir in greens; season to taste with salt and pepper and cook, stirring, until the greens just wilt and are bright green, about 2 minutes. Remove from heat and stir in about 1 teaspoon fresh lemon juice and serve immediately.

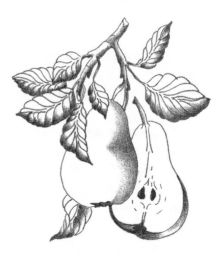

YUMMY CHICKPEA AND SPINACH SALAD

I grew up eating chickpeas not knowing how good they were for me, or that they were loaded with fiber, protein, and folate . . . I just knew I loved them. This hearty salad has nutrient-dense greens and . . . antioxidant-rich artichokes, so I was all in. This is one of my favorite recipes from those early veg days.

Makes 3–4 servings

1 cup dried chickpeas, soaked for
   1 hour with 1 tablespoon baking
   soda
1 bay leaf
1 cup oil-marinated artichoke hearts, cut
   into quarters
1 small red onion, thinly sliced into half-
   moons
3–4 cups baby spinach, rinsed well
12–14 oil-cured black olives, pitted
2 tablespoons balsamic vinegar
1 teaspoon fresh lemon juice
Sea salt
Cracked black pepper
6–7 tablespoons extra-virgin olive oil

Drain chickpeas and rinse very well. Place in a saucepan with 3 cups spring or filtered water and the bay leaf. Bring to a boil, cover, and reduce heat to low. Cook until beans are soft, about 45 minutes. Remove bay leaf and discard. Drain well and set aside to cool before proceeding.

Combine beans with artichoke hearts, onion, spinach, and olives.

Whisk together balsamic vinegar, lemon juice, and salt and pepper to taste. Stream oil into the mixture, whisking constantly to create an emulsified dressing.

Toss salad with dressing to coat and serve with crusty warm bread for a light lunch or dinner.

◆ **Note**

Chickpeas have a mind of their own and do not always cook easily. I learned this trick of soaking them in baking soda while in Israel, and it has served me well. The chickpeas cook in under an hour every single time, no pressure cooking, no stress.

SCRAMBLED CHICKPEAS AND BROCCOLI

I know what you're thinking. Scrambled chickpeas? This recipe is such a treat and so easy to make. The earthy spice of the curry provides more than heat. Naturally antiseptic, anti-inflammatory, and healing, curry is said to aid in the relief of arthritic symptoms as well as provide vitamins B6, A, C, and K.

Makes 3–4 servings

6–8 fingerling or new potatoes,
   unpeeled, cubed

Extra-virgin olive oil

3 cloves fresh garlic, minced

1 medium red onion, diced

Sea salt

1½ teaspoons curry powder

1 (15-ounce) can or 1½ cups cooked
    organic chickpeas

¼ cup dry white wine

1 medium stalk fresh broccoli, broken
    into small florets, stem peeled, diced

Cracked black pepper

Juice of ¼ fresh lemon

Bring a pot of water to a boil with a pinch of salt. Cook potatoes until they can be pierced with a fork, about 5–7 minutes.

Place oil, garlic, and onion in a deep skillet over medium heat. When the onion begins to sizzle, add a pinch of salt and curry powder and sauté for 2–3 minutes. Add chickpeas and potatoes and stir to combine. Season lightly with salt and add wine. Cover and simmer 3–5 minutes. Add broccoli, cover, and cook until broccoli is bright green and crisp-tender, about 3 minutes. Stir in lemon juice just before serving.

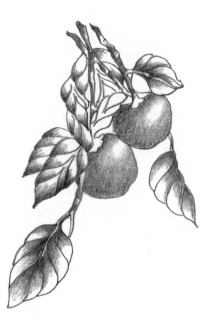

ASIAN LENTIL BURGERS WITH SAUTÉED ONIONS

With abundant folic acid as one of the calling cards of lentils, these high-fiber, protein-rich burgers are more than just fun to cook on the grill. While this recipe calls for cooking all ingredients from scratch, this is a great recipe for using up leftover cooked rice and lentils, too. New studies show that lentils can help significantly reduce heart disease risk when eaten once a week, so it's a good idea to have lots of ways to cook these babies.

Makes 4 servings

½ cup short-grain brown rice, soaked for 1 hour

¼ cup green or brown lentils, rinsed well

1½ cups spring or filtered water

1 bay leaf

2 tablespoons coarsely chopped roasted peanuts

2–3 tablespoons whole-wheat bread crumbs

2 tablespoons soy sauce

3–4 whole green onions, minced

1 tablespoon chia seeds, soaked in ¼ cup spring or filtered water for 30 minutes

Avocado oil

Sautéed Onions

Avocado oil

2 red onions, thinly sliced into half-moons

Soy sauce

2 teaspoons brown rice syrup

To make the burgers, drain rice and discard soaking water. Place rice, lentils, water, and bay leaf in a saucepan over medium heat. Bring to a boil, cover, and reduce heat to low. Cook until rice and beans are tender and the liquid has been absorbed, about 45 minutes. Remove bay leaf and discard.

Transfer mixture to a mixing bowl and mash with a fork. Add peanuts, bread crumbs, soy sauce, green onions, and soaked chia mixture and mix well. Form into four ½-inch-thick patties.

Cover the bottom of a skillet with oil and place over medium heat. When the oil is hot, lay burgers in pan and cook for about 5 minutes per side, turning once to ensure even browning. Transfer the burgers to a serving plate.

While the burgers cook, sauté the onions. Place a small amount of oil and onion in a skillet over medium heat. When the onion begins to sizzle, add a generous splash of soy sauce and rice syrup and sauté until the onions are soft and beginning to brown at the edges, about 7–10 minutes.

To serve, top burgers with sautéed onions.

TOFU FRIED RICE

This main course will stick to your ribs, satisfy hungry families, and can be on the table in no time. Loaded with fiber, protein, antioxidants, and essential nutrients, this is one main course you will create over and over again.

Makes 3–4 servings

Avocado or olive oil

2 cloves fresh garlic, minced

½ yellow onion, thinly sliced into half-
    moons

Soy sauce

1 stalk celery, thinly sliced on the
    diagonal

1 medium carrot, julienned

12 snow peas, thinly sliced on the
    diagonal

½ block extra-firm tofu, cut into small
    cubes

1 cup cooked brown rice

2 whole green onions, thinly sliced on
    the diagonal

Juice of ¼ fresh lemon

Place oil, garlic, and onion in a skillet or wok over medium heat. When the onion begins to sizzle, add a splash of soy sauce and sauté onions until just tender, about 2 minutes. Add celery and a splash of soy sauce and sauté for 1 minute. Add carrot, snow peas, and a splash of soy sauce and sauté for 1 minute. Stir in tofu and sea-son lightly with soy sauce. Spread cooked rice over vegetables evenly. Season lightly with soy sauce and add ¼ cup water to the skillet. Cover, reduce heat to low, and cook for 5 minutes or until liquid is absorbed. Stir in green onion and lemon juice and serve.

◆ Notes

You may also use packaged, frozen, precut veggies for this recipe to save time and work. The mixture of vegetables can be varied.

You may also use leftover rice that you cooked the day before or use packaged cooked brown rice for this recipe.

◆ Variation

You may use seasoned baked tofu, sold in many markets, to bring more intense flavor to this dish or to infuse the dish with a flavor your family likes: Indian, barbecue, Italian, Thai, etc.

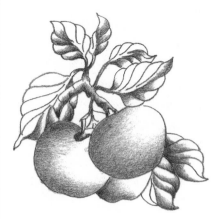

FRIED TOFU AND VEGETABLES

I love this recipe. It's rich-tasting, colorful, and completely versatile. It's a great source of protein and antioxidants and is low in fat. Change up the veggies to suit your family's desires.

Makes 4–5 servings

½ cup avocado oil

2 tablespoons soy sauce

2 tablespoons brown rice syrup

1 pound extra-firm tofu, cut into 1-inch cubes

Avocado oil

1 small leek, split lengthwise, rinsed free of dirt, thinly sliced

2–3 cloves fresh garlic, minced

1-inch piece fresh ginger, cut into very thin matchstick pieces

Soy sauce

1 medium zucchini, julienned

1 medium carrot, julienned

1 medium yellow squash, julienned

8 fresh shiitake mushrooms, thinly sliced

1 roasted red bell pepper, thinly sliced

1 tablespoon tomato paste

Generous pinch crushed red pepper flakes

¼ cup spring or filtered water

2–3 whole green onions, thinly sliced on the diagonal

Place oil, soy sauce, and syrup in a skillet over medium heat. Lay tofu cubes in oil, but don't overcrowd the pan. Cook in the hot oil until golden brown, turning once to ensure even browning. Remove from oil; set aside.

Place a small amount of oil, leek, garlic, and ginger in a skillet or wok over medium heat. When the leeks begin to sizzle, add a splash of soy sauce and sauté for 1–2 minutes. Stir in zucchini, carrot, and yellow squash with a splash of soy sauce and sauté for 2 minutes. Stir in shiitake and red bell pepper. Sauté for 1–2 minutes.

Puree tomato paste with red pepper flakes and the water. Stir this liquid into the veggie mixture. Gently stir in tofu. Cook, stirring, for 4–5 minutes. Remove from heat and stir in green onions and serve.

TEMPEH SALAD

Everyone loves tuna salad, but it's soooooo fishy. And with tuna being contaminated with mercury and fish becoming, in my view, a controversial food source, this satisfying salad, made from a fermented soy product, is the perfect alternative.

Makes 4–5 servings

2 cups spring or filtered water

2 tablespoons soy sauce

1 teaspoon garlic powder

8 ounces tempeh

½ red onion, minced

2 stalks celery, diced

3 natural dill pickles, diced

3–4 fresh chives, minced

1 tablespoon granulated kelp

⅓ cup vegan mayonnaise (Vegenaise)

1 tablespoon fresh orange juice

Sea salt

Cracked black pepper

Sweet paprika

Place water, soy sauce, and garlic powder in a saucepan and bring to a boil over medium heat. When the mixture boils, place tempeh in the broth and cook for 15 minutes. Remove tempeh and cool to room temperature before proceeding.

Crumble tempeh into a mixing bowl and mix in onion, celery, pickles, chives, and kelp. Fold in mayo and orange juice, salt and pepper to taste, with a touch of paprika for color. Serve chilled or at room temperature as a salad, on sandwiches, or on crackers.

THAI TEMPEH

This main dish is just yummy. There really is no other way to describe it. It's packed with nutrients, protein, and hot spice to stimulate circulation, which promotes heart health. It's easy, versatile, and is just gorgeous.

Makes 3–4 servings

Avocado oil

8 ounces tempeh

½ cup spring or filtered water or vegetable broth

1 teaspoon soy sauce

3 cloves fresh garlic, minced

2 serrano peppers, minced (with seeds for more heat, without seeds for mild taste)

1 teaspoon freshly grated ginger

½ cup unsweetened low-fat coconut milk

4 whole green onions, thinly sliced on the diagonal

1 teaspoon fresh lime juice

2–3 sprigs fresh flat-leaf parsley, coarsely chopped

Place avocado oil to cover the bottom of a flat-bottomed skillet over medium heat. Brown the tempeh on both sides, about 3 minutes per side. Remove tempeh. In the same skillet, add water, soy sauce, garlic, serranos, and ginger. Slice tempeh into strips and add to the skillet. Cook, covered, over medium-low heat until all the liquid has been absorbed into the tempeh, about 3–4 minutes. Stir in coconut milk, green onions, and lime juice and simmer 2–3 minutes more. Remove from heat and stir in parsley.

◆ **Note**

You may use cilantro in place of the parsley, but I personally hate the taste of cilantro, so I never use it.

STIR-FRIED CORN AND TEMPEH

This simple main course has it all and can almost stand on its own as a meal. With a whole grain, plenty of protein, and veggies, this is a nutrient-dense and satisfying main course. Serve it with a crisp salad and a light soup for a complete meal.

Makes 3–4 servings

Avocado oil
5–6 thin slices fresh ginger, finely
 julienned
2 cloves fresh garlic, thinly sliced
1 small leek, halved lengthwise, rinsed
 free of dirt, sliced thinly diagonally
Soy sauce
1 roasted red pepper, sliced into ribbons
1 (8-ounce) package tempeh, cut into
 cubes
1 cup frozen corn kernels
1 cup watercress, rinsed well, hand-torn
 into bite-size pieces

Place a generous amount of oil in a skillet or wok, along with ginger, garlic, and leek, over medium heat. When the leek begins to sizzle, add a splash of soy sauce and sauté for 1–2 minutes. Stir in pepper and tempeh cubes, season lightly with soy sauce, and stir-fry for 3–4 minutes, allowing the tempeh to brown on the edges. Stir in corn, season to taste with soy sauce, and stir-fry until the corn is just heated through. Remove from heat and stir in watercress. Transfer to a serving platter and serve hot.

LENTIL TOMATO SALAD

Chilled or warm, this richly flavored lentil dish is satisfying as a light main course or a side dish because it's loaded with protein, fiber, and heart-healthy compounds.

Makes 4–5 servings

1 cup dried lentils (preferably baby
 Italian or French), rinsed well
3 cups spring or filtered water
1 bay leaf
Extra-virgin olive oil
3 cloves fresh garlic, minced
½ medium red onion, diced
Sea salt
Cracked black pepper
3–4 sprigs fresh basil, leaves removed,
 coarsely chopped
3 sprigs fresh dill, minced
2 cups diced tomatoes (canned or fresh)
Red wine vinegar

Place lentils, water, and bay leaf in a saucepan over medium heat. Bring to a boil, cover, and reduce heat to low. Cook until lentils are soft, but not mushy, about 45 minutes. Drain any remaining water and set aside.

Place a small amount of oil, garlic, and onion in a skillet over medium heat. When the onion begins to sizzle, add a pinch of salt and pepper and sauté for 2–3 minutes. Stir in basil, dill, and tomatoes and season to taste with salt and pepper. Simmer for 3–4 minutes to develop flavors. Remove from heat and stir in cooked lentils and a splash of red wine vinegar. Serve warm or chilled.

LENTIL TIMBALES

Timbales are an Italian tradition of meat, eggs, pasta, and cheese all cooked together in molds. Mine is ridiculously delicious with the texture of a rich pâté. And since this recipe has no saturated fat and is lower in calories than meat and dairy dishes, you can enjoy it without guilt.
Makes 6 servings

Extra-virgin olive oil
1 yellow onion, diced
3 cloves fresh garlic, minced
Sea salt
Cracked black pepper

1 cup thinly sliced cremini mushrooms
  (about 10 large mushrooms)
3 tablespoons mirin or sweet white wine
½ cup whole-wheat bread crumbs
½ cup silken tofu
1 cup cooked lentils
2 tablespoons tomato paste
½ teaspoon minced fresh rosemary
½ teaspoon rubbed, dried sage
2–3 tablespoons arrowroot powder
1 cup cooked wild rice

Sautéed Mushrooms
Extra-virgin olive oil
1 cup sliced cremini mushrooms
Sea salt
3–4 sprigs fresh chives, minced, for
  garnish
Juice of ¼ fresh lemon

Preheat oven to 350°F. Lightly oil 6 ramekins and place them in a shallow baking dish.

Place a small amount of oil, onion, and garlic in a skillet over medium heat. When the onion begins to sizzle, add a pinch of salt and pepper and sauté for 2–3 minutes. Stir in mushrooms, a pinch of salt, and mirin or wine. Sauté for 2–3 minutes.

Transfer mushroom mixture to a food processor and add bread crumbs, tofu, lentils, and tomato paste. Puree until smooth. Add herbs, arrowroot, and salt and pepper to taste and puree until smooth.

Transfer to a mixing bowl and fold in

cooked rice. Spoon the mixture evenly into the ramekins, filling completely to the tops. Set the ramekins back in the baking dish with water to half cover the dishes. Bake, uncovered, until the tops are browned and crispy at the edges and the centers are firm to the touch. Remove from oven and allow to cool for 10 minutes. Run a knife around the rims and invert the ramekins onto serving plates or onto a platter.

While the timbales cool, sauté the mushrooms. Place oil and mushrooms in a skillet over medium heat and sauté until golden, about 7–10 minutes. Season lightly with salt and sauté for 1 minute more. Remove from heat and stir in chives and lemon juice.

To serve, spoon sautéed mushrooms over timbales and serve hot.

SEARED SEITAN WITH MUSHROOMS

This main course is hearty and full of flavor. I have served this dish to hard-core carnivores to rave reviews. With wheat gluten as its protein source, this dish combines with shiitake mushrooms to help the body digest and muscles relax.

Makes 3–4 servings

Avocado oil
¾ pound seitan, sliced into ½-inch-thick pieces

½ red onion, thinly sliced into half-moons
8–10 fresh shiitake mushrooms, thinly sliced
Sea salt
Cracked black pepper
Generous pinch dried thyme
2 tablespoons whole-wheat pastry flour
½ cup spring or filtered water or vegetable broth
2–3 sprigs fresh flat-leaf parsley, coarsely chopped, for garnish

Place about 2 tablespoons oil in flat-bottomed skillet over medium heat. When the oil is hot, lay the seitan slices in the skillet. Cook the seitan for about 3 minutes per side, spooning oil from the pan over the slices as they cook. Remove from the pan and set aside. In the same pan, sauté onions and mushrooms with a pinch of salt until soft, about 3 minutes. Remove from pan and set aside.

Place 2 tablespoons of oil in the same skillet over medium heat. Add thyme and flour, stirring continuously to make a roux. Slowly stir in water or broth and cook, stirring to incorporate the ingredients. Stir in cooked vegetables. Season with salt and pepper to taste.

Arrange seared seitan on a platter and spoon mushroom gravy over top. Garnish with fresh parsley and serve.

◆ **Note**

Made from wheat gluten, seitan is pure protein and can be found in natural food stores and some gourmet food stores. It is not to be used if you have gluten sensitivity. You may also use tempeh in this recipe.

CURRIED CHICKPEAS AND POTATOES

A quick and tasty main course, this will leave you with no excuses to order take-out. This spicy stew will satisfy you on many levels, but don't let the ingredient list scare you. It's lots of little pinches of spices and you can omit any that you wish and still have a great nutrient-dense stew.

Makes 3–4 servings

1 tablespoon avocado oil
1 red onion, diced
3 cloves fresh garlic, minced
1-inch piece fresh ginger, finely minced
Sea salt
½ teaspoon cumin
½ teaspoon turmeric
¼ teaspoon crushed red pepper flakes
¼ teaspoon chipotle powder
2 cups diced new or fingerling potatoes, unpeeled
1 cup canned organic chickpeas, rinsed well
1 cup spring or filtered water
Fresh lemon juice to taste

2–3 sprigs fresh flat-leaf parsley, coarsely chopped

Place oil in a deep skillet over medium heat. Add onions, garlic, and ginger and a pinch of salt. Sauté for 2 minutes. Stir in spices to coat the onions. Add potatoes and cook, stirring, until the potatoes are browned at the edges and tender, about 6 minutes. Add chickpeas and water. Season to taste with salt. Bring to a boil, cover, reduce heat to low, and cook until all liquid has been absorbed, about 7–10 minutes. Remove from heat, stir in lemon juice and parsley, and serve.

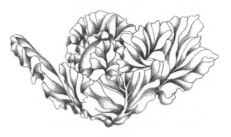

CANNELLINI PICCATA

You know chicken piccata, right? You won't miss the bird once you have tasted this recipe. With no saturated fat or other nasty stuff we know comes in chicken, these spicy beans are satisfying, and studies show that eating cannellini beans once a week can help reduce the risk of heart disease. And with hot spice to stimulate circulation, you have a heart-healthy winner.

Makes 3–4 servings

2 tablespoons extra-virgin olive oil

1 red onion, diced

3 cloves fresh garlic, minced

Sea salt

Cracked black pepper

Crushed red pepper flakes

Grated zest of 1 fresh lemon

10 button mushrooms, brushed free of dirt, coarsely chopped

2 tablespoons dry white wine

4 tablespoons whole-wheat pastry flour

1½ cups spring or filtered water

1 (15-ounce) can organic cannellini beans (or 2 cups cooked)

3–4 sprigs fresh basil, leaves removed, coarsely chopped

2–3 sprigs fresh flat-leaf parsley, coarsely chopped

Place oil, onion, and garlic in a deep skillet over medium heat. When the onion begins to sizzle, add a pinch of salt and pepper, a generous pinch of red pepper flakes, and lemon zest. Sauté for 2–3 minutes. Stir in mushrooms and wine and sauté for 2–3 minutes. Add flour, stirring to coat the veggies, but avoid lumps. Add water, stirring until thickened, about 3 minutes. Add beans, salt, pepper, and more red pepper flakes to taste. Cook over low heat, uncovered, stirring frequently until bubbling and thick, about 5 minutes. Remove from heat and stir in basil and parsley. Serve hot over pasta or as a side dish.

GRILLED EGGPLANT AND CANNELLINI BEANS

Eggplant is a nightshade, meaning it can be a little on the acidic side, but its ample bioflavenoids may be helpful in preventing stroke and hemorrhages. It is also said to prevent heart disease, so combined with cannellini beans, this is one heart-healthy side dish.

Makes 3–4 servings

½ cup extra-virgin olive oil

2–3 cloves fresh garlic, minced

Sea salt

Generous pinch crushed red pepper flakes

1 tablespoon fresh lemon juice

3 small eggplants, sliced into ½-inch
pieces

Extra-virgin olive oil
1 red onion, diced
Sea salt
Cracked black pepper
1 (14-ounce) can cannellini beans,
drained and rinsed well
2–3 sprigs fresh basil, leaves removed,
shredded
Juice of ¼ fresh lemon

Place ½ cup oil, minced garlic, salt to taste, red pepper flakes, and lemon juice in a saucepan over low heat. Heat a grill pan over medium heat. Brush eggplant slices with oil mixture and grill 4–5 minutes per side, brushing with oil mixture as you turn and grill slices.

While the eggplant grills, heat a small amount of oil and onion in a skillet. When the onion begins to sizzle, add a pinch of salt and pepper and sauté for 2–3 minutes. Stir in beans, season with salt to taste, reduce heat, and cook, stirring occasionally, until beans are warmed through, about 5 minutes. Remove from heat and stir in basil and lemon juice.

To serve, arrange eggplant slices on a plate with beans mounded on top.

◆ **Note**
Normally, I soak eggplant in salted water before cooking so I can remove some of the acid in it. But in this recipe, I use small eggplants so that step can be eliminated.

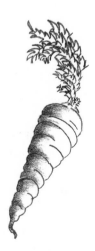

QUINOA AND BEAN CHILI

I love this recipe. It's protein-packed because of the quinoa and beans; it's spicy and delicious, so it stimulates circulation; and it's loaded with veggies, so it's antioxidant-rich. It's basically perfect nutrition.

Makes 3–4 servings

2 tablespoons avocado or extra-virgin olive oil

3 cloves fresh garlic, minced

1 red onion, diced

1 jalapeño pepper, minced, seeds and spines included

Sea salt

Crushed red chili flakes

Smoked paprika

2 stalks celery, diced

1 medium carrot, diced

1 red bell pepper, seeded, diced

1 (14-ounce) can diced tomatoes

2 tablespoons tomato paste

½ cup quinoa, rinsed well

1 (14-ounce) can organic black beans, drained and rinsed well

Spring or filtered water

2–3 sprigs fresh flat-leaf parsley, coarsely chopped

Place oil, garlic, onion, and jalapeño in a soup pot over medium heat. When the onion begins to sizzle, add a pinch of salt, crushed red pepper flakes, and smoked paprika. Sauté for 2–3 minutes. Stir in celery and a pinch of salt and sauté for 1 minute. Stir in carrot and a pinch of salt and sauté for 1 minute. Stir in pepper and a pinch of salt and sauté for 1 minute. Add tomatoes, tomato paste, quinoa, and beans and stir well. Add 1½ cups water. Cover and bring to a boil. Reduce heat to low and cook until quinoa is soft, about 15 minutes. Season to taste with salt and adjust heat with chili flakes if more is desired. Simmer for 2–3 minutes more. Serve garnished with parsley.

MEXICAN BEAN FONDUE DIP

Popular in Europe . . . and the United States in the '70s, fondue dips are fun, social, and delicious. They are also loaded with fat and calories. This spicy vegan version gives you all the delight and none of the saturated fat. It's so yummy, there's no need to tell anyone it's healthy.

Makes 4–5 servings

1 can organic red kidney beans, drained and rinsed well

1 can spicy tomato sauce

½ red onion, finely diced

2 cloves fresh garlic, minced

½ teaspoon chili powder

Sea salt

Cracked black pepper

4 ounces vegan cheddar cheese (Follow Your Heart brand melts very well)

Organic corn tortilla chips

Place all ingredients in a saucepan over low heat. Cook, stirring, until the mixture is creamy and melted. Adjust seasonings to taste. Keep the mixture hot and serve with chips.

BUTT-KICKING-DELICIOUS LASAGNA

I love this lasagna. It's a bit of work and takes some time, but it's so delicious and loaded with veggie nutrients, you won't care. It also freezes very nicely, so make a big batch and you will have it for those meals when you want something a bit fancy, but just don't have the time.

Makes 6–8 servings

Extra-virgin olive oil
1 red onion, diced
2 cloves fresh garlic, minced
Sea salt
6–8 cremini mushrooms, thinly sliced
2 tablespoons dry white wine
2 stalks fresh broccoli, broken into small florets
2 medium carrots, diced
2 roasted red bell peppers, diced
1 cup fresh or frozen corn

1 package firm tofu, hand crumbled
Generous pinch chili powder
1 teaspoon dried oregano
2 recipes Pomodoro Presto (or unsweetened tomato sauce)
2 boxes dried whole-wheat lasagna noodles
16 ounces frozen spinach, thawed and drained
2 sweet potatoes, cooked and mashed
6 ripe plum tomatoes, thinly sliced into rounds
1 cup blanched almonds, ground into a coarse meal

Preheat oven to 375°F and lightly oil a 9 x 13-inch baking dish.

Place a small amount of oil, onion, and garlic in a skillet over medium heat. When the onion begins to sizzle, add a pinch of salt and sauté for 2–3 minutes. Add mushrooms, wine, and salt to taste. Sauté for 2–3 minutes more. Transfer to a large mixing bowl.

In the same skillet, add a small amount of oil and sauté broccoli, with a pinch of salt, for 2–3 minutes. Stir in carrots and a pinch of salt and sauté for 2–3 minutes more. Transfer to the mushroom mixture. Stir peppers and corn into the mixture. Mix in the crumbled tofu, spices, and salt to taste.

Assemble the lasagna. Cover the bottom of the baking dish with sauce. Lay noodles to cover, with more sauce on top (this is to avoid having to precook the noodles). Spread the tofu mixture over the sauce and top with more noodles. Spoon sauce over the noodles. Cover the sauce with frozen spinach and more sauce. Cover with noodles and more sauce. Spread sweet potatoes over sauce. Spoon sauce over top followed by another layer of noo- dles. Spoon final layer of sauce over top. Arrange sliced tomatoes over top. Cover and bake for 45 minutes. Remove cover and sprinkle with almonds to cover. Return to oven for 15 minutes more. Allow to stand for 15 minutes before slicing into squares and serving hot.

NATURE'S PERFECT FOODS

I could wax rhapsodic about the wonders of vegetables and all the nutrients and energy they bring to our lives. But I won't. I will say just this . . . eat your veggies. They will change your life.

SWEET POTATO CHIPS

I know you're thinking that these chips will taste healthy, but man, I gotta tell you. You will love them. And I love that sweet potatoes are loaded with antioxidants and carotenoids, so the fun comes with a benefit! And they are fat-free, so enjoy!
Makes 3–5 servings

1 large sweet potato, scrubbed but not
    peeled, very thinly sliced
Sea salt
Chili powder

Preheat oven to 200°F and line 2 baking sheets with parchment.

Arrange potato slices on baking sheets, but do not let them touch, if possible. Sprinkle lightly with salt and chili powder. Bake, uncovered, for 50 minutes. The slices will dehydrate and wrinkle as they bake. Turn the chips over and bake for another 30–40 minutes, until the edges are lightly browned, but the centers of the chips are still orange. Remove from oven and transfer chips to cooling racks. They may still be soft when they come out of the oven, but will crisp as they cool. Store in an airtight container. They will stay fresh for 3–4 days.

◆ **Note**

Use a mandolin for perfectly thin slices if you are not confident with a knife.

SAUTÉED ZUCCHINI CROSTINI

I love crostini as a starter course. It's the type of dish that makes every meal more special. And while no one thinks of zucchini as a nutrient powerhouse, it is: a great source of vitamin A and flavenoids and so low in calories, you can use it as much as you like.

Makes 3–4 servings

1 whole-grain baguette, sliced
    diagonally
Extra-virgin olive oil
Garlic powder
Paprika

Zucchini Topping
Extra-virgin olive oil
2 cloves fresh garlic, minced
½ red onion, thinly sliced into half-
    moons
Sea salt
1 medium zucchini, sliced in half
    lengthwise and thinly sliced in half-
    moons
6–8 cherry tomatoes, halved

Preheat oven to 350°F and line a baking sheet with parchment.

Arrange bread slices on baking sheet and drizzle lightly with olive oil. Sprinkle lightly with garlic powder and paprika and bake until crisp and browned at the edges, about 5–7 minutes.

While the bread bakes, make the topping. Place oil, garlic, and onion in a skillet over medium heat. When the onion begins to sizzle, add a pinch of salt and sauté for 2–3 minutes. Add zucchini; season to taste with salt and sauté until just limp, about 3–4 minutes. Remove from heat and stir in cherry tomatoes.

To serve, arrange bread on a platter and mound zucchini mixture on top. Serve warm or at room temperature.

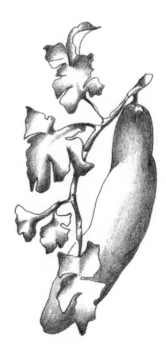

PRONTO POMODORO AND PANE

Visions of a Tuscan summer come in each spoonful of this simple, richly flavored Italian tradition. Usually made with fresh tomatoes and cooked for a long time, this version is ready in minutes but is still a rich source of lycopene, an essential nutrient for reproductive health.

Makes 3–4 servings

Extra-virgin olive oil
2–3 cloves fresh garlic, finely minced
2 (28-ounce) cans of diced tomatoes
2 cups spring or filtered water
Sea salt
Cracked black pepper
1 small loaf whole-grain sourdough
    bread (pane, in Italian), coarsely
    crumbled
1 small bunch fresh basil, finely minced

Place a small amount of oil and the garlic in a soup pot and turn the heat to medium. As soon as the garlic begins to sizzle (do not burn it), add the tomatoes and the water. Bring to a boil, add several pinches of sea salt and pepper and the bread. Stir well, cover, and return to a boil. Reduce heat to low and cook for 15–20 minutes, until the bread is quite soft. Season to taste with salt; stir in fresh basil and serve.

VEGETABLE BREAD SALAD WITH WHITE BEANS

This salad is a meal in itself. With whole-grain bread, lots of veggies, and beans, this baby gives new meaning to "A Big Salad."

Makes 3–4 servings

1 red onion, thinly sliced into half-moons
Red wine vinegar

½ loaf whole-grain baguette, cut into
    cubes
½ cup frozen organic corn kernels
3 firm but ripe tomatoes, diced, with
    their seeds
1 cucumber, unpeeled and diced, with its
    seeds
2 sprigs fresh basil, leaves shredded
3 cups baby arugula
12–16 oil-cured black olives, pitted
1 (14-ounce) can Great Northern beans
    or chickpeas, drained and rinsed well
8 tablespoons extra-virgin olive oil
3 tablespoons balsamic vinegar
Sea salt
Cracked black pepper

Place onion in a shallow bowl and cover with red wine vinegar. Marinate for 10 minutes.

While the onion marinates, combine the balance of the salad ingredients in a large mixing bowl.

Pour oil over salad and toss to coat. Add vinegar and salt and pepper to taste (take care with salt as there are olives in the salad). Toss to combine. Serve chilled or at room temperature.

STUFFED TOMATOES

When they are in season, I want fresh tomatoes in . . . everything! This recipe is easy enough for a weekday dinner and lovely enough for a fancy Saturday night meal al fresco in the garden. I love that the tomatoes are a rich source of antioxidants; the whole-wheat couscous provides fiber; and the herbs give us essential vitamins and minerals.

Makes 4 servings

4 large ripe tomatoes
1 cup spring or filtered water
½ cup oil-packed sun-dried tomatoes, minced
Sea salt
1 cup whole-wheat couscous
⅓ cup shredded vegan mozzarella (Daiya or Follow Your Heart)
3–4 sprigs fresh basil, leaves coarsely chopped
2 tablespoons coarsely chopped fresh mint
Cracked black pepper
Extra-virgin olive oil

Preheat oven to 375°F.

Cut the top third off each tomato and hollow out the inside, reserving tops and pulp. Invert tomatoes on a towel to drain them.

Bring water, sun-dried tomatoes, and a generous pinch of salt to a boil. Remove from heat and stir in couscous. Cover and set aside until all the liquid is absorbed, about 5 minutes. When the couscous is ready, stir in vegan cheese, basil, mint, and salt and pepper to taste. Gently fold in reserved pulp. Very gently spoon couscous mixture into each tomato and place in a shallow baking dish. Place the tops back on each tomato. Bake until heated through, about 25 minutes.

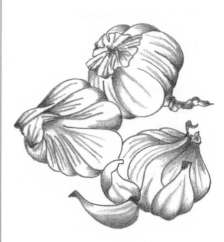

VEGGIE LETTUCE WRAPS

Lettuce wraps are so lovely as a light lunch, a starter course, or a side dish. These are packed with protein and satisfaction. And making them at home ensures that you know what's in them and can eliminate the fat, sugar, and salt that are the cornerstones of a lot of takeout.

Makes 3–4 servings

Avocado oil

2 cloves fresh garlic, minced

1 small leek, split lengthwise, rinsed free of dirt, diced

5–6 thin slices fresh ginger, minced

Soy sauce

2 cups minced seitan

2 teaspoons brown rice syrup

½ teaspoon arrowroot powder

Brown rice vinegar

2 cups mung bean sprouts

Several leaves romaine lettuce, rinsed, trimmed, left whole

Place oil, garlic, leek, and ginger in a skillet or wok over medium heat. When the leek begins to sizzle, add a splash of soy sauce and sauté for 1–2 minutes. Stir in seitan, brown rice syrup, and soy sauce to taste. Sauté for 2–3 minutes to heat seitan. Stir in arrowroot to create a thin sauce over the seitan and veggies. Remove from heat and stir in a splash of vinegar and the sprouts. Transfer to a serving bowl and serve with lettuce on the side so people can make their own wraps.

◆ **Note**

Made from wheat gluten, seitan is pure protein and can be found in natural food stores and some gourmet food stores. It is not to be used if you have gluten sensitivity.

BABY CARROTS AND CRISPY POTATOES

This side dish is lovely comfort food after a long day. The fact that it's easy to make and packed with antioxidants and carotenoids makes it beyond perfect.

Makes 3–4 servings

Carrots

12 baby carrots, tops removed

2 sprigs fresh thyme

2 bay leaves

Sea salt

1 tablespoon brown rice syrup

Potatoes

12 red-skinned potatoes, unpeeled and quartered

Sea salt

Extra-virgin olive oil

Cracked black pepper

Grated zest of 1 lemon

2 cloves fresh garlic, peeled, halved

2 sprigs fresh thyme

P lace carrots in a pan with water to just cover. Add thyme, bay leaves, a generous pinch of salt, and rice syrup. Bring to a boil, reduce heat to low, and cook until just tender, about 8 minutes.

While the carrots cook, cook the potatoes. Place them in a deep skillet with water to just cover and a generous pinch of salt. Bring to a boil, reduce heat to low, and cook until just tender, about 8 minutes.

When the carrots are tender, remove thyme and bay leaves, drain, and set aside.

When the potatoes are tender, drain them well and return them to the same skillet over high heat. Drizzle about 2 tablespoons of olive oil over the potatoes. Toss the potatoes to coat them with oil. Add salt and pepper to taste, lemon zest, garlic cloves, and thyme. Toss well and, using a masher, press the potatoes into the skillet. Do not mash them; just press them down. Toss them every 2–3 minutes to evenly brown and crisp them.

When the potatoes are ready, remove the thyme sprigs, toss with cooked baby carrots, and serve.

CRUNCHY TUSCAN KALE SALAD

Seriously, I never thought I could like raw kale, but in this salad, the textures and flavors shine. This is no ordinary salad, and is a great source of fiber; vitamins C, A, and K; and folic acid. Because the kale is raw, no enzymes are lost.

Makes 3–4 servings

1 bunch Tuscan kale (also called lacinato or dinosaur, but regular kale will work)

1 teaspoon extra-virgin olive oil

¾ cup coarse bread crumbs

1 clove fresh garlic, mashed

½ teaspoon sea salt

⅛ teaspoon cracked black pepper

Pinch crushed red pepper flakes

3 tablespoons extra-virgin olive oil

Juice from ½ fresh lemon

R inse the kale leaves and towel-dry. Shred the kale leaves, removing the stems if they are thick.

Place a teaspoon of oil in a skillet over medium heat. Sauté the bread crumbs until golden brown, about 3 minutes. Set aside.

Mix together garlic, salt, pepper, red pepper, oil, and lemon juice. Adjust seasonings to your taste and mix well.

Toss kale with bread crumbs and dressing to coat. Allow to marinate for about 5 minutes before serving.

CUCUMBER SALAD

A refreshing salad that goes well with any hearty meal. Usually, cucumbers are mixed with dill, but I chose to go with basil to make for a slightly different take on this easy, satisfying salad. Cooling to the body, cucumbers are rich sources of silica, which results in beautiful skin.

Makes 3–4 servings

2 cucumbers, unpeeled and thinly sliced
1 red onion, thinly sliced into half-moons
10–12 cherry tomatoes
2–3 sprigs fresh basil, leaves shredded
¼ cup extra-virgin olive oil
2 teaspoons balsamic vinegar
Sea salt
Cracked black pepper

Combine cucumbers with red onion and tomatoes. Stir in basil, oil, balsamic vinegar, and salt and pepper to taste. Serve chilled or at room temperature.

◆ **Note**

The key to this salad is to slice the veggies very thinly. If you can't do it with your knife, use a mandolin.

MARINATED EGGPLANT BRUSCHETTA

This is another winning starter. And the cool thing is you can make the marinated eggplant and keep it in the fridge for as long as a month, using it as you like in this recipe, in salads, on sandwiches, or in pasta dishes.

Makes 8–10 servings

2 eggplants, peeled, halved, thinly sliced into long matchstick pieces
4 ounces apple cider vinegar
2 cloves fresh garlic, minced
Pinch dried oregano
½ cup minced fresh flat-leaf parsley
Generous pinch crushed red pepper flakes
Sea salt
Cracked black pepper
4 ounces extra-virgin olive oil

1 whole-grain baguette, sliced on the diagonal

Prepare the eggplant while bringing a large pot of water to a boil. Add 2 ounces vinegar to the water and the eggplant. Cook eggplant for 2 minutes. Using a slotted spoon, transfer eggplant to a kitchen towel and wrap tightly to dry.

Place eggplant in a mixing bowl with remaining vinegar, garlic, oregano, parsley, crushed red pepper flakes, salt and pepper to taste, and oil. Toss well. Adjust seasonings to taste. Transfer to a glass jar and refrigerate. You may use immediately or allow to marinate.

To serve, toast bread slices in a 350°F oven until crisp, about 7 minutes. Transfer to a tray and top with eggplant.

WHOLE POACHED ARTICHOKES

Rich in antioxidants, pantothenic acid, and other essential nutrients, artichokes are said to be an aphrodisiac and a diuretic, and for the mere twenty-five calories in a whole uncooked artichoke, you get sixteen essential nutrients as well as fiber.
Makes 4 servings

4 globe artichokes
Extra-virgin olive oil
8 whole cloves fresh garlic, peeled
Sea salt

Trim the artichokes by removing the stem at the base so the artichokes stand upright. Peel the stem and set aside.

Using kitchen scissors, trim the tips of each leaf, removing the prickly end. When you get to the top third of the artichoke, slice it completely off with a

sharp knife. Repeat with the remaining artichokes. Arrange them in a pan that holds them tightly and can be covered. Add about an inch of water to the pan. Drop garlic cloves in the pan. Place artichoke stems on top of each artichoke. Drizzle with olive oil and sprinkle lightly with salt. Cover pan and bring to a boil. Reduce heat to low and cook for an hour. The artichokes are done when you can easily pluck a leaf from the bottom. Lift the artichokes out of the pan and transfer to a platter. Remove garlic cloves to the platter and raise the heat to high. Reduce the liquid to a syrup. Spoon syrup over the artichokes and serve.

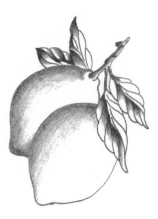

ROASTED WINTER SQUASH

This simple side dish is sweetly satisfying, warming, and comforting. Loaded with antioxidants and carotenoids and requiring little prep, this dish just needs the time to bake and you are on your way. Relaxing to the spleen, stomach, and pancreas, this dish can help you manage sweet cravings.
Makes 3–4 servings

1 small winter squash, halved, seeded,
    cut into 1-inch cubes
Extra-virgin olive oil
Sea salt
Cracked black pepper
Juice of ½ fresh lemon

Preheat oven to 375°F. Cut squash and arrange it in a shallow baking dish, avoiding overlap, if possible. Drizzle generously with olive oil and season to taste with salt and pepper. Toss to coat. Cover tightly with foil. Bake for 45 minutes. Remove cover and return to oven for 10 minutes more. Drizzle with lemon juice just before serving.

GOOD-FOR-WHAT-AILS-YOU STEW

This stew brings together Mother Nature's finest cleansing veggies. I love this stew during cold and flu season because not only can it help prevent sniffles, aches, and pains, but the ingredients can also help you feel better faster.
Makes 3–4 servings

1-inch piece kombu
2 dried shiitake mushrooms, soaked until
    tender
1 cup diced fresh daikon
1 cup diced burdock
1 cup diced winter squash
1 cup diced carrot
Soy sauce
Juice of ¼ fresh lemon
3–4 sprigs fresh flat-leaf parsley,
    coarsely chopped

Layer the veggies in a heavy pot in the order listed. Add ⅓ cup spring or filtered water and a splash of soy sauce and bring to a boil over medium heat. Reduce heat to low and cook until carrot is soft, about 20 minutes. Season to taste with soy sauce and simmer, uncovered, until any remaining liquid cooks away. Stir gently to incorporate lemon juice and parsley and serve hot.

◆ **Note**

Kombu is a sea vegetable that can be purchased at natural food stores.

STUFFED LOTUS ROOT

This is the best party snack! Most people don't think of this strange veggie as party food, but once you make this dish, you will change your mind. Some of the ingredients are a wee bit exotic, but worth searching out.

Makes 5–6 servings

1 lotus root, washed, ends trimmed

Filling
4 tablespoons almond butter
4 tablespoons barley miso

Avocado oil, for frying

Place whole lotus root in a pressure cooker with ½ inch of water. Seal the lid and bring to full pressure. Reduce heat to low and cook for 5 minutes. Force pressure down and remove lotus root carefully. Set aside to cool enough to handle.

While the lotus root cools, make the filling by mixing the ingredients together. Transfer filling to a flat saucer. Holding the lotus root so that one of the cut sides is immersed in the filling, begin to turn the lotus root as you press it into the filling. You will see the filling travel up into the many chambers of the veggie. When the lotus root is filled, slice it thinly.

Heat about ½ inch oil in a skillet over medium heat. When the oil is hot, quickly fry the lotus slices until crispy, about 2 minutes. Drain on paper and serve hot.

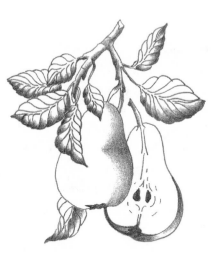

SPICY TEMPURA SWEET POTATOES

There's nothing quite like deep frying to get people to eat their veggies, right? In this recipe, a light, crisp batter combines nicely with the natural sweet flavor of the sweet potatoes. Served with a tart dipping sauce, this is food heaven . . . and loaded with carotenoids for health, but no one needs to know.

Makes 5–6 servings

2 sweet potatoes, unpeeled and thinly
   sliced on the diagonal

Batter
1 cup whole-wheat pastry flour
½ cup semolina flour
Sea salt
Generous pinch chili powder
1 teaspoon baking powder
1 tablespoon kuzu, dissolved in 3
   tablespoons spring or filtered water
Sparkling water

Dipping Sauce
Soy sauce
Fresh lime juice

Avocado oil for frying

Slice the sweet potatoes and cook them in boiling water for 3 minutes. Transfer to a kitchen towel and dry them completely.

Make the batter by combining flours, salt, spices, and baking powder. Stir in dissolved kuzu and enough sparkling water to create a thin batter, as for pancakes. Set aside for 5 minutes.

Make the dipping sauce by whisking together equal amounts of soy sauce and lime juice.

Heat 2 inches oil in a deep pot over medium heat. When the oil is hot, dip sweet potato slices in batter and fry until golden, about 2 minutes. Drain well and serve with dipping sauce on the side.

Note that you can keep the sweet potatoes that are fried in a warm oven so they stay crisp while you fry the balance of them.

◆ **Note**
Kuzu can be found in natural food stores and works in recipes very much like cornstarch. Said to be alkalizing to the intestines, kuzu creates creamier results than either arrowroot or cornstarch.

BROCCOLI PÂTÉ

This simple, fresh pâté is lovely on crackers at parties and is a great way to get your kids to try out some veggies. Since broccoli is a fabulous source of calcium, it's important that you find ways to work it into your diet to ensure strong bones in your future.

Makes 5–6 servings

1 head broccoli, broken into florets, stem peeled and diced
1 teaspoon brown rice syrup
2 tablespoons sesame tahini
2 teaspoons soy sauce
½ cup pine nuts
1–2 teaspoons avocado oil
1 teaspoon fresh lemon juice

Lightly steam the broccoli until just bright green, about 2 minutes. Drain well and allow to cool.

Place broccoli, syrup, tahini, soy sauce, and pine nuts in a food processor. Puree, streaming oil slowly into the mixture to create a smooth, creamy consistency. Add lemon juice and puree until smooth. Transfer to a serving bowl and serve at room temperature or chilled with crackers or chips.

CREAMY CAULIFLOWER DIP

Cauliflower is so versatile and mild, we forget that it's a powerful source of cancer-fighting antioxidants and is essential to good health. This creamy dip will have your family loving this humble veggie.

Makes 4–5 servings

2 russet potatoes, peeled, cubed
1 head cauliflower, broken into small florets
Avocado oil
2 cloves fresh garlic, minced
1 yellow onion, diced
1 teaspoon curry powder
Sea salt
1 teaspoon brown rice syrup
¼ cup vegan sour cream or plain soy yogurt
Generous pinch nutmeg
3–4 sprigs fresh flat-leaf parsley, coarsely chopped

Bring a pot of water to a boil. Cook potatoes and cauliflower until soft, about 15 minutes. Drain well and transfer to a mixing bowl. Using a fork, mash the veggies into a coarse paste. Set aside.

Place a small amount of oil, garlic, and onion in a skillet over medium heat. When the onion begins to sizzle, add curry powder and a light seasoning of salt and sauté for 4–5 minutes. Transfer to the cauliflower mixture and mix in sea salt to taste, syrup, sour cream or yogurt, nutmeg, and parsley. Mix very well. Serve warm with crackers or toasted whole-wheat pita bread.

CRISP WATERCRESS SALAD

This salad is brilliant at any time of year and has so much interesting flavor and texture . . . and with watercress being a rich source of vitamins A, C, E, and K, as well as calcium and potassium, and at only eleven calories per cup, this peppery green is invaluable to health.

Makes 2–3 servings

¼ cup extra-virgin olive oil
½ teaspoon sea salt
¼ teaspoon cracked black pepper
2 teaspoons fresh lemon juice

1 bunch watercress, rinsed well, hand shredded into bite-size pieces
2 tangerines, peeled, sectioned
½ cup almonds
½ cup raisins (organic, if possible)

Combine dressing ingredients in the bottom of your salad bowl. Add watercress, tangerines, almonds, and raisins and toss to coat ingredients with dressing.

◆ **Variations**

You may use pear or apple slices, unsweetened dried cranberries, hazelnuts, walnuts, or pine nuts. You can change the salad completely by adding cherry tomatoes and cucumbers or olives and leaving out the fruit.

THE MOTHER OF ALL TOMATO SALADS

There is nothing fresher, easier, or yummier than a tomato salad. If this baby takes you more than three minutes to put together, well, I will be stunned. And with olive oil in the dressing, your body absorbs the precious lycopene 60 percent better than without it.

Makes 4–5 servings

2 containers cherry or grape tomatoes, rinsed and dried
¼ cup extra-virgin olive oil
1 tablespoon balsamic vinegar
Generous pinch dried oregano
1 small red chili pepper, seeded, finely minced
1 clove fresh garlic, very finely minced
Sea salt
Cracked black pepper

Place the tomatoes in a mixing bowl. Whisk together oil, vinegar, oregano, chili, and garlic with salt and pepper to taste. Toss dressing with tomatoes to coat and serve at room temperature or chilled.

KICK-ASS SAUTÉ

This sauté is like rocket fuel. It keeps the body warm and gives us lots of nutrients for energy, and its spicy flavor stimulates circulation so you have stamina and endurance to spare. A rich source of folic acid, this dish can result in strong red blood and heart health.

Makes 3–4 servings

Avocado oil
1 jalapeño pepper, with seeds and
    spines, minced
4–5 whole green onions, cut into 1-inch
    pieces
Soy sauce
5–6 thin slices fresh ginger, minced
4 cloves fresh garlic, minced
5-inch piece burdock, cut into fine
    matchstick pieces
5-inch piece carrot, cut into fine
    matchstick pieces
5-inch piece parsnip, cut into fine
    matchstick pieces
3–4 sprigs fresh flat-leaf parsley,
    coarsely chopped
Juice of ¼ fresh lemon

Place a small amount of oil, pepper, and green onions in a skillet over medium heat. When the onions begin to sizzle, add a splash of soy sauce and cook for 1 minute. Add ginger and garlic and stir well. Add burdock and a splash of soy sauce and sauté for 2 minutes. Add carrot and a splash of soy sauce and sauté for 2 minutes. Add parsnip and a splash of soy sauce and cook for 2 minutes. Season to taste with soy sauce and sauté for 2–3 minutes more. Remove from heat and stir in parsley and lemon juice. Serve immediately.

APPLE-BRAISED GREENS

Mixing more bitter-tasting greens with good olive oil and a bit of fruit makes them so yummy your loved ones will never complain about eating their veggies again. And the benefits of the apple cider vinegar for digestion make this dish just perfect.

Makes 3–4 servings

2 tablespoons extra-virgin olive oil
3 cloves fresh garlic, minced
2 ripe but firm apples, unpeeled and
    thinly sliced
Sea salt
Cracked black pepper
1 bunch dark leafy greens (kale, collards,
    broccoli rabe, etc.), rinsed well and cut
    into bite-size pieces
1 tablespoon apple cider vinegar

Place oil, garlic, and apples in a deep skillet over medium heat. When the apples begin to sizzle, add a pinch of salt and pepper and sauté for 1–2 minutes, just until the apples begin to wilt. Stir in the greens and a light seasoning of salt, and cook, stirring, just until the greens turn a deep green and wilt, about 2–3 minutes. Remove from heat and gently stir in vinegar. Serve immediately.

Place a small amount of oil, garlic, and onion in a deep skillet over medium heat. When the onion begins to sizzle, add a pinch of salt, pepper, and crushed red pepper flakes. Sauté for 2–3 minutes. Stir in tomatoes and a light seasoning of salt and sauté for 3 minutes. Stir in greens and a light seasoning of salt and sauté until the greens just wilt, about 3 minutes. Serve hot.

ITALIAN-STYLE GREENS

When I was a kid, we ate sautéed greens from the garden nearly every day. They changed with the seasons, but my mother knew she could count on us to eat our veggies if she made them this way. Hope it works with your kids because the antioxidants, fiber, and chlorophyll are essential to their good health.

Makes 3–4 servings

Extra-virgin olive oil
2 cloves fresh garlic, thinly sliced
½ red onion, thinly sliced into half-
　　moons
Sea salt
Cracked black pepper
Crushed red pepper flakes
2 ripe tomatoes, thinly sliced into half-
　　moons
1 bunch dark leafy greens (kale,
　　collards, broccoli rabe, etc.), rinsed
　　well

RAW BEET AND PEAR SALAD

I love this salad because it's packed with flavor and nutrients like iron and is oh-so-easy. And because it's sweet, even the pickiest eater will go for it. This is a great salad to get the kids in on, too.

Makes 3–4 servings

2 beets, peeled
3 unpeeled pears (I like red pears, but
　　use whatever you like)
Small handful mint leaves, shredded
3 cups baby spinach
½ cup coarsely chopped walnut pieces

Dressing
3 tablespoons extra-virgin olive oil
1 tablespoons fresh lemon juice
1 tablespoon brown rice syrup
Sea salt
Cracked black pepper

Prepare the beets by cutting them in half lengthwise and slicing them into very thin half-moon pieces. Transfer to a mixing bowl. Prepare the pears by cutting them in half, removing the cores, and then slicing very thinly lengthwise. Combine with beets. Stir in mint, spinach, and walnuts.

Whisk together dressing ingredients with salt and pepper to taste. Toss with salad and serve immediately.

Place oil, syrup, salt, and pepper in a flat-bottomed skillet over medium heat. Once the ingredients are warmed through, stir them to combine. Arrange carrots and squash in the skillet, being careful to avoid overlap. Cover, reduce heat to low, and cook until the veggies are soft in the center and browned on the edges, about 20 minutes. Remove from heat and stir in lemon juice and parsley, stirring gently to avoid breaking the veggies. Serve hot.

PERFECTLY BRAISED CARROTS AND WINTER SQUASH

This side dish is gorgeous . . . sweet, satisfying, warming. Even kids love this one. And the fact that it's rich in antioxidants and carotenoids, can help with eyesight, is high in fiber so they stay satisfied, and helps curb sugar cravings is why you'll love this dish that they love.

Makes 3–4 servings

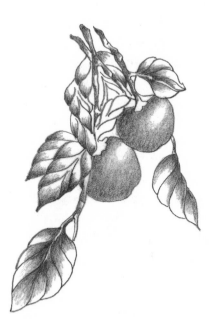

2–3 tablespoons extra-virgin olive oil

1 tablespoon brown rice syrup

1 teaspoon sea salt

¼ teaspoon cracked black pepper

2 medium carrots, cut into large dice

2 cups large-dice winter squash

Juice of ¼ fresh lemon

2–3 sprigs fresh flat-leaf parsley, coarsely
   chopped

BRAISED ASPARAGUS

The perfect side dish is quick and yummy . . . so yummy that you might actually get your family to eat some veggies, especially if you get the kids involved by letting them snap off the ends of the asparagus. The fact that it's a great source of folate, vitamin C, and potassium, as well as being prized as an aid in controlling homocysteine, means these slender stalks are heart-healthy, too.
Makes 3–4 servings

1 bunch asparagus
4 tablespoons extra-virgin olive oil
1 tablespoon balsamic vinegar
1 teaspoon sea salt
½ teaspoon cracked black pepper

Snap the ends off the asparagus where they naturally break.

Place oil in a flat-bottomed skillet. Add vinegar, salt, and pepper. Mix well to combine and coat the bottom of the skillet. Arrange asparagus spears in the oil mixture, avoiding overlap. Cover and place skillet over medium heat. When you hear a sizzling sound, reduce heat to low and braise asparagus until it's bright green and lightly browned, about 5 minutes. About halfway through the cooking, gently shake the pan to turn the asparagus and ensure even cooking. Serve hot with lemon slices as garnish, if desired.

SEA VEG SAUTÉ

This dish combines sweet veggies with the strong flavor of arame for a dramatic dish that is rich in valuable calcium in combination with the other minerals we need to absorb and use this valuable nutrient.
Makes 3–4 servings

½ cup arame, rinsed well and left to
    soften
Avocado oil
1-inch piece fresh ginger, minced
1 small leek, halved lengthwise, rinsed
    free of dirt, thinly sliced
Soy sauce
1 medium carrot, finely julienned
½ cup fresh or frozen corn kernels
Dry white wine
½ bunch fresh chives, minced

Rinse the arame several times, until the water runs clear-ish. Set aside. In about 5 minutes, the arame will soften enough to cook.

Place a small amount of oil, ginger, and leek in a skillet over medium heat. When the leek begins to sizzle, add a splash of soy sauce and sauté for 2 minutes. Stir in carrots and corn and spread veggies evenly in the skillet. Top with arame and add enough white wine to half cover the ingredients and a light seasoning of soy sauce. Cover, reduce heat to low, and cook until the wine has reduced to a syrup. Remove from heat and stir in chives. Serve hot.

For Love of the Sea ... Vegetables

When we think of sea vegetables, we think of the slimy stuff that wraps around our feet at the Jersey Shore ... not as a food source. In fact, sea vegetables provide us with concentrated mineral nutrition and are an important—but small—part of a healthy whole foods diet.

Sea vegetables come in many varieties, and they all offer something special to our health. Calcium-rich hiziki and arame, antioxidant-rich wakame/alaria, keratin-rich kombu/kelp, potassium-rich dulse, and magnesium-rich nori are the most commonly used and easily found sea plants.

Sea veggies are an acquired taste, but one I recommend you acquire. Loaded with minerals and vitamins essential to health, sea veggies make for strong blood, bones, and vascular strength. They are rich sources of calcium, potassium, magnesium, iron, protein, and fiber, to name just a few of the valuable nutrients we receive from eating these strongly flavored vegetables, but remember that a little goes a long way. Sea veggies are also rich sources of sodium, combined with the concentrated amounts of other nutrients, especially minerals, so only about 5 percent of our daily diet need come from these vegetables.

So, a bit of nori to garnish a soup or a nori roll in your week, a touch of wakame in soup, a small square of kombu cooked in with beans or grains or a richly flavored side dish once a week or so will give us all the nutrition we need. Vary your sea veggies just like those from land to get the full spectrum of what they have to offer.

GINGERED SEA VEGGIE SALAD

Wakame is mild, so the strongly flavored dressing will stand out. But make no mistake; wakame is no wimp in the nutrient department. Studies show that it aids in preventing heart disease, preserving bone density, and lowering triglycerides.

Makes 4–5 servings

½ cup loosely packed wakame flakes
1 tablespoon brown rice vinegar
2 teaspoons fresh lime juice
2 teaspoons brown rice syrup
1 teaspoon finely grated ginger, juice
    squeezed and reserved, pulp
    discarded
2 teaspoons soy sauce
1 tablespoon light sesame oil
2 tablespoons lightly pan-toasted tan
    sesame seeds

2 cups baby arugula

Place the wakame in a small mixing bowl. Whisk together vinegar, lime juice, syrup, ginger juice, soy sauce, and sesame oil. Adjust seasonings to your taste. Toss wakame with dressing and allow to marinate for 10–15 minutes.

Toss marinated sea vegetables with sesame seeds and arugula. Serve at room temperature or chilled.

◆ **Note**

Pan-toast sesame seeds by heating a dry skillet over medium heat and cooking the seeds, stirring constantly, until golden and fragrant.

SUMMER SEA VEG SALAD

This raw sea vegetable salad is great on hot summer days when we need to replace minerals because we are sweating more. Using dulse helps keep potassium levels stable so you sail through hot, humid days.

Makes 3–4 servings

1 large cucumber, unpeeled and thinly
    sliced into rounds
2 cups cherry tomatoes, halved
1 ripe but firm avocado, pitted and diced
3–4 sprigs fresh basil, coarsely chopped
2 cups baby spinach, rinsed well
½ cup torn dulse leaves
Avocado oil
Soy sauce
Cracked black pepper
Juice of ½ fresh lime

Combine cucumber, tomatoes, avocado, basil, spinach, and dulse in a salad bowl. Whisk together oil, soy sauce, pepper, and lime juice. Adjust seasonings to your taste. Toss dressing gently with salad, taking care not to break avocado. Serve at room temperature or chilled.

BRAISED ENDIVE AND PINE NUTS

This elegant side dish only looks fancy. It's so easy to make . . . and so delicious, you will make it one of your go-to recipes. The delicate bitter taste of the endive helps cleanse the liver so you metabolize nutrients more efficiently, meaning it aids the body in stabilizing weight.
Makes 3–6 servings

3 tablespoons extra-virgin olive oil
1 tablespoon balsamic vinegar
1 teaspoon sea salt
½ teaspoon cracked black pepper
3 Belgian endive, split lengthwise
½ cup pan-toasted pine nuts
2–3 sprigs fresh basil, coarsely chopped

Place oil, vinegar, salt, and pepper in a flat-bottomed skillet over medium heat. When the mixture is warmed through, lay the endive halves, cut side down, in the oil. Cover and reduce heat to medium low. Cook until the top sides of the endive are sweating and slightly wilted and the cut sides are browned, about 10–12 minutes.

While the endive cooks, heat a dry skillet over medium heat and cook pine nuts, stirring, until lightly browned and fragrant, about 3 minutes. Set aside.

To serve, arrange endive, cut side up, on a platter and sprinkle with pine nuts and fresh basil.

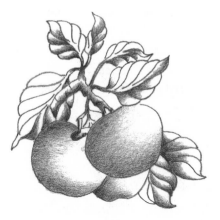

BITTER GREEN SALAD WITH SWEET ORANGE DRESSING

Bitter greens, while great for aiding the liver in its work, are, well, bitter. So I pair them with a sweet dressing that lights up the salad with its delicate orange flavor. The olives provide pantothenic acid, iron, vitamin E, and monounsaturated fats for heart health, so don't skimp on them.

Makes 3–4 servings

4 cups mixed bitter greens, dandelion, frisee, escarole, watercress, arugula, etc., rinsed well and hand torn into bite-size pieces
2 ruby grapefruits, peeled and sectioned
½ cup slivered almonds
10–12 oil-cured black olives, pitted and halved

Dressing
4 tablespoons extra-virgin olive oil
2 tablespoons fresh orange juice
1 teaspoon fresh orange zest
1 teaspoon apple cider vinegar
1 teaspoon brown rice syrup
Sea salt
Cracked black pepper

Combine salad ingredients in a bowl.

Whisk together dressing ingredients with salt and pepper to taste. Take care to use salt lightly, as the salad contains olives. Toss salad with dressing and serve immediately.

You can make the salad and dressing in advance, but do not dress the salad or add the almonds until ready to serve.

POTATO SALAD

My mother never made potato salad with mayonnaise. We made it with potatoes, lots of veggies, and olive oil. I didn't experience our mayo-laden version until I was an adult. I still prefer my mother's recipe, but I have also given you the option of making this all-American with vegan mayo.

Makes 3–4 servings

2 pounds red-skinned potatoes, unpeeled and cut into chunks
2 stalks celery, diced
1 roasted red bell pepper, diced
12–14 cherry tomatoes, halved
12 black oil-cured olives, pitted
3 tablespoons capers, drained but not rinsed
Extra-virgin olive oil
Red wine vinegar
Sea salt
Cracked black pepper
Sweet paprika
2 sprigs fresh basil, leaves removed, shredded

Place potatoes in a pot with water to just cover. Bring to a boil over medium heat. Reduce heat to low and cook until the potatoes are just tender, about 20 minutes. Drain well; transfer to a mixing bowl and cool slightly. Gently mix in vegetables, olives, and capers.

Drizzle salad generously with olive oil and add vinegar, salt, and pepper to taste. Gently fold dressing into potato mixture until ingredients are coated. Transfer to a serving dish and sprinkle the top with paprika and basil.

All-American Mayo Dressing

¾ cup vegan mayonnaise (Vegenaise)
¼ cup natural pickle relish
1 tablespoon Dijon mustard
1 teaspoon brown rice syrup
1 teaspoon sea salt
½ teaspoon cracked black pepper
¼ teaspoon hot sauce

Make the dressing by mixing together mayo, relish, mustard, syrup, salt, pepper, and hot sauce. Adjust seasonings to your taste.

CRISPY TORTILLAS WITH GUACAMOLE

I love this dish. It's fun, so kids will eat it. It's packed with nutrients, like omega-3 fatty acids, so you want the kids to eat it. It's delicious, so everyone wants to eat it. And by gently frying your own tortillas, you control the fat and salt in everyone's "chips."

Makes 3–4 servings

Tortilla Chips
12 whole-grain tortillas
Extra-virgin olive oil (in a spray bottle)
⅛ teaspoon paprika (optional)
¼ teaspoon sea salt
⅛ teaspoon chili powder (optional)

Guacamole
3 ripe avocados (Haas are most common)
Juice of 1 fresh lemon or lime
½ red onion, finely minced
1 jalapeño pepper, seeds removed, finely minced
1 clove fresh garlic, crushed and finely minced
2 plum tomatoes, seeded and diced
½ cup frozen organic corn, thawed
Sea salt
2–3 sprigs fresh flat-leaf parsley or cilantro, coarsely chopped

To make the guacamole, halve avocados and remove pit. Mash in a mixing bowl to form a creamy texture.

Stir in balance of ingredients with sea salt to taste. Mix very well. Cover tightly with plastic and chill for 15 minutes to allow the flavors to develop.

Heat your broiler to 350°F or high. Line a baking sheet with parchment paper.

Spray each tortilla with oil on one side and sprinkle with spices and salt. Stack the tortillas and slice them into wedges, halves, quarters, and then eighths. Arrange on baking sheet, avoiding overlap (you may need more than one baking sheet), and broil until crisp, about 5 minutes.

◆ **Note**

Trader Joe's and some supermarkets sell guacamole "kits" with all the ingredients you need in one package. It's cool.

Extra-virgin olive oil
Sea salt

Preheat oven to 425°F.

Cut the butternut squash into home fries shapes. You can use a crinkle cutter or just slice them into french fry shapes. Transfer the squash pieces to a mixing bowl and drizzle lightly with oil. Toss to coat. Sprinkle lightly with salt and toss again. Transfer to a baking sheet and spread the pieces so there is no overlap. Bake until crisp and browned on the edges, about 40 minutes, turning the pieces at 20 minutes. Serve hot.

◆ **Variation**

You can add cayenne or chili pepper to create a spicy taste or a pinch of cinnamon to bring out the sweetness.

FRENCH FRIES

You wouldn't think butternut squash could make crispy, satisfying fries, but you would be wrong. Richly flavored and crunchy, these babies are loaded with antioxidants and carotenoids and are oh-so-satisfying.

Makes 3–4 servings

1 butternut squash, peeled, halved
   lengthwise, seeded

CRISPY BAKED KALE CHIPS

I know what you're thinking. Here it is, the healthy chip recipe. I thought that, too, when Dr. Will Klevos first told me about this. But I have found that even the most ardent greens-haters love it. And since leafy greens provide vitamins C, A, and K, along with iron, calcium, protein, potassium, magnesium, chlorophyll, manganese, and other essential nutrients, you really want to get them into your family's tummies . . . a lot . . . however you can.

Makes 4–5 servings

1 bunch kale, rinsed well, spun dry,
    hand-torn into bite-size pieces
Extra-virgin olive oil
Sea salt
Cracked black pepper

Preheat oven to 350°F and line a baking sheet with parchment paper.

Place kale in a mixing bowl and lightly drizzle with olive oil. Toss with your hands so the oil coats the leaves but doesn't drown them. Arrange on baking sheet, avoiding overlap, and bake for 15–20 minutes until the kale is seriously crisp, but still green. Do not let the leaves brown or they will be bitter. Remove from oven, toss lightly with salt and pepper, and serve.

You can spice things up with a little chili powder in place of the black pepper. You can eliminate both and just use salt as well.

◆ **Note**

The secret to perfect "chips" is to get the kale super dry, by spinning it after washing. And the second is to salt the chips when they come out of the oven. Salting before will cause the kale to "bleed" water and just get soggy.

SIMPLE STEAMED GREENS

Really? A recipe for steamed greens? You'd be surprised at the number of people who can't do this. And steamed greens done right are so delicious, so nutrient-packed that I felt compelled to share. Just greens, naked with no dressing. Try it.

Makes 3–4 servings

1 medium-size bunch dark leafy greens
    (kale, collards, baby bok choy, etc.),
    rinsed well, left whole

Place a small amount of water in a wide skillet over medium heat. Place a bamboo or metal steaming tray over the boiling water with greens in the tray. Cover and steam until bright green and crisp-tender, about 3 minutes. Carefully turn greens if needed to ensure even steaming.

You may also steam greens by immersing a metal steamer in a deep pot over an inch of water and placing greens in the steamer. Cook until bright green and tender, about 3 minutes.

Cool greens slightly before slicing into bite-size pieces. Serve hot or at room temperature.

HUSH PUPPIES

I know, who thought hush puppies were so popular? It turns out they are in the top one hundred favorite foods of Americans. So here is a dairy-free, egg-free, guilt-free . . . and flavorful vegan version. The addition of chia seeds adds iron, omega-3, calcium, and protein to these American faves. A great side dish to chili, soups, or stews or great as snacks.

Makes about 24 pups

1 tablespoon chia seeds
⅔ cup unsweetened almond milk
1¼ cup yellow cornmeal
½ cup whole-wheat pastry flour
½ teaspoon sea salt
¼ teaspoon cracked black pepper
3 teaspoons baking powder
½ yellow onion, minced
½ cup fresh or frozen corn kernels
4 whole green onions, minced
1 jalapeño, finely minced (keep seeds if you want these spicier; remove them for a more mild flavor)
Avocado oil, for frying

Whisk the chia seeds into the almond milk and set aside for 15 minutes, stirring occasionally. The mixture will thicken.

While the chia soaks, whisk together cornmeal, flour, salt, pepper, and baking powder. Fold in onions, corn, green onions, and jalapeño. When the chia has thickened, stir it into the cornmeal mixture, creating a thick batter that can be formed.

Form the batter into 1–2-inch spheres.

Heat 2 inches of oil in a deep skillet or wok over medium heat. When the oil is hot, fry the hush puppies until golden brown. Drain and serve.

LEMON-SCENTED BRUSSELS SPROUTS WITH ROASTED WALNUTS

There's something so sexy about brussels sprouts. I love their compact shape, their strong flavor, but mostly I love their intense nutrition profile, like containing a unique fiber that can help lower cholesterol and protect DNA. Combining them with protein-packed nuts and sweetly roasting them will change your mind about these underappreciated veggies.

Makes 4–5 servings

1 pound brussels sprouts, bases trimmed
Extra-virgin olive oil
2 teaspoons brown rice syrup
Sea salt
Cracked black pepper
Grated zest of 1 fresh lemon
Juice of ½ fresh lemon
1 cup walnut pieces, pan-roasted

Preheat oven to 375°F.

Place trimmed brussels sprouts in a mixing bowl. Drizzle lightly with oil, syrup, salt and pepper to taste, and lemon zest. Mix well and transfer to a large baking dish, arranging to avoid overlap. Cover tightly with foil and bake for 45 minutes. Remove cover and return to oven to brown for 7–10 minutes more.

While the sprouts bake, pan-toast the walnuts by heating a dry skillet over medium heat and cooking the nuts, stirring, until fragrant and lightly browned, about 4 minutes. Set aside.

To serve, gently toss the sprouts with lemon juice and walnuts. Serve hot.

SWEET ENDINGS

Sweet is the flavor we love; we crave it. But it can do us in if the quality of our treats is less than optimal. These sweet endings will satisfy you without compromise to your health.

As you have seen, there are a lot of options for adapting recipes, so once you have mastered the basics of natural baking, you can begin to alter some family favorites to be healthier. The recipes here will build a great foundation as you discover the techniques and ingredients needed for success.

Gluten-Free Baking

A lot of people ask about making my desserts gluten-free. I will go on record as saying that I am not a fan of most of the gluten-free mixes on the market. Many of them contain compromised ingredients and leave a funny aftertaste in your mouth from the vegetable gums they use. So, I bake from scratch.

I have had the most success with substituting quinoa flour for whole-wheat pastry and semolina flours in most recipes. Piecrusts can be challenging, but I solved that by adding to the crust a tablespoon of chia seeds that were soaked in a small amount of the cold water for 15 minutes. That mixture behaves like an egg and binds the crust.

I have tried other gluten-free flours without as satisfying a result as with quinoa flour, but if you have successfully baked with rice flour or millet flour, then go for it. Quinoa flour yields light and delicate results that most closely resemble the original recipe.

Experiment for your own results.

BLUEBERRY PEACH PIE

There's nothing quite like pie to make any day just a little more special. This one is a summer favorite in my house, and the lutein and antioxidants in the berries are a great reason to turn on the oven on even the hottest day.

Makes 6–8 servings

Crust
1 cup whole-wheat pastry flour
¼ cup semolina flour
Sea salt
½ cup avocado oil
Cold water

Filling
6–8 firm but ripe peaches, peeled, halved, pitted, and thinly sliced
1 pint blueberries, rinsed well and towel-dried
2 tablespoons avocado oil

¼ cup brown rice syrup
Pinch sea salt
⅛ teaspoon grated nutmeg
Grated zest of 1 fresh lemon
4–5 tablespoons arrowroot flour

Topping
½ cup ground almond meal
¼ cup whole-wheat pastry flour
⅓ cup granulated maple syrup
¼ cup avocado oil

Preheat oven to 350°F and lightly oil a 9-inch pie plate.

Prepare the crust by mixing flours with salt. Using a fork, cut the oil into the flour to form the texture of wet sand. Slowly add cold water until the crust gathers together. Knead dough about 4 times to pull it together. Roll the crust out evenly between 2 sheets of parchment paper to a size about an inch larger than your pie plate. Remove the top sheet of parchment and invert the crust over the pie plate. Without stretching the dough, press the crust into place, allowing the excess to hang over the rim of the plate. Pull up the excess and, pressing the first finger of one hand and the thumb and first finger of the other hand together, pleat the top of the crust decoratively. Pierce the crust in several places with a fork and bake for 5 minutes. Remove from oven and set aside.

Make the filling by simply tossing the fruit with the oil, syrup, salt, nutmeg, lemon zest, and arrowroot. The arrowroot should coat the fruit thoroughly. Spoon the fruit mixture abundantly and evenly into the crust.

Make the topping by combining all the ingredients to create a crumbly texture. Sprinkle on top of the fruit, covering completely.

Bake the pie on a baking sheet for 50–60 minutes, until the topping is browned, the filling is bubbling, and the crust is golden. Remove from oven and allow to cool to warm before slicing. Serve warm, at room temperature, or chilled.

◆ **Note**

You can use a frozen whole-wheat piecrust for this recipe.

PECAN PIE

A good pecan pie is just the best thing ever. But it's usually loaded with sugar and calories, making it less than desirable when you are eating a healthy diet, even as an indulgence. Well, this version is still an indulgence, but there's no simple sugar and it's truly delicious.

Makes 6–8 servings

Crust
1 cup whole-wheat pastry flour
¼ cup semolina flour
Sea salt
½ cup avocado oil
Cold water

Filling
¼ cup avocado oil
1½ cups pecan pieces coarsely chopped
1¾ cups unsweetened almond milk
¾ cup brown rice syrup
1 teaspoon pure vanilla extract
Pinch sea salt
3 tablespoons arrowroot powder
4 tablespoons agar flakes

2 cups pecan halves
⅓ cup brown rice syrup
1 teaspoon grated orange zest

Preheat oven to 350°F and lightly oil a 9-inch pie plate.

Prepare the crust by mixing flours with salt. Using a fork, cut the oil into the flour to form the texture of wet sand. Slowly add cold water until the crust gathers together. Knead dough about 4 times to pull it together. Roll the crust out evenly between 2 sheets of parchment paper to a size about an inch larger than your pie plate. Remove the top sheet of parchment and invert the crust over the pie plate. Without stretching the dough, press the crust into place, allowing the excess to hang over the rim of the plate. Pull up the excess and, pressing the first finger of one hand and the thumb and first finger of the other hand together, pleat the top of the crust decoratively. Pierce the crust in several places with a fork and bake for 20 minutes. Remove from oven and set aside.

Make the filling by combining all ingredients in a saucepan over medium heat. Cook, stirring as it comes to a boil. Reduce heat to low and cook, stirring, for 5 minutes, until the agar is dissolved and the mixture has thickened. Spoon evenly into pie shell. Arrange pecan halves decoratively over the top of the pie. Bake for 12–15 minutes.

Remove pie from oven. Heat remaining syrup and orange zest to a high rolling boil. Quickly spoon over the pecans on top of the pie. Allow to cool for at least 30 minutes so the pie sets before slicing into wedges.

COCONUT CREAM PIE

Is it wrong to dream of coconut cream pie as a vegan? That rich, creamy, oh-so-coco-nutty dessert is sooooo decadent and delicious . . . and damaging to your health, right? Not anymore.

Makes 6–8 servings

Crust
1 cup whole-wheat pastry flour
¼ cup semolina flour
Sea salt
½ cup avocado oil
Cold water

Coconut Filling
⅓ cup brown rice syrup
Pinch sea salt
6 tablespoons arrowroot powder
14 ounces coconut milk (regular or low-fat)
½ teaspoon pure vanilla extract
½ teaspoon coconut extract
6 ounces silken tofu, pureed
1 cup unsweetened shredded coconut

Preheat oven to 350°F and lightly oil a 9-inch pie plate.

Prepare the crust by mixing flours with salt. Using a fork, cut the oil into the flour to form the texture of wet sand. Slowly add cold water until the crust gathers together. Knead dough about 4 times to pull it together. Roll the crust out evenly between 2 sheets of parchment paper to a size about an inch larger than your pie plate. Remove the top sheet of parchment and invert the crust over the pie plate. Without stretching the dough, press the crust into place, allowing the excess to hang over the rim of the plate. Pull up the excess and, pressing the first finger of one hand and the thumb and first finger of the other hand together, pleat the top of the crust decoratively. Pierce the crust in several places with a fork and bake until lightly browned, 20–25 minutes. Remove from oven and set aside.

Place syrup, salt, arrowroot, and coconut milk in a saucepan over medium heat. Cook, stirring constantly, until the mixture thickens, about 4 minutes. Stir in extracts, tofu, and ⅔ cup coconut. Mix very well to combine. Spoon mixture into cooled pie shell and sprinkle the top with reserved coconut. Chill until set, about an hour.

DECADENT NUTTY CHOCOLATE FUDGE

Who doesn't love fudge? Who doesn't hate what fudge can do to your waistline? In this recipe, we combine dark chocolate with spices to make the chocolate taste more chocolatey, creating the healthiest fudge you will ever enjoy . . . yum!
Makes 8–10 pieces

1 cup raw cashews or cashew butter (make sure to pour the oil out of the jar)
¼ cup unsweetened cocoa powder
Pinch sea salt
Scant pinch ground cinnamon
Scant pinch chili powder
Scant pinch cracked black pepper
⅓ cup brown rice syrup
2 tablespoons cold vegan buttery spread (Earth Balance)
½ teaspoon pure vanilla extract
½ cup coarsely chopped walnut pieces

Place cashews in a food processor and puree about 5 minutes or until a dense "butter" forms (it will look like Play-Doh). Add cocoa, salt, and spices and puree again. Add syrup, buttery spread, and vanilla and puree until thick and smooth. It will become a ball in the processor.

Transfer to a dry work surface and knead the walnuts into the fudge mixture. Shape mixture into a 1-inch-thick square; wrap in plastic and chill for about 3 hours before cutting into squares.

BLACK FOREST CAKE

Black forest cake is a classic, richly flavored chocolate cake that makes any occasion a bit more special. In my vegan version, I have created a moist chocolate cake and a sumptuous cherry topping that is sure to please.

Makes 8–10 servings

Cake
2 tablespoons chia seeds or meal
2 cups unsweetened almond milk
3 cups whole-wheat pastry flour
1 cup semolina flour
1½ cups unsweetened cocoa powder
4 teaspoons baking powder
2 teaspoons baking soda
Generous pinch sea salt
½ teaspoon ground cinnamon
⅔ cup avocado or light olive oil
1 cup brown rice syrup
2 teaspoons brown rice vinegar

Frosting
2 cups non-dairy dark chocolate chips
⅔ cup avocado oil
4 tablespoons brown rice syrup
Pinch sea salt
2 tablespoons pure vanilla extract

Cherry Topping
1 quart fresh cherries, pitted
4 tablespoons brown rice syrup
½ cup cherry juice
Pinch sea salt

Preheat oven to 350°F and lightly oil two 9-inch round cake pans. Cut a round of parchment that will fit into the bottoms of each pan.

Make the cakes by soaking chia seeds or meal in ½ cup of the almond milk for 15 minutes or until slightly thickened, stirring occasionally.

Combine flours, cocoa powder, baking powder and soda, salt, and cinnamon. Mix in oil, syrup, vinegar, and chia mixture. Mix well. Slowly add almond milk to form a smooth, spoonable batter.

Divide batter evenly into cake pans and bake until set and the tops of the cakes spring back to the touch, about 35 minutes. Remove from oven and allow to cool for 10 minutes before inverting cakes onto wire racks to cool completely.

Make the frosting while the cakes cool. Over a double boiler, melt chocolate with oil, syrup, and salt. Whisk until smooth and creamy. Remove from heat and whisk in vanilla extract. Transfer to a bowl and cover tightly. Place in the freezer for 15 minutes to thicken the frosting.

To make the topping, place all ingredients in a saucepan over medium-low heat. Simmer until liquid has reduced and thickened, about 15 minutes. Allow to cool before using.

To assemble the cakes, slice them in half horizontally with a serrated knife and carefully separate them. Take one of the cake layers and crumble it into coarse crumbs.

Place a cake layer on a serving plate with parchment tucked under the edges to protect the plate from getting dirty. Remove frosting from freezer and whip vigorously with a hand beater until creamy and fluffy. Spread a layer of frosting on the cake. Top with another cake layer, another layer of frosting, and a last layer of cake. Frost the cake top and sides, but do not worry about it being smooth. Press cake crumbs into the side of the cake to cover the frosting. Spoon cherry topping over the top of the cake right to the edges. Allow to stand for 15 minutes before serving.

BUTTERY PECAN SHORTBREAD

Shortbread cookies are moist, buttery, and lovely. And loaded with calories and saturated fat. In these cookies, we use a healthier fat and protein-packed pecans to make them all the better for you.

Makes 24–36 cookies

1 cup coarsely chopped pecans
2 cups whole-wheat pastry flour
Generous pinch sea salt
Generous pinch ground cinnamon
1 cup vegan buttery spread (Earth Balance)

½ cup brown rice syrup
1 teaspoon pure vanilla extract

Chocolate glaze (optional)
6 ounces non-dairy dark chocolate, coarsely chopped

Mix pecans with flour, salt, and cinnamon. In a separate bowl, using a hand mixer, whip the vegan buttery spread, syrup, and vanilla until smooth and fluffy, 2–3 minutes. Combine with flour mixture to create a soft dough. Gather into a ball, wrap in plastic wrap, and chill for 1 hour before proceeding.

Preheat oven to 350°F and line 2 baking sheets with parchment paper.

Divide the dough in half. Rewrap one half and return to the fridge. Roll the other half between 2 sheets of parchment into a ¼-inch-thick circle. Dip a round cookie cutter or a glass into flour and cut the dough into round shapes. Arrange on baking sheet. You do not need room for the cookies to spread, so you can fit a lot on the sheet. Reroll dough to use it up. Place the filled cookie sheet in the fridge while rolling out the other half of the dough.

Bake the cookies until deeply browned, 13–15 minutes for a crisp shortbread, 11–13 minutes for a softer cookie. Remove from oven and immediately transfer to a wire rack.

To make the chocolate glaze if using, simply melt the chocolate over a double boiler, whisking until smooth. Dip one end of each cookie into the chocolate and return them to the wire rack to cool and for the chocolate to set.

LIFE BY CHOCOLATE CAKE

We have all heard of "death by chocolate." But what about life by chocolate? Sounds good? Then you will love this richly flavored chocolate cake. The secret to "life"? Dark chocolate and chia seeds, of course.

Makes 8–10 servings

1 tablespoon chia seeds or meal

1 cup warm water

1 cup whole-wheat pastry flour

¼ cup semolina flour

⅓ cup unsweetened cocoa powder

2 teaspoons baking powder

1 teaspoon baking soda

Pinch sea salt

⅓ cup avocado oil

½ cup brown rice syrup

1 teaspoon pure vanilla extract

1 teaspoon apple cider vinegar

1 (3.5-ounce) non-dairy dark chocolate bar (at least 70 percent), coarsely chopped

Ganache

½ cup brown rice syrup

4 tablespoons vegan buttery spread (Earth Balance)

2 tablespoons unsweetened almond milk

2 tablespoons unsweetened cocoa powder

2 teaspoons pure vanilla extract

Preheat oven to 350°F and lightly oil a standard Bundt pan.

Soak chia in warm water until slightly thickened, at least 15 minutes.

Combine flours, cocoa powder, baking powder and soda, and salt in a mixing bowl. Add oil, syrup, vanilla, vinegar, and chia mixture. Mix, slowly adding warm water if needed to create a smooth, spoonable batter. Fold in chocolate chunks. Spoon evenly into prepared pan and bake until the top springs back to the touch, about 35–40 minutes.

Remove from oven and allow to cool for 7–10 minutes before inverting cake onto a serving plate.

While the cake cools, make the glaze. Combine syrup, vegan buttery spread, milk, and cocoa in a saucepan over low heat. Cook, stirring, until the mixture melts and is creamy. Remove from heat and stir in vanilla.

When the cake cools completely, spoon the ganache over the cake, allowing it to run down the sides.

PEANUT BUTTER DROPS

If these cookies got any easier, then they would make themselves. No excuses for not baking healthy treats now!

Makes 24–36 cookies

1 cup whole-wheat pastry flour
½ cup semolina flour
Pinch sea salt
½ teaspoon baking powder
1 cup creamy or crunchy natural peanut butter
¼ cup avocado oil
½ cup brown rice syrup
1 teaspoon pure vanilla

Preheat oven to 350°F and line 2 baking sheets with parchment paper.

Mix the dry ingredients together well. Mix in peanut butter, oil, syrup, and vanilla to form a stiff dough. With wet hands, form 2-inch balls. Arrange on baking sheets, leaving room for the cookies to spread. With a wet fork, make a crisscross pattern on top of each cookie. Bake for 16–18 minutes. Take the cookies from the oven while they are still soft and immediately transfer them to a cooling rack.

Substitute nut butters or use sunflower butter as desired to create different versions of this cookie.

SICILIAN FRUIT COOKIES

These are my husband's favorite cookies. They are my healthier version of a cookie that his Auntie Pina makes for him when we are in Sicily visiting the family. Instead of traditional candied fruit, I use natural dried fruit with delicious results.

Makes 24–30 cookies

½ cup (1 stick) vegan butter (Earth Balance), softened
½ cup brown rice syrup
1 teaspoon pure vanilla extract
1 cup whole-wheat pastry flour
½ cup semolina flour
Pinch sea salt
Pinch ground cinnamon
1 teaspoon baking powder
¼ cup slivered almonds
¼ cup pine nuts
½ cup golden raisins

Place the vegan buttery spread, syrup, and vanilla in a mixing bowl and whip with a hand mixer until creamy and fluffy.

Mix together flours, salt, cinnamon, baking powder, almonds, pine nuts, and raisins to form a soft dough.

Form the dough into a 3-inch-thick log. It will be long. Wrap it in plastic and chill for 1 hour before proceeding.

Preheat oven to 350°F and line 2 baking sheets with parchment paper.

Unwrap the chilled dough and, using a wet knife, slice the log into ½-inch-thick pieces. Lay the cookies on the baking sheets, leaving some room for them to spread. Bake for 18 minutes. Remove the cookies from the oven while they are still soft and transfer to a cooling rack. Cool completely before storing.

COOL CHOCOLATE MOUSSE

This is so easy, so creamy, rich, and chocolatey, you will make it all the time. You are four ingredients away from a most excellent antioxidant-rich dark chocolate mousse.

Makes 2 servings

1 package silken tofu
⅔ cup cocoa powder
1½ teaspoons pure vanilla extract
1 cup pitted Medjool dates

Combine all ingredients in a food processor and puree until smooth and creamy. Spoon into 2 individual dishes and chill completely. Serve topped with chopped nuts, shredded coconut, or fresh raspberries.

VANILLA CAKE

This basic cake will take you anywhere you want to go, baking-wise, that is. From cakes to cupcakes to flavored cakes, fruited cakes, spiced cakes . . . once you master this one, the world is your bake shop! Made from whole-grain flours, it will yield healthy, light, and moist results.

Makes 1 standard Bundt cake

1½ cups whole-wheat pastry
     flour
½ cup semolina flour
Pinch sea salt
2 teaspoons baking powder
1 teaspoon baking soda
⅓ cup avocado oil
½ cup brown rice syrup
1 teaspoon pure vanilla extract
½–1 cup unsweetened almond
     milk

Mix flours, salt, baking powder, and soda together. Mix in oil, syrup, and vanilla. Slowly add almond milk to create a smooth, spoonable batter. Spoon into prepared pan and bake until the top of the cake springs back to the touch, about 35–40 minutes.

Remove from oven and allow to cool for 7–10 minutes before inverting the cake onto a serving plate.

BOMBSHELL BLONDIES

Blondies are just as rich as brownies, but different . . . just like blondes and brunettes. Who has more fun? You decide.
Makes 16 bars

¾ cup cooked or canned pumpkin
⅓ cup avocado oil
½ cup brown rice syrup
¼ cup unsweetened almond milk
1 teaspoon pure vanilla extract
1 cup whole-wheat pastry flour
½ cup semolina flour
Pinch sea salt
Generous pinch ground cinnamon
Pinch ground ginger
½ teaspoon baking powder
½ cup coarsely chopped walnuts
½ cup non-dairy dark chocolate chips
  (optional)

Preheat oven to 350°F and lightly oil an 8 x 8-inch brownie pan.

Using a hand mixer, whip together pumpkin, avocado oil, syrup, almond milk, and vanilla. Fold in flours, salt, spices, and baking powder to form a smooth batter. Fold in nuts and chocolate, if using. Bake until a toothpick comes out mostly clean (these are meant to be moist), between 25–35 minutes. Do not overbake.

Allow blondies to cool for a full 30 minutes before slicing into squares so the flavors can develop as the blondies cool. Store in a sealed container.

BERRY CRUMBLE

A simple dessert that can be made with any fruit, it's satisfying, delicious, antioxidant-rich, and oh-so-easy to make for any meal.
Makes 4 individual crumbles

Crumble Topping
½ cup almond meal (purchased or whole
  almonds ground in a food processor)
2 teaspoons avocado oil
⅓ cup brown rice syrup

Filling
2 cups mixed fruit (fresh or frozen
  berries, chopped apples, pears,
  peaches, or plums)
2 teaspoons arrowroot flour
2 tablespoons brown rice syrup
Grated zest of 1 organic lemon

Preheat oven to 350°F and lightly oil four 3-inch ramekins. Place them on a baking sheet.

Combine the topping ingredients, mixing by hand to create the texture of wet sand. Set aside.

Mix fruit with arrowroot, rice syrup, and lemon zest, tossing gently to coat the fruit. Spoon fruit evenly into the ramekins. Sprinkle topping over each ramekin, covering completely and evenly.

Bake for 20–25 minutes, until the fruit is bubbling and the topping is browned.

HOT FUDGE SUNDAES

Decadent and delicious, this treat will win you raves . . . and no one will even guess it's vegan.

Makes 4 sundaes

Hot Fudge Topping
½ cup coconut cream
2–3 tablespoons brown rice syrup
5 ounces dark chocolate, coarsely chopped
½ teaspoon ground cinnamon
1 teaspoon pure vanilla extract

1 quart vegan vanilla ice cream (I love Coconut Bliss, Rice Dream, Soy Delicious)

Coarsely chopped nuts, for garnish (I love pistachios, but whatever you love works)

Make the sauce. In a saucepan, heat the coconut cream through. Remove from heat and stir in syrup and chocolate until melted and smooth. Stir in cinnamon and vanilla. Adjust sweetness to your taste.

Spoon ice cream into bowls and spoon sauce over top. Sprinkle with nuts and serve.

◆ **Variation**
You may also add chopped fresh fruit or berries to these sundaes.

◆ **Note**
The sauce can be made ahead of time and stored in the fridge. Gently heat before using.

QUICK CHOCOLATE PUDDING

Okay, this dessert is so easy and delicious you'll be tempted to make it every night. It still has calories, so as healthy as it is, it will land right on your butt if you eat too much of it. But man, it's tempting . . . and loaded with antioxidants from dark chocolate.

Makes 3–4 servings

2 cups unsweetened almond milk
1 tablespoon kuzu
2 tablespoons arrowroot
3–4 tablespoons unsweetened cocoa powder
Pinch sea salt
Generous pinch ground cinnamon
4 tablespoons brown rice syrup
5 tablespoons coarsely chopped dark chocolate, divided
1 teaspoon pure vanilla extract

Mix the kuzu with 2 tablespoons of the almond milk, dissolving it completely. Set aside. Whisk together arrowroot, cocoa, salt, and cinnamon in a saucepan. Add 1 cup almond milk and rice syrup, whisking until smooth. Stir in balance of almond milk and 3 tablespoons chopped chocolate. Cook, stirring constantly, over low heat until the chocolate melts and the mixture is smooth, 3–4 minutes. Stir in kuzu and cook, stirring until the mixture is thickened, which will happen fast. Remove from heat and stir in vanilla. Spoon into desired serving dishes and cover with plastic wrap, making sure the plastic touches the top of the pudding to prevent a skin. Chill, if desired. (If you do not wish to chill the pudding, just allow it to cool down a bit before garnishing so the chopped chocolate does not melt.)

To serve, remove from fridge and stir each pudding, as they may separate as they chill. Garnish with chopped chocolate and serve.

◆ **Note**

Kuzu can be found in natural food stores and works in recipes very much like cornstarch. Said to be alkalizing to the intestines, kuzu creates creamier results than either arrowroot or cornstarch, hence the use of it with arrowroot in this dish.

DOWN-AND-DIRTY EASY TRUFFLES

These are not totally quick, but they are so easy to make and so delicious. And since most of your time is simply spent waiting for them to set in the fridge, I advise you to make them the night before you plan to enjoy them.

Makes 24 truffles

12 ounces dark chocolate, finely chopped
1 tablespoon brown rice syrup
¾ cup unsweetened almond milk
Generous pinch ground cinnamon
1 tablespoon pure vanilla extract
2 tablespoons silken tofu, pureed
¼ cup unsweetened cocoa powder

Place a couple of inches of water in a deep pot and bring to a boil. Place chocolate and rice syrup in a glass bowl and set aside. In a small saucepan, bring almond milk and cinnamon to a gentle boil and pour it over the chocolate. Place the chocolate mixture over the boiling water and whisk until the chocolate is smooth and creamy. Remove from heat and mix in vanilla and tofu. Cover tightly with plastic and refrigerate until well set, as long as 3 hours.

When the mixture is set, remove from fridge. Make your hands as cold as possible so you don't melt the truffles. (Run them under cold water and dry them). Using a teaspoon, take 1 teaspoon of the truffle mixture and form ¾-inch balls and place them on a parchment-lined cookie sheet.

Place the tray of formed truffles in the fridge for 20 minutes. To coat them with cocoa, roll each truffle in your hands for a couple of seconds to warm the surface. Toss in the cocoa powder to coat and return to the baking sheet. Do not worry if there is too much cocoa on the truffles. Return to the fridge for 20 minutes. Shake off any excess cocoa and place each truffle in a miniature foil candy cup.

These will keep, in a sealed container, in the fridge for about 2 weeks.

MOIST, YUMMY BANANA BREAD

Banana bread is one of the greatest comfort foods of all time. Sweet, delicate, moist, and delicious, this egg- and dairy-free version is just as delicious as the one Mom used to make. I add chocolate chips to mine for that extra bit of luxury.

Makes 1 standard loaf

5 organic, very ripe bananas
⅔ cup brown rice syrup
1 teaspoon pure vanilla extract
⅓ cup avocado oil

1¾ cups whole-wheat pastry flour
¼ cup semolina flour
Pinch sea salt
Pinch ground cinnamon
2 teaspoons baking powder
1 teaspoon baking soda
⅓ cup coarsely chopped walnuts
½ cup non-dairy dark chocolate chips

Preheat oven to 350°F and lightly oil and flour a standard (9 x 5 x 2¾-inch) loaf pan.

Peel bananas and place in a large mixing bowl. Using a hand mixer, whip them with syrup, vanilla, and oil until smooth and creamy. Mix in flours, salt, cinnamon, baking powder, and soda to form a spoonable cake batter. If the batter seems too stiff, slowly add water to create the consistency you need. Fold in walnuts and chocolate chips. Spoon batter evenly into prepared loaf pan and bake for 45–55 minutes, until a toothpick comes out clean and the top of the bread springs back to the touch. Allow to cool for 10 minutes before removing from pan and cooling on a wire rack.

THE BEST CHOCOLATE CHUNK COOKIES

No kidding, the best—ever. Vegan, not vegan, healthy or not, everyone who tastes these says they are the best.

Makes 28–30 cookies

½ cup (1 stick) vegan butter (Earth
    Balance), softened
½ cup brown rice syrup
1 teaspoon pure vanilla extract
¼ cup coconut sugar

1¼ cups whole-wheat pastry flour
¼ cup semolina flour
Pinch ground cinnamon
Pinch sea salt
½ teaspoon baking soda
½ cup coarsely chopped pecans
1 (3.5-ounce) bar dark chocolate (70
    percent or more), coarsely chopped

Preheat oven to 350°F and line 2 baking sheets with parchment paper.

Using a hand mixer or a whisk, blend the buttery stick with syrup, vanilla, and coconut sugar until creamy. Mix in flours, cinnamon, salt, and baking soda to form a stiff cookie dough. Fold in nuts and chocolate until incorporated through the batter. Wet a teaspoon and your fingers, and spoon cookie dough onto the lined sheets, allowing room for the cookies to spread (about a dozen cookies per standard sheet). Bake for 18 minutes. Remove from oven and allow cookies to stand for 2 minutes on the sheet tray. Transfer to a wire rack to cool completely.

GOOPY ICE CREAM SANDWICHES

You will not buy any junk-food treats after you taste these babies!

Makes 4 sandwiches

Chocolate Glaze
1 cup non-dairy dark chocolate
    chips
2 teaspoons brown rice syrup
⅓ cup unsweetened almond milk

8 Best Chocolate Chunk Cookies
    (at left)
1 pint vanilla soy or other vegan ice
    cream, softened

To make the glaze, place the chocolate chips in a heat-resistant bowl. Bring syrup and almond milk to a rolling boil. Pour over chocolate and whisk until smooth. Cover with plastic and cool slightly.

Make the sandwiches by scooping softened ice cream onto the underside of a cookie. Place another cookie on top and press slightly to spread the ice cream. Dip one-half of the ice cream sandwich into chocolate glaze.

Place the ice cream sandwiches on a baking sheet lined with parchment paper and place them in the freezer for 15–30 minutes to set the chocolate.

ALICIA'S PEANUT BUTTER PIE

I got this recipe from my pal Alicia Silverstone. When I first tasted this, I could not believe how incredibly yummy it was. You will love it. And being from her book, The Kind Diet, *you know it will be kind to your health.*

Makes 1 pie, 8 servings

1 vegan chocolate cookie crust
(Arrowhead Mills makes one)
1 (10-ounce) bag grain-sweetened non-dairy chocolate chips
½ cup soy or hemp milk (do not use rice or nut milk)
1¼ cups unsweetened peanut butter, divided
1 (12.3-ounce) box silken tofu (firm)
¼ cup maple syrup
1–2 teaspoons vanilla extract to taste

Preheat oven to 375°F.
Bake the cookie crust for 4–5 minutes just to make it a bit crispy. Cool completely.

Melt the chocolate chips in the top of a double boiler set over simmering water. If you don't have a double boiler, place a stainless steel bowl over boiling water and melt the ingredients in it. Whisk in the milk until combined and smooth. With a measuring cup, scoop out about ¼ cup of the chocolate mixture, then pour the remainder into the cookie crust. Place the filled cookie crust in the refrigerator to cool completely.

While the filling chills, combine 1 cup peanut butter, the tofu, syrup, and vanilla extract in a food processor or blender; process until very smooth, scraping down the sides of the bowl as needed. Pour the peanut butter mixture on top of the chilled chocolate filling in the cookie crust, smoothing it over the pie as you pour. Return the filled cookie crust to the refrigerator to chill for 1 hour or until firm.

To serve, return the reserved chocolate filling to the double boiler or stainless steel bowl and stir in the remaining ¼ cup peanut butter. Stir until the chocolate and peanut butter are very well combined and very warm. If the mixture seems too thick to drizzle, add some soy milk until it is runny enough to pour. Decoratively drizzle the mixture over the chilled pie in zigzags or swirls or use a small spatula to spread it smoothly over the whole pie. Refrigerate for 15–20 minutes before serving.

ORANGE-GLAZED ITALIAN DONUTS

Is there anything better than fried dough? I think not, and as a kid, my life was all about "zeppole," fried Italian donuts. Here is my version . . . healthier, although still fried . . . so not entirely guilt-free.
Makes 12–16 donuts

2 cups water
3 tablespoons brown rice syrup
3 tablespoons extra-virgin olive oil
1½ cups whole-wheat pastry flour
½ cup semolina flour
Pinch sea salt
3 teaspoons baking powder
1 teaspoon baking soda
¼ cup sparkling wine or water
Oil, for frying

Orange-Scented Glaze
½ cup brown rice syrup
Grated zest of 2 oranges
2 teaspoons fresh orange juice

To make the zeppole, bring the water, syrup, and oil to a boil. Whisk together flours, salt, baking powder, and soda. Mix in boiling water mixture and stir well. Add wine or water and mix well. Add wine or water as needed to create a soft, but not sticky, dough.

Oil a cutting board and turn dough onto it. Pat down flat and fold dough to create 3 layers. Flatten it and repeat this process 3 more times.

Cut off one-third of the dough and roll out the thickness of your thumb. Pinch off teaspoon-size pieces and fry in hot oil until golden and puffy. Drain on paper.

Whisk together syrup with orange juice and zest and drizzle on zeppole.

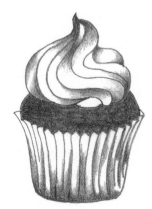

PERFECT CHOCOLATE CUPCAKES

These are moist, chocolatey, sweet, light, and . . . perfect. Since they contain chia, you can have your cake and . . . your omega-3's, iron, and protein, too!

Makes 12 cupcakes

1½ tablespoons chia seeds or
   meal
½ cup unsweetened almond milk
1½ cups whole-wheat pastry flour
½ cup semolina flour
⅔ cup cocoa powder (organic, fair trade,
   if possible)
Generous pinch sea salt
Generous pinch ground cinnamon
2 teaspoons baking powder
1 teaspoon baking soda
½ cup unsweetened shredded
   coconut
½ cup avocado oil
⅔ cup brown rice syrup
1 teaspoon pure vanilla extract
1 teaspoon brown rice vinegar
Unsweetened almond milk
½ cup coarsely chopped walnuts
½ cup coarsely chopped non-dairy
   baking chocolate

Chocolate Glaze
1 cup non-dairy dark chocolate
   chips
2 teaspoons brown rice syrup
⅓ cup unsweetened almond milk

Preheat oven to 350°F and lightly oil a 12-cup muffin tin or use cupcake papers.

Soak chia meal or seeds in almond milk for 5 minutes or until it thickens slightly.

Mix together all dry ingredients, whisking to ensure the ingredients are well combined. Mix in oil, syrup, vanilla, and vinegar. Stir in chia–almond milk mixture. Slowly mix in additional almond milk to create a thick, smooth batter. Fold in nuts and chocolate. Spoon into prepared cups to fill three-fourths full. Bake for 25 minutes or until the tops of the cupcakes spring back to the touch. Cool before frosting.

Make the glaze by placing the chocolate chips in a heat-resistant bowl. Bring syrup and almond milk to a rolling boil. Pour over chocolate and whisk until smooth. Cover with plastic and cool slightly. When the cupcakes are cooled, spread frosting on top of each one.

CHOCOLATE CHEESECAKE

I don't really love faux things like lasagna and cheesecake, but this recipe is just amazing and I had to share it. If you love cheesecake, you will love this one . . . and enjoy it without compromise to your health. It's a bit of work, but it's worth it.

Makes 8–10 servings

Crust

1¼ cups whole-grain graham crackers, crushed into a meal

2 teaspoons brown rice syrup

Pinch sea salt

4 tablespoons vegan buttery spread (Earth Balance)

Chocolate Filling

2 cups brown rice syrup

¼ cup water

8 ounces dark chocolate (60–70 percent or higher), coarsely chopped

2 pounds silken tofu

⅓ cup unsweetened cocoa powder (not Dutch-processed)

16 ounces vegan soy cream cheese (room temperature)

1 teaspoon pure vanilla extract

Generous pinch sea salt

Preheat oven to 350°F and lightly oil a 9-inch springform pan, taking care to oil the sides and the lip of the bottom.

To make the crust, stir together all crust ingredients. The ingredients should hold together. Press the crust onto the bottom and 1 inch up the sides of the pan. Bake until set, 10–12 minutes. Cool completely before proceeding with recipe.

To make the filling, heat rice syrup for 5 minutes over low heat. Remove from heat and stir in water. Whisk well. Return to heat and cook over medium-low heat, stirring constantly, for 2–3 minutes more. Remove from heat and whisk in chopped chocolate until smooth. Cool slightly.

Puree tofu and cocoa powder in a food processor until smooth. Add soy cream cheese and puree until smooth and creamy. Add vanilla, salt, and fudge sauce until the mixture is fully incorporated.

Pour filling into crust and bake on the middle rack of the oven until the top of the cake is shiny but still slightly wobbly when the pan is gently shaken, about an hour. Turn off heat and leave the cake in the oven for another hour.

Run a knife around the top edge of the cake to loosen, but cool the cake completely in the pan on a rack. The cake will continue to set as it cools. Release the pan's latch and transfer to a plate. Serve at room temperature or chilled.

BROWNIES

My pal Dennis thought I'd lost my mind when I first served these. He thought I had pulled the wool over his eyes and made Duncan Hines brownies. It's in the zucchini, man! It adds moisture and antioxidants.

Makes 16

1½ cups whole-wheat pastry
    flour
½ cup semolina flour
½ cup maple syrup granules
½ cup cocoa powder
Generous pinch sea salt
Generous pinch ground cinnamon
1 teaspoon baking soda
2 cups finely grated zucchini
½ cup avocado oil
⅔ cup brown rice syrup
2 teaspoons pure vanilla extract
½ cup non-dairy, grain-sweetened
    chocolate chips
½ cup chopped walnuts (or other nuts)

Preheat oven to 350°F and lightly oil a 10-inch-square pan.

Mix dry ingredients together, whisking to combine. In a small bowl, mix together zucchini, oil, syrup, and vanilla. Combine the wet and dry ingredients to form a thick batter. Fold in chocolate chips and walnuts.

Spoon batter into prepared pan and bake for 35 minutes or until the center of the brownies bounce back to the touch. Remove from oven and allow to cool in the pan for 10 minutes before cutting into squares. Serve frosted or not.

Frosting
½ cup non-dairy, grain-sweetened
    chocolate chips
2 tablespoons brown rice syrup
Almond milk (unsweetened)

Place the chocolate and rice syrup in a heat-resistant bowl. Bring about ⅔ cup almond milk to a rolling boil and slowly pour over chocolate while whisking. Use only enough almond milk to create a thick, smooth frosting. You may have heated more almond milk than you need. Just cool it down and return it to the container for later use. Whisk the frosting until smooth.

Once the brownies have cooled completely, spread frosting on top of each one.

MUFFINS

This basic muffin recipe will work for any muffin you could want to create . . . apple, banana nut, blueberry, cranberry, pumpkin, and with a couple of adjustments you can make corn muffins, bran muffins, or any other kind of whole-grain muffins you can imagine.

Makes 12 muffins

½ cup unsweetened almond milk

1 tablespoon chia seeds

¼ cup avocado oil

½ cup unsweetened applesauce

⅔ cup brown rice syrup

1 teaspoon pure vanilla extract

1½ cups whole-wheat pastry flour

½ cup semolina flour

Generous pinch sea salt

Scant pinch cinnamon

1 tablespoon baking powder

2 teaspoons baking soda

Soak chia seeds in almond milk, stirring frequently, for 15 minutes before making muffins.

Preheat oven to 350°F and line a standard muffin tin with papers or lightly oil and flour.

Whisk together oil, applesauce, rice syrup, milk, and vanilla until emulsified. In a separate bowl, whisk together flours, salt, cinnamon, baking powder and soda. Fold in wet ingredients to create a smooth batter. Divide batter evenly among the muffin cups, making them each about three-quarters full. Bake until the centers of the muffins spring back to the touch, about 35 minutes. Cool on a wire rack.

Variations: To create bran muffins, substitute bran for semolina flour. For corn muffins, substitute ½ cup cornmeal for semolina flour. To add fruit, add ½ cup blueberries, cranberries, chopped apples, pears, peaches, or cherries. For pumpkin muffins, substitute cooked or canned pumpkin for the applesauce. For banana muffins, you would substitute ½ cup mashed bananas for the applesauce. To add nuts, simply fold in ½ cup of the chopped nuts of your choice to any recipe.

SWEET ALMOND CHOCOLATE MILKSHAKE

Who doesn't love milkshakes? But nobody loves the saturated fat, calories, artificial flavors and colors, and, well, growth hormones in the milk . . . that's if they use milk at all! These are so delicious and easy, you'll feel like you have a soda fountain in your kitchen!

Makes 1–2 servings

1 large banana, chopped and frozen

¾ cup unsweetened almond milk

1 teaspoon pure vanilla extract

3 tablespoons dark cocoa powder

1 cup strawberries, fresh or frozen

Place all ingredients in a blender and puree until smooth and thick. Enjoy immediately.

◆ **Note**

If you don't want to use or don't like bananas, use a cup of ice cubes to create the milkshake texture we all love.

ACKNOWLEDGMENTS

As I complete this latest book with Penguin Group (USA), I feel compelled to thank John Duff before all others. For the past fifteen years, he has proven to be a thoughtful, committed, and passionate publisher and editor. He has driven me to be the best I can be; to write the best books I can. With his wisdom and finesse, friendship, humor, and mentoring, he shapes my words into the books people enjoy. I thank you, John. And to all the people at Penguin, thank you. It's been quite a ride.

I am, above all other things, a cooking teacher enjoying a twenty-year career that's still going strong. In that time I have met some of the most extraordinary people. I have shared what I know, and in return, each and every student who has graced my kitchen has given me a piece of their life experiences and taught me so much. Each one of you has made me a better teacher and a better person. Thank you.

We all have our little circle of friends who are family. They surround us with love and are deeply woven into the fabric of our lives. They are, in my case, a small but mighty group who has seen me through good and bad times, have cried and celebrated with me, and are always there no matter what. Cynthia and Dennis, Mary, Tina, Susie, Patrick, Charlene, Michele and Kevin, Deb, Patrecia, Lois, the Island God, Jennifer, Girl Wonder, Art, Andy, Chris, Oz, Larry, Uncle Sandy, Mark, Dan and Robyn, Salvatore and Anna, Peter and Sheila, John and Jan: there are no words to express how much I truly love you all.

I have been blessed with the joy of amazing young people in my world. Their energy, passion, exuberance, and idealism keep me inspired: Ben, Sara, Alex, Alicia, David, Little Jen, Caitlin, and Emma; you guys are the future, and I rest a little easier knowing it's all in your hands.

My work is demanding and taxing: from schlepping cases of produce for classes and seminars, to the "joy" of modern air travel. Thanks, Anthony and Joanne, for keeping me strong, fit, and flexible for the life I choose to lead.

To my colleagues, Neal Barnard, MD; Marilu Henner; T. Colin Campbell, PhD; Bill Tara; Bernardo Merizalde, MD; Dr. Will Klevos; Patrick Riley; David Steinman (my hero); the entire staff at the Restaurant School at Walnut Hill College, especially Danny Liberatoscioli: I thank you for your wisdom, your support, and your generosity.

Finally, to my husband, Robert. After twenty-seven years of being together night and day, day and night, you still take my breath away. Your kindness, optimism, passion, love, and pure soul make life worth living. I am not sure how I feel about marriage as a concept, but with you, it's perfection. I could not do what I do without you. I love you.

SOURCES

1. Another Nice Mess We've Gotten Ourselves Into

A BRIEF HISTORY OF FOOD

Mark, "A Brief History of Obesity," *Lose That Tyre*, July 25, 2008, www.losethattyre
.co.uk/search/history-on-obesity-and-processed-foods.

Mintz, Steven, "Food in America," *Digital History*, www.digitalhistory.uh.edu/history
online/food.cfm.

HUMANS ARE MEANT TO COOK

"Eat Less Processed Food, Say Experts," *BBC News*, March 3, 2003, http://news.bbc.co
.uk/2/hi/health/2814253.stm.

"Processed Foods to Blame for Obesity and Chronic Disease," Healing Search, March 3,
2003, www.healingsearch.com/_ReportPages/processed_foods_to_blame.htm.

Wald, Jonathan, "Lawyers Revise Obesity Lawsuit Against McDonald's," CNN.com,
February 21, 2003, http://articles.cnn.com/2003-02-21/justice/obesity.lawsuit_1_
samuel-hirsch-filet-o-fish-obesity-lawsuit?_s=PM:LAW. Accessed July 20, 2011.

2. How Fast Food Has Changed Our Nation

FAST-FOOD DECEPTION

"Fast Food," *Tuberose*, www.tuberose.com/Fast_Food.html.

"Food processing," Wikipedia, http://en.wikipedia.org/wiki/Food_processing.

Komlos, John, and Marek Brabec, "The Trend of Mean BMI Values of US Adults, Birth Cohorts 1882–1986 Indicates That the Obesity Epidemic Began Earlier Than Hitherto Thought," National Bureau of Economic Research, April 2010, www.nber.org/papers/w15862.pdf.

"McFast-Food Conquers America: Global Perspectives on Fast-Food History," American Forum for Global Education, www.globaled.org/curriculum/ffood4.html.

WHO'S CALLING THE SHOTS ON OUR DIETARY GUIDELINES

"Dietary Guidelines for Americans," Center for Nutrition Policy and Promotion, 2010, www.cnpp.usda.gov/Publications/DietaryGuidelines/2010/PolicyDoc/Chapter4.pdf.

MY PYRAMID MEETS MYPLATE

"Agriculture Subsidies: Further Reading," Law Library: American Law and Legal Information, http://law.jrank.org/pages/4201/Agriculture-Subsidies.html.

Apgar, Toni, "Consumers in Wonderland," *Vegetarian Times*, February 1994, http://books.google.com/books?id=lAgAAAAAMBAJ&lpg=PA4&ots=bkUem_lQdB&dq=%22consumers%20in%20wonderland%22%20apgar&pg=PA4#v=onepage&q=%22consumers%20in%20wonderland%22%20apgar&f=false.

"MyPlate," U.S. Department of Agriculture, www.choosemyplate.gov.

"Power Plate," Physicians Committee for Responsible Medicine, http://pcrm.org/health/diets/pplate/power-plate.

3. What's Really Going into Our Food?

THE SCOURGE OF PROCESSED FOODS

Olver, Lynne, "FAQs: Cakes," *Food Timeline*, 2000, www.foodtimeline.org/foodcakes.html.

WHAT'S REALLY IN THE "FOOD" YOU ARE EATING?

"All the Health Risks of Processed Foods—In Just a Few Quick, Convenient Bites," SixWise.com, www.sixwise.com/newsletters/05/10/19/all-the-health-risks-of-processed-foods----in-just-a-few-quick-convenient-bites.htm.

"Artificial Food Coloring Dangers," *Science News*, May 9, 2008, http://science-news.org/artificial-food-coloring/artificial-food-coloring-dangers.

"Preservatives and Additives," *Freedomyou*, excerpted from *North American Diet*, by Ron Lagerquist, International Bible Society, 1984, www.freedomyou.com/nutrition_book/enriched_fortified_synthetic_food.htm.

"The Six Thousand Hidden Dangers of Processed Foods (and What to Choose Instead)," *Body Ecology*, October 18, 2007, http://bodyecology.com/articles/hidden_dangers_of_processed_foods.php.

A DAY IN YOUR LIFE WITH PROCESSED FOODS

Fraser, Jessica, "Avoiding High-Carb Processed Foods Cuts Heart Disease Risk in Women by 30 Percent," *Natural News*, November 10, 2006, www.naturalnews.com/021039.html#ixzz1OH3Cf1rt.

"Identifying Whole Grain Products," Whole Grains Council, www.wholegrainscouncil.org/whole-grains-101/identifying-whole-grain-products.

Langer, Gary, "Poll: What Americans Eat for Breakfast," *Good Morning America*, May 17, 2005, http://abcnews.go.com/GMA/PollVault/story?id=762685. Accessed June 20, 2011.

EATING WELL ALL DAY LONG

"Anatomy of a Big Mac," *Health Basics*, August 2, 2010, www.healthbasics.net/blog/2010/08/02/anatomy-of-a-big-mac.

"American cheese," Wikipedia, http://en.wikipedia.org/wiki/American_cheese.

Groch, Judith, "Convenience Foods Save Little Time, Lack Nutrients," *MedPage Today*, August 8, 2007, www.medpagetoday.com/PrimaryCare/DietNutrition/dh/6368.

SOME SWEET TALK ABOUT SWEETENERS

Bray, George A., MD, "Fructose: Is It Bad for Our Health?" Pennington Biomedical Research Center, March 2008, www.pbrc.edu/pdf/bray-final-paper-080508.pdf.

Bray, George A., Samara Joy Nielsen, and Barry M. Popkin, "Consumption of High-Fructose Corn Syrup in Beverages May Play a Role in the Epidemic of Obesity," *American Journal of Clinical Nutrition*, Vol. 79, no. 4 (April 2004): 537–43, www.ajcn.org/content/79/4/537.full.

Casel, Andrew, "Why U.S. Farm Subsidies Are Bad for the World," *Philadelphia Inquirer*, May 6, 2002, www.commondreams.org/views02/0506-09.htm.

"Corn Refiners Association: HFCS Is Not the Cause of Obesity," *Science Blog*, March 24, 2004, www.scienceblog.com/community/older/archives/K/2/pub2598.html.

"Finger Points to Corn Syrup in Obesity Epidemic," International Congress on Obesity, August 29, 2002, www.innovations-report.de/html/berichte/medizin_gesundheit/bericht-12472.html.

King, Patricia, "Blaming It on Corn Syrup," *Los Angeles Times*, March 24, 2003, http://articles.latimes.com/2003/mar/24/health/he-fructose24.

Pollan, Michael, "The (Agri)Cultural Contradictions of Obesity," The Way We Live Now, *New York Times*, October 12, 2003, www.nytimes.com/2003/10/12/magazine/12WWLN.html.

100 PERCENT BEEF (OR CHICKEN OR THE OTHER WHITE MEAT): WHAT'S
REALLY IN THAT STUFF?

Chek, Paul, "You Are What You Eat—Animal Products," *Holistic Health Blog*, June 20, 2007,
http://joshrubin.wordpress.com/2007/06/20/you-are-what-you-eat-animal-products
-by-paul-chek.

Lichtenstein, A. H., E. Kennedy, P. Barrir, D. Danford, N. D. Ernst, S. M. Geundy, G. A.
Leveille, L. Van Horn, C. L. Williams, and S. L. Booth SL, "Dietary Fat Consumption and Health," *Nutrition Reviews* 56, 5, Pt. 2 (May 1998): S3–19, www.ncbi.nlm
.nih.gov/pubmed/9624878.

6. Get Smart About What You're Eating

HOW TO READ A LABEL

"How to Read a Food Label," Department of Food and Nutrition Services, www.health
care.uiowa.edu/fns/nutritional/foodlabel.htm.

"How to Understand and Use the Nutrition Facts Label," U.S. Food and Drug Administration, www.fda.gov/food/labelingnutrition/consumerinformation/ucm078889
.htm.

GMOS (GENETICALLY MODIFIED ORGANISMS)

"Say No to GMOs!" www.saynotogmos.org/fda.htm.

ORGANIC OR NON-ORGANIC, THAT IS THE QUESTION

Green Patriot, www.greenpatriot.us.

7. The Chemistry of Food and How It Affects You

ACID AND ALKALINE BALANCE

"Acid/Base Balance," *Tuberose*, http://tuberose.com/Acid_Base_Balance.html.

Cohen, Robert, "Early Sexual Maturity and Milk Hormones," *Health 101*, www.health101
.org/art_Milk_and_Girls.htm.

THE GLYCEMIC INDEX

Ciok, J., and A. Dolna, "Carbohydrates and Mental Performance—The Role of Glycemic
Index of Food Products," *Pol Mrkuriusz Lek* 20, 117 (March 2006): 367–70, www
.ncbi.nlm.nih.gov/pubmed/16780278.

Stevenson, E. J., C. Williams, L. E. Mash, B. Phillips, and M. L. Nute, "Influence of High-
Carbohydrate Mixed Meals with Different Glycemic Indexes on Substrate Utilization During Subsequent Exercise in Women," *American Journal of Clinical Nutrition*
84, 2 (August 2006): 354–60, www.ncbi.nlm.nih.gov/pubmed/16895883.

10. Stocking a Healthy Kitchen

THE PANTRY

The Olive Oil Source, www.oliveoilsource.com.

11. The Basic Tools

CUTTING BOARDS

Cliver, Dean O., PhD, "Plastic and Wooden Cutting Boards," UC–Davis Food Safety Laboratory, http://faculty.vetmed.ucdavis.edu/faculty/docliver/Research/cutting board.htm.

POTS AND PANS

"Are You Exposing Your Family to Toxic Fumes from Non-Stick Cookware?" *Mercola*, www.mercola.com/Downloads/bonus/dangers-of-nonstick-cookware/report.aspx.

13. Changing Ingredients Because There's No Substitution for Health

BUTTER

The Olive Oil Source, www.oliveoilsource.com.

BIBLIOGRAPHY

Aihara, Herman, *Acid and Alkaline* (California: Georges Ohsawa Macrobiotic Foundation, 1986).

Colbin, Annemarie, *The Natural Gourmet* (New York: Ballantine, 1989).

Critser, Greg, *Fatland: How Americans Became the Fattest People in the World* (Boston: Houghton Mifflin, 2003).

Gagne, Steve, and John David Mann, *Energetics of Food* (New Mexico: Spiral Science, 1990).

Marks, Susan, *Finding Betty Crocker: The Secret Life of America's First Lady of Food* (New York: Simon & Schuster, 2005).

Masson, Jeffrey Moussaieff, *The Face on Your Plate* (New York: W. W. Norton & Co. Inc., 2009).

Nestle, Marion, *Food Politics* (Berkeley: University of California Press, 2002).

Nestle, Marion, *What to Eat* (New York: North Point Press, 2006).

Pollan, Michael, *In Defense of Food* (New York: Penguin Press, 2008).

Pollan, Michael, *Food Rules* (New York: Penguin Press, 2009).

Pollan, Michael, *The Omnivore's Dilemma* (New York: Penguin Press, 2006).

Schlosser Eric. *Fast Food Nation: The Dark Side of the All-American Meal* (New York: Houghton Mifflin, 2001).

Spencer, Colin, *The Heretic's Feast: A History of Vegetarianism* (London: Fourth Estate, 1993).

Steinman, David, *Diet for a Poisoned Planet* (New York: Running Press, 2006).

Tara, William, *Natural Body, Natural Mind* (Philadelphia: X Libris, 2009).

INDEX

Page numbers in **bold** indicate tables; those in *italics* indicate illustrations.

ABOUT THE AUTHOR

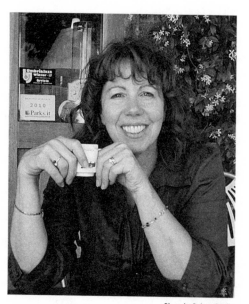

Photo by Robert Pirello

In 1983, **Christina Pirello**, Emmy Award–winning host of the national public television series *Christina Cooks*, was diagnosed with terminal cancer and fought her way back to robust good health through her zest for life and an alternative nutritional approach.

Today, Christina has set out on a mission to educate and inform about the impending and potentially catastrophic health crises facing our culture. Christina's mission has led her to teach and lecture internationally, from natural food stores to corporate boardrooms; from inner-city high schools, elementary schools, and universities to hospitals and wellness and senior centers; as well as in Israel, Croatia, Italy, and Spain.

In an effort to bring her message to a wider audience, Christina's national public television series *Christina Cooks* was launched in 1997. Today, this motivational, educational, and increasingly popular program airs nationally on more than 250 public television stations.

In 2008, Christina founded the Christina Pirello Health Education Initiative, a nonprofit organization dedicated to changing America's relationship with food through community outreach, media programs, and in-school programs designed to teach our kids to make healthier choices.

In January 2009, Christina, along with other nutrition experts, offered testimony to the U.S. Senate subcommittee working to revise the food pyramid guidelines for healthy eating.

Christina founded the Christina Pirello School of Natural Cooking and Integrative Health Studies at the Restaurant School at Walnut Hill College in Philadelphia and also sits on the boards of directors of the Farm Market Trust, the Philadelphia Green Council, the Green City Youth Council, and the Chefs' Council of Chefs for Humanity. She is on the faculty of the Restaurant School at Walnut Hill College.

She is a contributor to the *Huffington Post*/AOL, Examiner.com, *One Green Planet*, and *VegNews*.

Christina's first book, *Cooking the Whole Foods Way*, was named the healthiest cookbook of the decade by Washington, DC–based Physicians' Committee for Responsible Medicine. She is the author of *Christina Cooks, Glow, Cook Your Way to the Life You Want, This Crazy Vegan Life*, and *I'm Mad as Hell and I'm Not Going to Eat it Anymore!*

To learn more about Christina Pirello and the Christina Pirello Health Education Initiative, visit www.christinacooks.com and www.christinapirello.org.

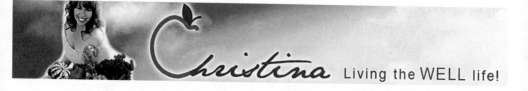

The food industry is more sophisticated than most in its ability to direct attention away from unpleasant or unpopular truths. Large food manufacturers, fast food empires, and even some in the natural foods trade would prefer us not to think too deeply about the food we eat. The Chemical Kitchen feeds America, and the cost of service is very high indeed.

—Bill Tara

For more information, recipes, recommended resources, inspiring stories and to keep up-to-date on the latest scoop on food, check out www.christinacooks.com.

There is a lot of work to do if we are to save ourselves and future generations from the health crises we face. We control very little in life, but we do control the food choices we make.

Join Me in the Fight to Save Our Kids' Health

In the last several decades, the addition of hydrogenated fats, high-fructose corn syrup, chemical and artificial additives too numerous to list, together with questionable manufacturing and farming practices, has contributed to more and more of our kids today suffering from adult diseases. Obesity, diabetes, heart disease, and even bone loss in the late teens and early twenties have become more and more prevalent. As reported in many medical journals, the unnatural phenomenon of early onset puberty (attributable to the widespread use of growth hormones in factory-farming practices) is creating a generation of kids who may not live as long as their parents.

A Sense of Purpose

The purpose of the Christina Pirello Health Education Initiative is to change our relationship with food. With education as its foundation, the goal of the Initiative is to provide a number of specifically designed programs to the schools, the community, and the food industry.

As public demand for more healthy food choices has increased, many mainstream food manufacturers are actively seeking help in creating higher-quality, more healthful foods. Through the work of this nonprofit, I work with schools, consumer groups, chefs, medical experts, and manufacturers to change the system from within.

For ways you can help take up the cause of our kids' health, head over to www.christinapirello.org.